Uterine Fibroids

Nash S. Moawad
Editor

Uterine Fibroids

A Clinical Casebook

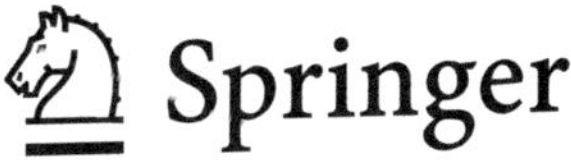 Springer

Editor
Nash S. Moawad, MD, MS, FACOG
Minimally Invasive Gynecologic Surgery
Department of Obstetrics and Gynecology
University of Florida
Gainesville, FL, USA

Additional material to this book can be downloaded from http://extras.springer.com

ISBN 978-3-319-58779-0   ISBN 978-3-319-58780-6   (eBook)
https://doi.org/10.1007/978-3-319-58780-6

Library of Congress Control Number: 2017951903

Printed on acid-free paper

This Springer imprint is published by Springer Nature
The registered company is Springer International Publishing AG
The registered company address is: Gewerbestrasse 11, 6330 Cham, Switzerland

To
My wife Stephanie, my amazing daughters Mary and Christi, and to my parents
For their abundant support, love, understanding, sacrifices, and for their inspiration

To
Professor Sir Magdi Yacoub
Who has always been a role model and an inspiration to pursue my dreams

Foreword

Fibroids remain one of the most ubiquitous and difficult-to-treat disorders in modern gynecology. As a result, a multitude of treatments, both surgical and nonsurgical, continue to be developed. Selection of the most appropriate treatment for an individual woman has always been dictated by symptomatology, fibroid size and location, and desired outcome. As the number of treatment options rapidly increases, it has become progressively more difficult for clinicians to stay abreast of all of the new approaches. This book fills an important knowledge gap for clinicians by showcasing a comprehensive array of state-of-the-art approaches and putting them into perspective. Dr. Moawad has recruited an impressive number of highly qualified experts from throughout the country and the world to share their insights and perspectives. Certainly, this thought-provoking book will be of great interest to clinicians everywhere as they strive to provide their patients the best, most up-to-date treatment for symptomatic uterine fibroids.

North Carolina, USA					William W. Hurd, MD, MPH

Preface

It is with great pleasure and honor that I introduce this unique clinical casebook on uterine fibroids, written by world experts in the field, for practitioners in obstetrics and gynecology, gynecologic surgeons, reproductive endocrinology and infertility specialists, residents and fellows, medical students, and allied health practitioners. This book starts with three introductory chapters about the pathogenesis, histopathology, classification, and symptomatology of uterine fibroids; the impact of fibroids on fertility; and current state-of-the-art, evidence-based management options for fibroids. Following this comprehensive introduction, each chapter presents a unique clinical scenario. The case presentations encompass various locations of fibroids, including different types of submucosal, intramural, and subserosal fibroids, a cervical fibroid, a broad ligament fibroid, the prolapsed myoma, a fibroid with "red flags," and the "innumerable fibroids." Each chapter guides the reader in a real-life exercise of exploring the possible treatment options, and how to navigate the decision-making process and guide the patient in understanding the risks and benefits of each approach and supporting evidence. This is followed by a detailed explanation of the treatment of choice with practical tips and tricks for the surgical management when indicated. All current treatment options are reviewed, from expectant management to hysteroscopic, laparoscopic, robotic, open and vaginal myomectomy, nonsurgical options, and hysterectomy. Complementary and alternative management options and expectant management are discussed as well for selected patients. Issues such as tissue extraction, hemostasis, effect on fertility, and the potential value of robotics are also discussed.

I would like to take this opportunity to express my deep gratitude to my esteemed colleagues and friends who shared their expertise, time, and effort and contributed to the success of this book. I sincerely hope this book will be a great resource for the reader and a valuable asset to the clinical care of women with uterine fibroids.

Gainesville, FL   Nash S. Moawad, MD, MS, FACOG

Contents

Contributors

Sukinah Alfaraj, MD Division of Reproductive Endocrinology and Infertility, Department of Obstetrics and Gynecology, The University of British Columbia, Vancouver, BC, Canada

Ayman Al-Hendy, MD, PhD OB/GYN, Augusta University, Augusta, GA, USA

Ibrahim Alkatout, MD, PhD Department Obstetrics and Gynecology, University Clinics Schleswig-Holstein, Campus Kiel, Germany

Mohamed A. Bedaiwy, MD, PhD Division of Reproductive Endocrinology and Infertility, Department of Obstetrics and Gynecology, The University of British Columbia, Vancouver, BC, Canada

Maryam Baikpour, MD Department of Obstetrics and Gynecology, Duke University School of Medicine, Durham, NC, USA

Paula C. Brady, MD Center for Infertility and Reproductive Surgery, Department of Obstetrics, Gynecology and Reproductive Biology, Brigham and Women's Hospital, Boston, MA, USA

Paul C. Browne, MD OB/GYN, Augusta University, Augusta, GA, USA

Aarathi Cholkeri-Singh, MD, FACOG The Advanced Gynecologic Surgery Institute, Naperville, IL, USA

Gregory M. Christman, MD Division of Reproductive Endocrinology and Infertility, University of Florida College of Medicine, Gainesville, FL, USA

Randi Shae Connor, MD Department of Gynecologic Oncology, University Hospitals Seidman Cancer Center, Cleveland, OH, USA

Cyra Cottrell University of Florida College of Medicine, Gainesville, FL, USA

Anupama Deenadayal Mettler, MD, PhD Department Obstetrics and Gynecology, University Clinics Schleswig-Holstein, Campus Kiel, Kiel, Germany

Andrew Deutsch, MD, MS Department of Gynecology, Advocate Lutheran General Hospital, Park Ridge, IL, USA

Michael Diamond, MD Research Department, Augusta University, Augusta, GA, USA

Jennifer S. Eaton, MD, MSCI Department of Obstetrics and Gynecology, Duke University School of Medicine, Durham, NC, USA

Deepika Garg, MD Department of Obstetrics and Gynecology, Maimonides Medical Center, Brooklyn, NY, USA

Antonio R. Gargiulo, MD Center for Infertility and Reproductive Surgery, Department of Obstetrics, Gynecology and Reproductive Biology, Brigham and Women's Hospital, Boston, MA, USA

Richard Guido, MD, CIP Department of Obstetrics, Gynecology and Reproductive Sciences, University of Pittsburgh, Magee-Womens Hospital of the UPMC Health System, Pittsburgh, PA, USA

Hye-Chun Hur, MD, MPH Division of Minimally Invasive Gynecology, Beth Israel Deaconess Medical Center, Harvard Medical School, Boston, MA, USA

William W. Hurd, MD, MPH Department of Obstetrics and Gynecology, Duke University School of Medicine, Durham, NC, USA

Keith Isaacson, MD Minimally Invasive Gynecologic Surgery, Newton Wellesley Hospital, Harvard Medical School, Newton, MA, USA

Christa Lepik, MD Division of Reproductive Endocrinology and Infertility, Department of Obstetrics and Gynecology, The University of British Columbia, Vancouver, BC, Canada

Grace Liu, MD Department of Obstetrics and Gynaecology, Sunnybrook Health Sciences Centre, Toronto, ON, Canada

Antonio Malvasi, MD International Translational Medicine and Biomodelling Research Group, Department of Applied Mathematics, Moscow, Institute of Physics and Technology (State University), Moscow Region, Russia

Department of Obstetrics and Gynecology, GVM Care and Research, Santa Maria Hospital, Bari, Italy

Liselotte Mettler, MD, PhD Department Obstetrics and Gynecology, University Clinics Schleswig-Holstein, Campus Kiel, Germany

Charles E. Miller, MD, FACOG The Advanced Gynecologic Surgery Institute, Naperville, IL, USA

Nash S. Moawad, MD, MS, FACOG Minimally Invasive Gynecologic Surgery, Department of Obstetrics and Gynecology, University of Florida College of Medicine, Gainesville, FL, USA

Mona Omar, MD, PhD OB/GYN, Augusta University, Augusta, GA, USA

OB/GYN, Tanta University, Tanta, Egypt

William Parker, MD Department of Obstetrics and Gynecology, UCLA School of Medicine, Santa Monica, CA, USA

Elizabeth Plasencia, MD Department of Obstetrics and Gynecology, University of Florida College of Medicine, Gainesville, FL, USA

Kari Plewniak, MD Division of Minimally Invasive Gynecology, Beth Israel Deaconess Medical Center, Harvard Medical School, Boston, MA, USA

Leonardo Resta, MD, PhD Section of Pathological Anatomy, Department of Emergency and Organ Transplantation (DETO), University of Bari, Bari, Italy

Alice Rhoton-Vlasak, MD Department of Obstetrics and Gynecology, University of Florida College of Medicine, Gainesville, FL, USA

James Robinson, MD, MS, FACOG Director, Minimally Invasive Gynecologic Surgery, National Center for Advanced Pelvic Surgery, Washington Hospital Center, Washington, DC, USA

Carlos Rotman, MD, FACOG, FACS Department of Gynecology, Weiss Memorial Hospital, Chicago, IL, USA

Christina Salazar, MD Minimally Invasive Gynecologic Surgery, Newton Wellesley Hospital, Harvard Medical School, Newton, MA, USA

Stacey Scheib, MD Department of Gynecology and Obstetrics, Johns Hopkins University Hospital, Baltimore, MD, USA

James H. Segars, MD Department of Gynecology and Obstetrics, Johns Hopkins School of Medicine, Baltimore, MD, USA

Jonathan Y. Song, MD, FACOG, FACS Robotics and Minimally Invasive Surgery, Northwestern Medicine Delnor Hospital, TLC Medical Group, St. Charles, IL, USA

Radmila Sparić, MD Clinic for Gynecology and Obstetrics, Clinical Centre of Serbia, Belgrade, Serbia

Medical Faculty, University of Belgrade, Belgrade, Serbia

Aleksandar Stefanovic, MD, PhD Clinic for Gynecology and Obstetrics, Clinical Centre of Serbia, Belgrade, Serbia

Medical Faculty, University of Belgrade, Belgrade, Serbia

Mallory Stuparich, MD Department of Obstetrics, Gynecology and Reproductive Sciences, University of Pittsburgh, Magee-Womens Hospital of the UPMC Health System, Pittsburgh, PA, USA

Andrea Tinelli, MD, PhD Division of Experimental Endoscopic Surgery, Imaging, Technology and Minimally Invasive Therapy, Department of Obstetrics and Gynecology, Vito Fazzi Hospital, Lecce, Italy

Laboratory of Human Physiology, Department of Applied Mathematics, Moscow, Institute of Physics and Technology (State University), Moscow Region, Russia

Edgardo L. Yordan, MD, FACOG, FACS Department of Gynecology, Weiss Memorial Hospital, Chicago, IL, USA

Kristine Zanotti, MD Division of Gynecologic Oncology, Department of Obstetrics and Gynecology, University Hospitals Cleveland Medical Center, Cleveland, OH, USA

Chapter 1
Pathogenesis, Classification, Histopathology, and Symptomatology of Fibroids

Andrea Tinelli, Leonardo Resta, Radmila Sparić, Aleksandar Stefanović, and Antonio Malvasi

A. Tinelli, MD, PhD (✉)
Division of Experimental Endoscopic Surgery, Imaging, Technology and Minimally Invasive Therapy, Department of Obstetrics and Gynecology, Vito Fazzi Hospital, Lecce, Italy

Laboratory of Human Physiology, Department of Applied Mathematics, Moscow, Institute of Physics and Technology (State University), Moscow Region, Russia
e-mail: andreatinelli@gmail.com; andrea.tinelli@unisalento.it

L. Resta, MD, PhD
Section of Pathological Anatomy, Department of Emergency and Organ Transplantation (DETO), University of Bari, Bari, Italy
e-mail: leonardo.resta@uniba.it

R. Sparić, MD • A. Stefanović, MD, PhD
Clinic for Gynecology and Obstetrics, Clinical Centre of Serbia, Višegradska 26, 11000 Belgrade, Serbia

Medical Faculty, University of Belgrade,
Doktora Subotića 8, 11000 Belgrade, Serbia
e-mail: radmila@rcub.bg.ac.rs; stefanovic.gak@gmail.com

A. Malvasi, MD
International Translational Medicine and Biomodelling Research Group, Department of Applied Mathematics, Moscow, Institute of Physics and Technology (State University), Moscow Region, Russia

Department of Obstetrics and Gynecology, GVM Care and Research, Santa Maria Hospital, Bari, Italy
e-mail: antoniomalvasi@gmail.com

N.S. Moawad (ed.), *Uterine Fibroids*,
https://doi.org/10.1007/978-3-319-58780-6_1,
© Springer International Publishing AG 2018

Introduction

Uterine fibroids (leiomyomas or benign tumors of the smooth muscle) represent the most common form of benign mesenchymal disease of the female genital tract. Clinical studies report an incidence of 25–30% of the female population of childbearing age, with higher prevalence after 40 years and in black women [1].

The etiology of the fibroid's birth remains unknown. Cytogenetic studies have shown the presence of clonal chromosome rearrangements in over 60% of the myomas, more frequently in chromosomes 12 and 14, with the responsibility of different genetic loci [2].

The estrogen receptors are present in the myomatosic (fibroid) tissue, at a greater extent than in normal myometrium, as well as in the case of progesterone receptors: the action favoring the development of myomas by estrogen is demonstrated by the absence of myomas before puberty and by the significant reduction in volume with menopause, almost constantly [3].

The action of progesterone on these tumors has been seen in their tendency to increase in volume in the first trimester of pregnancy, increased mitotic activity of myomatosic cells in the secretive phase, conditions of higher rate of progesterone in the blood, and tendency to reduce their volume following the antiprogestin administration [4].

Epidemiology

Fibroids are one of the most common indications for gynecological surgery, with 40–60% of all performed hysterectomies for fibroids [5] (Fig. 1.1). Depending on the study population and diagnostic techniques implemented, fibroids' incidence has been estimated to be as high as 77% of women [1]. Epidemiological studies conducted in the USA documented that more than 80% of African-American and more than 70% of Caucasian women developed fibroids by 50 years of age [6]. Until the broad use of sophisticated up-to-date imaging

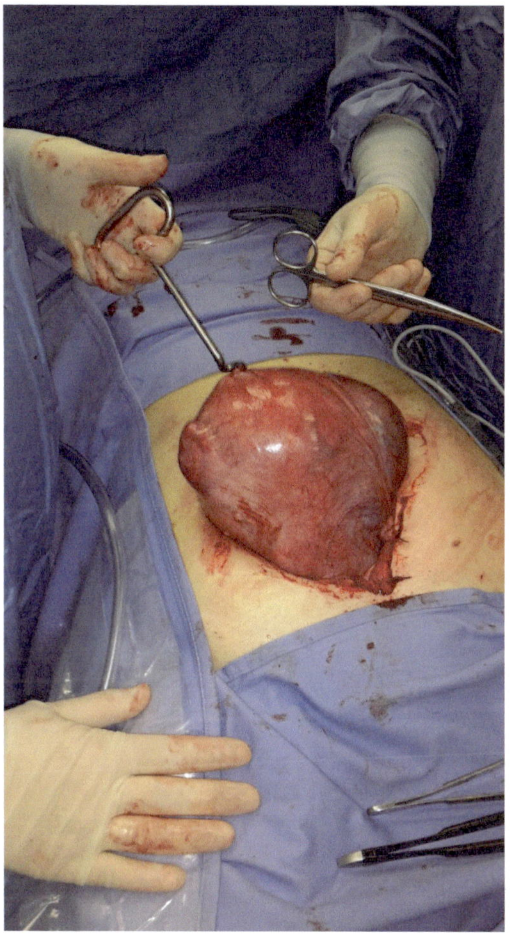

FIGURE 1.1 Laparotomic hysterectomy for a giant myomatosic uterus that reaches almost up to the diaphragm

techniques, mainly ultrasound, epidemiological studies that were focused on surgical and symptomatic cases largely reported lower fibroid prevalence [1]. Furthermore, racial disparities in fibroid incidence even now cause significant differences in fibroid prevalence throughout the world [1].

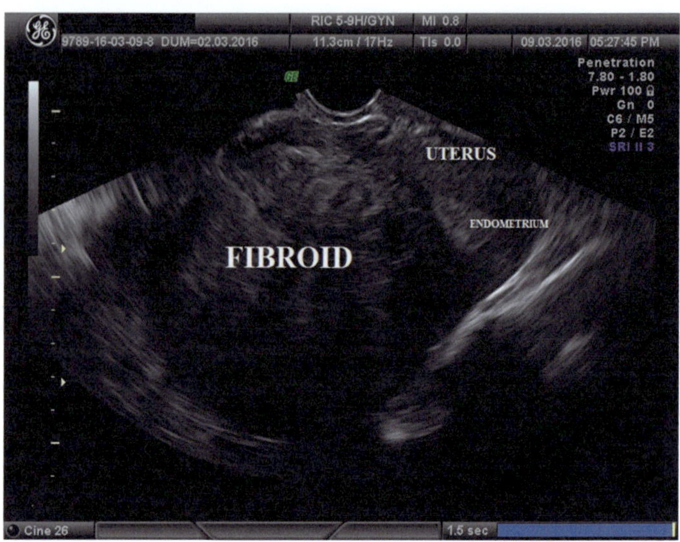

FIGURE 1.2 A transvaginal ultrasonographic scan showing a uterus with a posterior large fibroid of 9 cm in diameter

Nowadays, well-designed ultrasound screening studies (Fig. 1.2) are expected to provide the most reliable information on fibroid's true prevalence [7].

Despite paucity of the studies investigating epidemiological factors associated with fibroid onset and growth, not all the risk factors are fully defined and understood yet. Risk factors linked with fibroid formation include age, race, body mass index (BMI), heritage, reproductive factors, sex hormones, obesity, hypertension, and diabetes. Moreover, environmental and lifestyle factors such as diet, caffeine and alcohol consumption, smoking, physical activity, and stress have also been investigated as possible impact factors in fibroid development [1].

In spite of being a benign disease, uterine fibroids represent an immense health burden throughout the world, requiring more research in epidemiology, particularly in terms of modifiable risk factors and these that possibly represent new drugs for fibroid treatment.

Epidemiological studies clearly indicate that risk of fibroid formation is increasing throughout women's reproductive age, while their frequency decreases with menopause [1, 7]. In line with these observations, clinical reports' data indicate that incidence of symptomatic fibroids, requiring treatment, is the highest in perimenopausal years [1].

Fibroids are mostly frequent in the black race, indisputably, with up to three times greater incidence in blacks in comparison with whites [7]. Furthermore, black women are affected in younger age, more frequently with multiple fibroids and having more pronounced symptoms than other ethnic groups [1, 6]. Thus, rates of hospitalizations for fibroids are also higher for black women, and they have longer hospital stays and higher medical costs per day [7]. In these, treated by abdominal myomectomy (Fig. 1.3), both blood transfusion and postoperative complication rates are higher [6]. Fibroid growth rates in premenopausal years are also higher in black women, compared to white [7]. In African-Americans, the

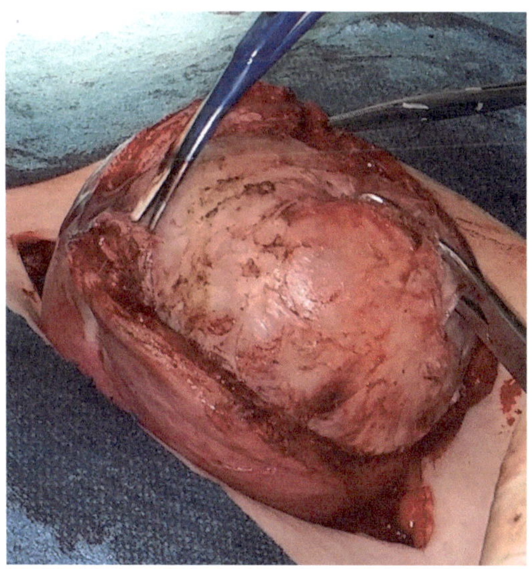

FIGURE 1.3 A laparotomic myomectomy, with a removal of a large fibroid of 12 cm in diameter

mean percentage of European ancestry has been documented to be associated with younger age in affected women [1]. Data on fibroid frequency in a younger woman come from reports on early pregnancy screening. Laughlin et al. [8] estimated, by ultrasound, fibroid incidence throughout various ethnic groups in the first trimester of pregnancy as follows: 18% in black women, 10% in Hispanic women, 8% in white women, and 13% in "others," consisting mostly of Asian women. Possible reasons for this observation might be differences in biosynthesis and/or metabolism of estrogens, receptor-associated factors, and genetic factors. Furthermore, different races exhibit diverse lifestyle habits, including dietary habits, and are documented to be exposed to various levels of stress [1, 9]. Nevertheless, clear causes for the observed ethnic variations are not fully understood yet.

Fibroid formation risk is clearly associated with numerous reproductive factors by both hormonal and non-hormonal mechanisms [7]. These include early age at menarche, less term pregnancies, lower parity, older age in last term pregnancy, and shorter time since last birth, while data on breast-feeding are still contradictory [1, 7]. Pregnancies that did not reach term seem to be unrelated to fibroid risk [7].

Association of both endogenous and exogenous hormones and fibroid development has been widely investigated, with conflicting results in terms of some of these. Fibroids occur exclusively during a woman's reproductive period, thus confirming their dependence of ovarian steroid hormones. Importance of estrogen and progesterone in fibroid formation and development has been confirmed both by experimental and clinical research [1]. In comparison with normal myometrium, fibroid cells have increased expression of steroid hormone and growth factor receptors, mostly regulated by estrogens [7]. Nevertheless, the exact mechanism on how estrogen and progesterone trigger fibroid formation is still unclear. Epidemiological studies indicated early menarche as one of the risk factors for fibroid onset and growth. Polycystic ovary syndrome is also positively associated with fibroids, indicating elevated levels of luteinizing hormone (LH) and insulin-like growth factor I (IGF-I), insulin resistance, and hyperandrogenism as possible causes for this observation [1].

Despite paucity of studies' relationship between myomas and oral contraceptive (OC) use, epidemiological data on it are still controversial, showing either absent or reduced risk of fibroid formation. Furthermore, there is a question of possible detection bias, as OC users may be undergoing gynecological exams more often than general population. Research conducted in the USA in African-American women failed to document the influence of both ingredients and hormonal strength of OC on fibroid occurrence, while the age of first OC use was associated with a slightly higher risk [1, 7]. The same study documented a lower risk in current users of progestin-only injectable. Data on duration of the OC use are also inconsistent [7]. Clear data on relationship between fibroids and use of levonorgestrel intrauterine contraceptive device are still missing [1]. Hormone replacement therapy after menopause is associated with fibroid growth, both in women using estrogens only and in those using combined therapy [7]. Moreover, exogenous hormones in food, like so-called phytoestrogens and those of artificial origin, possibly also enhance fibroid risk [1]. Fibroid formation risk is also increased in women prenatally exposed to diethylstilbestrol [7].

Some researchers indicated increased fibroid risk in obese women. A tween cohort study from Finland showed increased fibroid risk associated with higher body mass index (BMI), while an Italian study failed to document an association [1]. The possible explanatory mechanism for this observation might be increased levels of circulating estrogens, due to aromatization of androgens in fatty tissue [1]. The contributing factor in such cases is decreased production of sex hormone-binding globulin in the liver of obese women, causing increased bioavailability of both estrogens and androgens [1]. However, most of the circulating estrogens in premenopausal women originate from ovaries. A study from the USA revealed an inverse J-shaped pattern between BMI and fibroid risk, which appeared to be dependent on parity, extent of obesity, and detection bias. The relationship between BMI in obese women and fibroids has been found to be stronger in surgical cases [1].

Investigated lifestyle risks include diet, caffeine and alcohol consumption, smoking, physical activity, and stress. Due to numerous biases and confounding factors, results on dietary factors and fibroid occurrence are inconclusive. Nevertheless, a number of dietary factors have been documented to contribute to the growth of symptomatic fibroids. Food with higher glycemic index increases the fibroid risk, while data on soy food are still under investigation [1]. Fibroid incidence is increased in women having diet rich in red meat and dark meat fish, while it is decreased in those consuming a diet rich in fruit and vegetables [1, 7]. Particularly, intake of citrus fruits is in a strong inverse relationship with fibroid onset risk [1, 10].

Data on micronutrients, such as vitamins A, C, and E, as well as folate intake and fibroid risk, are still limited, while hypovitaminosis D is considered to be an important risk factor for fibroid formation, particularly pronounced in blacks [1, 11]. Experimental data indicate that 1,25-dihidroxyvitamin D inhibits fibroid growth [1, 10]. Fibroid risk is lower in both blacks and whites with sufficient vitamin D levels. Furthermore, fibroid cells express reduced levels of vitamin D receptors in comparison with normal myometrium [11]. Moreover, vitamin D is considered to be a potential regulator of fibroid growth, which requires further investigation as a potential candidate for treatment of uterine fibroids, as vitamin D analogs could represent a potential medical treatment option for fibroids [11]. Carotenoids found in many fruits and vegetables are strong antioxidants, out of which lycopene is the most potent. Experimental studies in animals documented that lycopene-supplemented diets reduce the number and size of fibroids in laboratory animals in a dose-dependent manner, while data from large USA epidemiological studies, both in blacks and whites, showed no associations between carotenoid intake and fibroid risk [1, 7, 10]. Diary consumption is found to be associated with reduced fibroid risk [8]. Data on intake of soy food are still inconclusive [1]. Some animal studies demonstrated an inhibitory effect of green tea extract gallactocatehin gallate on fibroid cell proliferation, but these substance effects require more research [1]. While coffee and caffeine consumption do not seem to influence the fibroid risk, alcohol intake increases it [1].

Given that these risk factors for myoma formation are modifiable, they require more research. Literature data on smoking are inconsistent [1]. Very few studies investigated the association of stress and physical activity and the risk of fibroid formation, and relevant data are mostly lacking. The risk is reduced in women who take physical exercise [1]. Stress has been recently demonstrated to be a potential risk factor as it possibly increases estrogen and progesterone levels [1, 7]. Furthermore, stress influences various health-related habits which possibly promote fibroid formation, both in terms of physical activity and dietary behavior.

Arterial hypertension and diabetes mellitus are also investigated in association with fibroid risk by several researches [1]. Several studies documented a positive association between fibroids and arterial hypertension [7]. A study from the Netherlands demonstrated that women with surgically treated uterine fibroids have greater hypertension risk, independent of common risk factors [12]. Moreover, authors suggested that women with fibroids are eligible for hypertension screening. The exact nature of association between high blood pressure and fibroids is not clear, as it is yet unknown if it is caused by detection bias or shared etiology. Data from the USA studies conducted in both blacks and whites found an inverse association between diabetes and fibroid formation, probably due to systemic vascular dysfunction in women with diabetes [1]. On the other hand, hypertension is considered to be a risk factor for fibroid formation [1].

Since the last century, uterine injury caused by either infection or irritation is postulated to be a possible risk factor for fibroid onset [1]. The expression of vascular endothelial growth factor-A, which is important for tumor growth and cell proliferation, is higher in fibroids than in normal endometrium [7]. In line with this are results on the positive association among use of perineal talc and Chagas disease and fibroid risk. Moreover, the relation between pelvic inflammatory disease (PID) episodes and surgically diagnosed fibroids has also been documented [1].

Data on environmental contaminants, such as phthalates, lead, mercury, and cadmium, and risk of fibroid formation are scarce. They could possibly be influential through various mechanisms, including endocrine disruption [7].

Pathogenesis of Uterine Fibroids

Uterine fibroids are thought to be monoclonal uterine mass that occurs via clonal expansion from a single mutated myometrial smooth muscle stem cell [13].

In the recent years, significant progress has been made in our understanding of fibroid tumorigenesis. A current model suggests that a distinct stem/reservoir cell-enriched population, designated as the leiomyoma-derived side population (LMSP), is responsible to sustain proliferation and tumor growth [14].

Hormones have been considered as the major promoter of fibroid growth. In addition, several pathogenic factors such as genetics, microRNA, growth factors, cytokines, and chemokines have a role in the fibroid development and growth [15].

The fibroid mechanical properties are another key feature of these benign tumors that may contribute to their growth. Fibroids are in fact stiff tumors characterized by an excessive deposition of disordered extracellular matrix (ECM) components, particularly collagen I, III, and IV, proteoglycans, and fibronectin [15].

Matrix metalloproteinases (MMPs) are implicated in fibroid remodeling with a higher activity of MMP-2 in fibroids than in surrounding myometrium [16].

Fibroids are also surrounded by a thin fibro-neurovascular pseudocapsule, which separates fibroids from normal peripheral myometrium (Fig. 1.4).

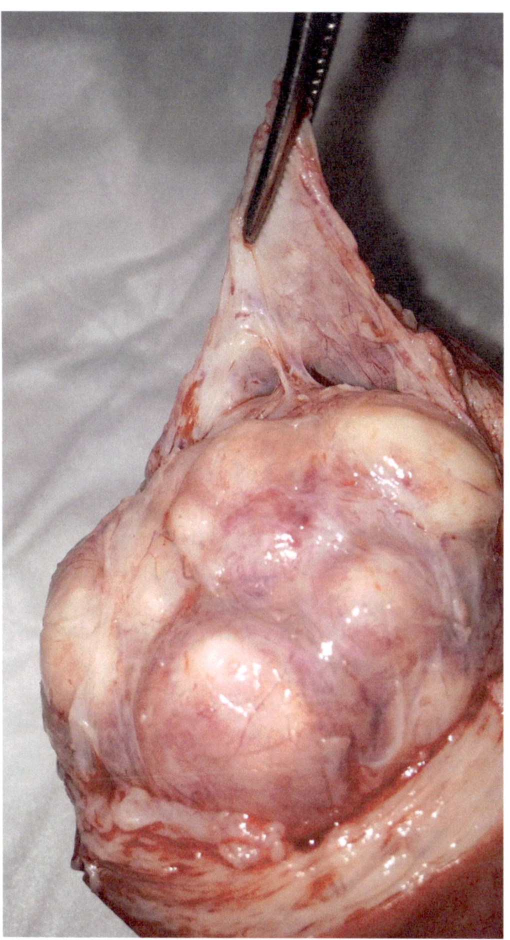

FIGURE 1.4 A uterine fibroid surrounded by a thin fibro-neurovascular structure of a few millimeters, the myoma pseudocapsule, taken with the anatomical forceps; it separates the fibroid from the normal peripheral myometrium

This means that the tumor microenvironment may greatly influence tumor growth and proliferation [17]. Uterine fibroid is a multifactorial and still enigmatic pathology. The genetic background seems to play an important role, with cytogenetic anomalies observed in about 40% of uterine fibroids.

Abnormal ECM expression, increased growth factors, cytokine and chemokine concentrations, and an extracellular disorganized matrix have been implicated in development and growth of uterine fibroids. Estrogens may exert their growth stimulatory effects on such tumors through the action of a complex network of cytokines, growth factors, or apoptosis factors and through different cellular mechanisms [18].

Biochemical and clinical studies also suggested that progesterone, progestin, and progesterone receptors (PR-A and PR-B) might increase proliferative activity in fibroids by enhancing the expression of growth factors (EGF, IGF-I) and apoptosis-related factors (TNF alpha, Bcl-2 proteins) [19].

Uterine fibroid cells typically show a high expression of cell-cycle regulator and anti-apoptotic proteins. This can trigger tumor growth and make cells resistant to apoptosis [20].

Lora and collaborators demonstrated that the ratio between PR-A and PR-B is similar in normal myometrium and fibroids, while p53 and p21 mRNA and protein levels are increased in fibroids [21].

Matsuo and collaborators showed that Bcl-2 protein, an apoptosis-inhibiting gene product, was abundantly expressed in fibroids compared with normal myometrium [22]. In this study, Bcl-2 protein expression in fibroid cells was upregulated by progesterone but downregulated by estradiol. The same group reported upregulation of expression of proliferating cell nuclear antigen (PCNA) in fibroids by progesterone and estradiol [22].

Wang and collaborators showed that protein and mRNA expression of bFGF and T-cadherin in uterine fibroid were present with significantly higher expression than that in adjacent normal myometrium and control normal myometrium. In addition, T-cadherin correlated well with bFGF. There was a relationship between T-cadherin and color Doppler flow imaging (CDFI) [23].

Data from genomic and proteomic studies demonstrated that many of the differences in fibroid's gene expression observed in the two ethnic groups might be attributed to differences in myometrial gene expression, as well as differences in fibroids vs. myometrium. Moreover, functional analysis of microarray and proteomic data revealed that many of the observed differences may be attributed to molecules with a role as transcriptional, translational, and signal transduction mediators, cell cycle and EMC regulators, cell-cell adhesion, and metabolic regulators. The current approach to diagnosis and treatment should evolve in the future and consider women with a greater genomic risk.

Somatic mutations involving the gene encoding the mediator complex subunit 12 (*MED12*) and the gene encoding the high-mobility group AT-hook 2 (*HMGA2*) are known to be associated to fibroids.

Mäkinen and collaborators [24] found that approximately 70% of fibroids contained heterozygous somatic mutations that affect *MED12*, a gene located on the X chromosome. Authors described that all mutations resided in exon 2 (codon 44), suggesting that aberrant function of this region of *MED12* contributes to tumorigenesis. Moreover, they also performed a pathway analysis, comparing eight tumors positive for *MED12* mutations with their respective normal tissues. Three pathways were found to be substantially altered in the tumors, namely, focal adhesion, extracellular matrix receptor interaction, and Wnt signaling pathways. This suggests that *MED12* mutations contribute to tumor development by altering specific cellular pathways [25].

MED12 belongs to a family of evolutionarily conserved transcriptional factors (mediator) that promote the assembly, activation, and regeneration of transcription complexes on core promoters during the initiation and reinitiation phases of transcription [26].

In detail, this gene codifies for a 26-subunit transcriptional regulator that bridges DNA regulatory sequences to the RNA polymerase II initiation complex. It is a subunit of the "kinase" module of the mediator complex, which also contains MED13, CYCLIN C, and Cyclin-dependent kinase 8 (CDK8).

It was also observed that activation of ERK signaling by *MED12* suppression may confer resistance to tyrosine kinase inhibitors including crizotinib, gefitinib, vemurafenib, selumetinib, and sorafenib, thus providing a link between suppression of *MED12* and drug resistance [27].

As demonstrated by Mäkinen and collaborators, *MED12* mutations alone are sufficient for driving tumor development. Authors analyzed whole exome sequencing data of 27 uterine fibroids (12 *MED12* mutation-negative and 15 *MED12* mutation-positive) and their paired normal myometrium. They searched for genes, which would be recurrently mutated. No such genes were identified in *MED12* mutation-negative uterine fibroids as well as *MED12* mutation-positive fibroids. These results highlight the unique role of MED12 mutations in genesis of uterine fibroids [28].

Although fibroids are believed to be chromosomally rather stable, cytogenetic rearrangements have been detected in 40–50% of fibroids. Studies found translocation between chromosomes 12 and 14, trisomy 12, translocation between chromosomes 6 and 10, and deletion of chromosomes 3 and 7, with multiple candidate genes [27].

Several signaling pathways are activated in uterine fibroids. The role of the wingless-type (Wnt) pathway in supporting tumor initiation of fibroids is well demonstrated. The Wnt pathway could mediate molecular and cellular mechanisms involved in tumor initiation. Wnt acts as a paracrine signal from estrogen/progesterone receptor-rich mature cells to activate the canonical β-catenin pathway in fibroid stem cells to stimulate self-renewal and proliferation, eventually leading to tumor growth [29].

Other studies have demonstrated a central role for the phosphoinositide 3-kinase–protein kinase B/AKT (PI3K/AKT) pathway leading to the activation of mammalian target of rapamycin (mTOR) in the pathogenesis of fibroids [30].

Histopathological Aspects of Uterine Fibroids

As abovementioned, uterine fibroid is a benign tumor that originates from the uterine smooth muscle and grossly appears as round, well-circumscribed (but not encapsulated),

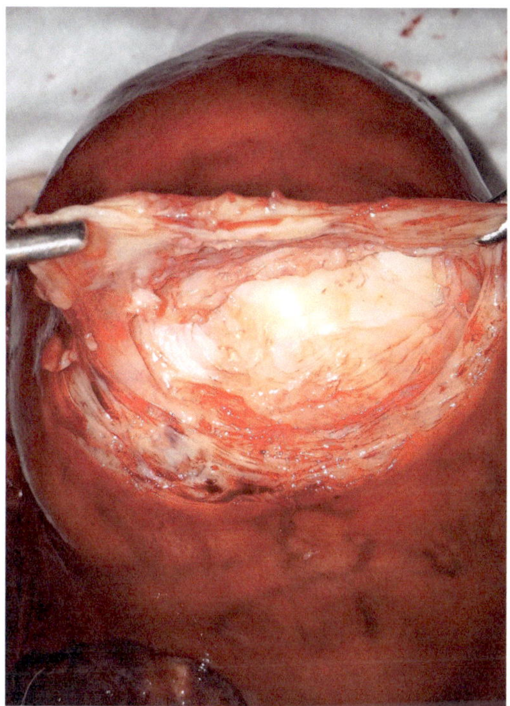

FIGURE 1.5 The fibromatosis of the uterus transversally incised after its removal, showing an inner uterine fibroid appearing as round, well-circumscribed white solid nodules

solid nodules (Fig. 1.5) that are white or tan and show whorled appearance on histological section. The size varies, from microscopic to lesions of considerable size, from a few millimeters to over 20 cm in diameter, felt by the patient herself through the abdominal wall.

Growth and location are the main factors that determine if a fibroid leads to symptoms and problems, so in uterine fibroids placing is very important to evaluate its clinical or surgical treatment.

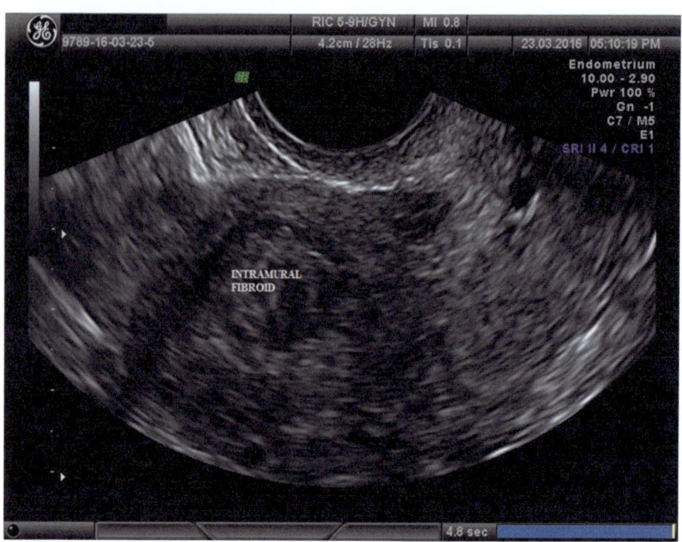

FIGURE 1.6 A transvaginal ultrasonographic scan showing an antevert uterus, with a uterine body intramural fibroid of 2 cm

As the traditional reported classification of fibroids, these tumors can be subserous, intramural, submucosal, or cervical.

Intramural fibroids are located within the wall of the uterus (Fig. 1.6) and are the most common type; unless large, they may be asymptomatic. Intramural fibroids begin as small nodules in the muscular wall of the uterus. With time, intramural fibroids may expand inwards, causing distortion and elongation of the uterine cavity (Fig. 1.7).

Subserosal fibroids are located underneath the peritoneal surface of the uterus (Fig. 1.8) and can become very large. They can also grow out in a papillary manner to become pedunculated fibroids (Fig. 1.9).

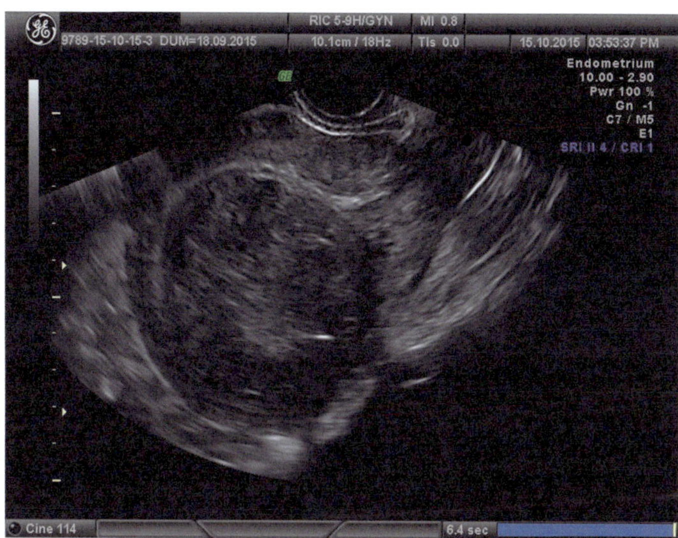

FIGURE 1.7 A transvaginal ultrasonographic scan showing a uterus with a fundal fibroid of 5 cm in diameter, causing distortion of the uterine cavity

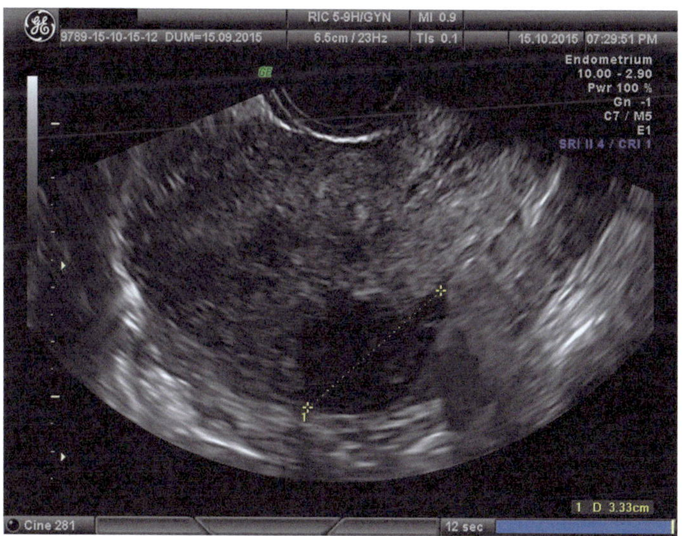

FIGURE 1.8 A transvaginal ultrasonographic scan showing a uterus with a posterior subserosal uterine body fibroid of 2.5 cm in diameter, located underneath the peritoneal surface of the uterus

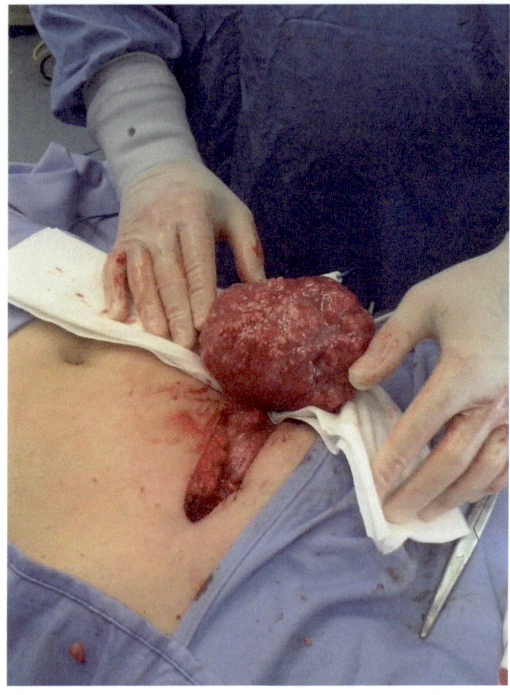

FIGURE 1.9 A laparotomic myomectomy of a fundal mitotically active pedunculated fibroid of 10 cm in diameter; fibroma expresses a highly irregular surface, is of mixed consistency (soft and hard), and grew up in the patient in less than a year

These pedunculated growths can actually detach from the uterus to become a parasitic leiomyoma (Fig. 1.10).

Submucosal fibroids are located in the muscle beneath the endometrium of the uterus and distort the uterine cavity; even small lesions in this location may lead to bleeding and infertility (Fig. 1.11).

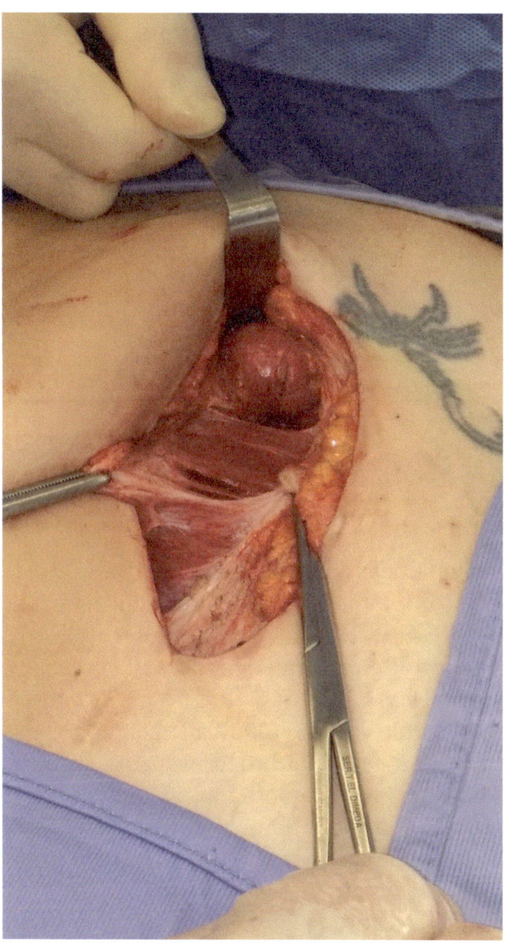

FIGURE 1.10 A rare image, taken during transversal suprapubic laparotomy, of parasitic uterine fibroid of 4 cm in diameter, grew up in the rectus abdominis muscle. The patient was operated with two previous myomectomies, after which he suffered pain and a palpable mass in the abdomen area

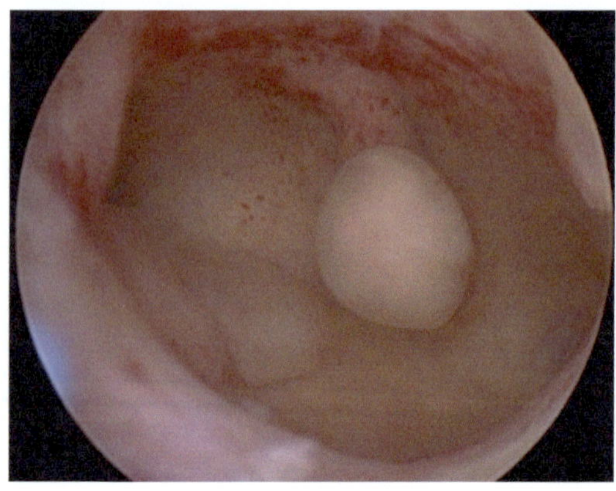

FIGURE 1.11 A hysteroscopic image of a small submucosal G0 fibroid; these fibroids, even small of diameter, may lead to bleeding and infertility

A pedunculated lesion within the cavity is termed an intra-cavitary fibroid and can be passed through the cervix (Fig. 1.12).

Cervical fibroids are located in the wall of the cervix (neck of the uterus) (Fig. 1.13).

Sometimes, fibroids are found in the supporting uterine structures (round ligament, broad ligament, uterosacral liga-ment) that also contain smooth muscle tissue.

To best standardize the fibroid location in the uterus, FIGO used the leiomyoma subclassification system of Wamsteker et al. of 1993 [31]. The system that includes the tertiary classification of leiomyomas categorizes the submucosal group and adds cat-egorizations for intramural, subserosal, and transmural lesions. Intracavitary lesions are attached to the endometrium by a nar-row stalk and are classified as type 0, whereas types 1 and 2 require a portion of the lesion to be intramural—with type 1 being less than 50% and type 2 at least 50%. The type 3 lesions are totally extracavitary but about the endometrium. Type 4 lesions are intramural leiomyomas that are entirely within the myometrium, with no extension to the endometrial surface or to the serosa. Subserosal (types 5–7) leiomyomas represent the

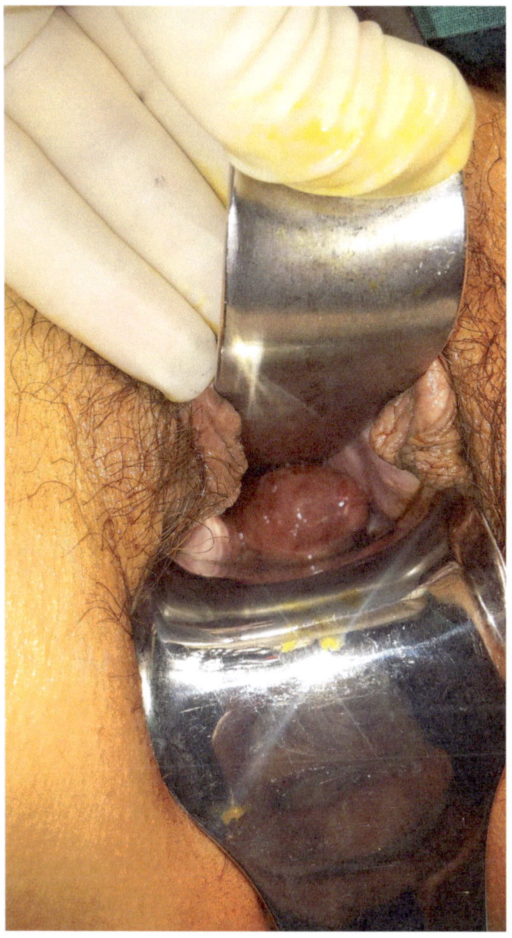

FIGURE 1.12 An intracavitary fibroid passed through the uterine cervix and expelled into the vagina

mirror image of the submucosal leiomyomas—with type 5 being at least 50% intramural, type 6 being less than 50% intramural, and type 7 being attached to the serosa by a stalk. The classification of lesions that are transmural would be categorized by their relationship to both the endometrial and the serosal surfaces.

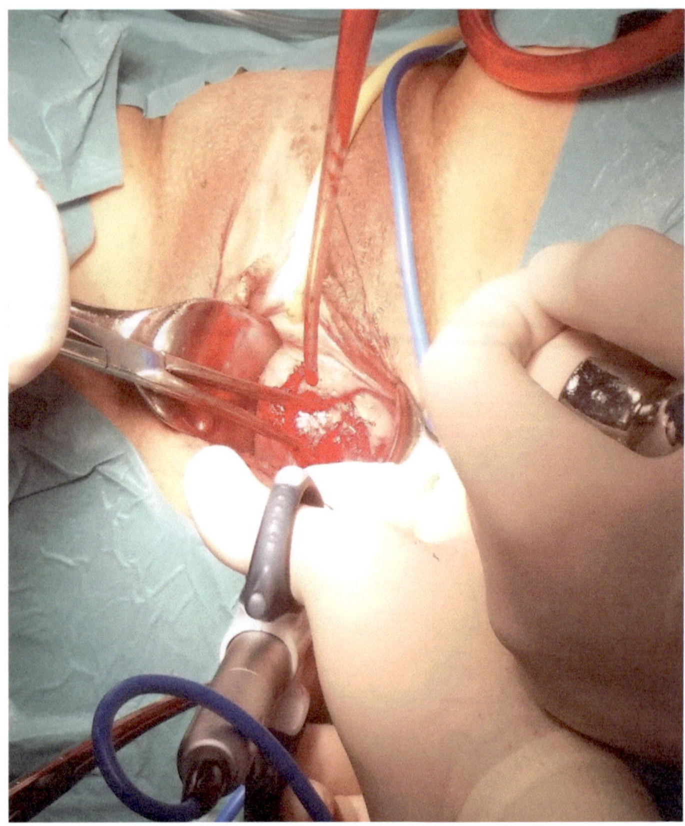

FIGURE 1.13 A transvaginal cervical myomectomy, with a removal of a cervical fibroid of 7 cm in diameter located in the anterior wall of the cervix

Discussing on histological characteristics, uterine fibroids can be single or multiple and induce symptoms depending on the size and location. Most fibroids start in the muscular wall of the uterus and, with further growth, some lesions may develop toward the outside of the uterus or toward the internal cavity. They can become large and interfere with pregnancy or cause inflammatory complications. Macroscopically they have a cutting tense-elastic surface (Fig. 1.14).

Microscopically the tumor is formed by smooth muscle cells separated by a more or less plentiful quantity of vascular

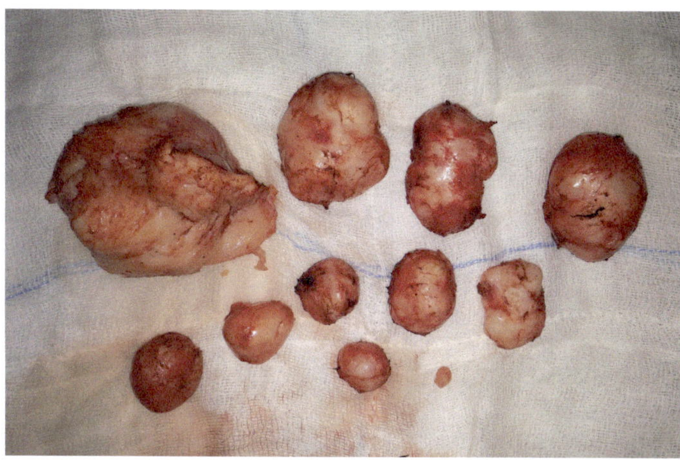

FIGURE 1.14 A collection of removed fibroid of different diameter by laparotomic myomectomy. Macroscopically they have a cutting tense-elastic surface

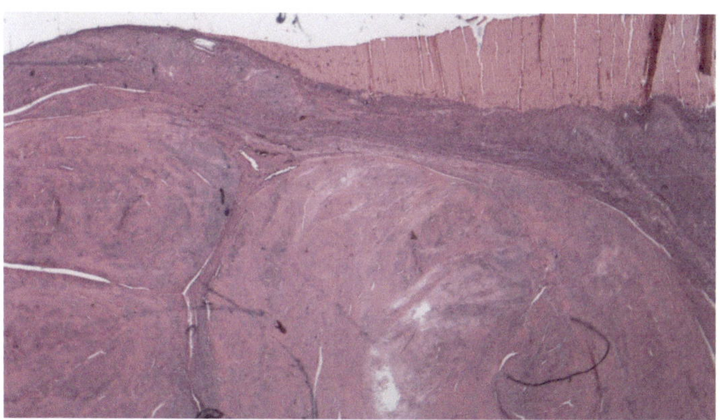

FIGURE 1.15 A histologic examination of fibroids, on a slide colored by hematoxylin and eosin, at 1X; microscopically the tumor is formed by smooth muscle cells separated by a more or less plentiful quantity of vascular connective tissue

connective tissue (Fig. 1.15). Malignant transformation of these tumors is a rare event, quite exceptional. In general, it appears that uterine leiomyosarcomas do not arise from benign leiomyomas, with rare exceptions [32].

The genetic origin of the malignant tumor has always been much discussed, since genetic evidence has been inconsistent over the years. In fact, it is still not well understood if uterine leiomyosarcoma arises de novo or whether there is karyotypic evolution from myomas to ULMS or the so-called sarcomatous degeneration. The consensus from genetic studies has been that most sarcomas arise independently [33]. On the contrary, histologic studies have found rare examples that appear consistent with progression from a leiomyoma to sarcoma [34].

Histological Variants of Fibroids

Uterine fibroids have many histological variants and aspects (Figs. 1.16, 1.17, 1.18, 1.19, 1.20, 1.21, 1.22, 1.23, 1.24, 1.25, 1.26, 1.27, 1.28, and 1.29), classified in the histopathological atlas [35]:

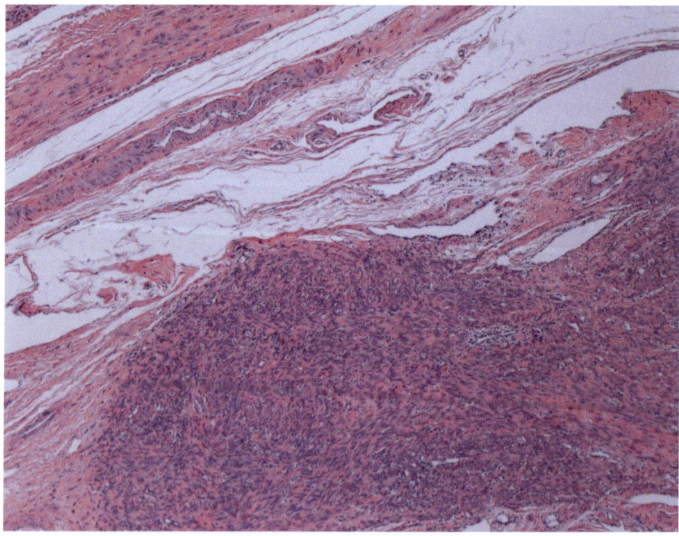

FIGURE 1.16 Leiomuscular proliferation of cells (simple leiomyoma), separate from the normal myometrium (*top left*) by a frame layer (pseudocapsule) rich in vessels. The arrangement of tumor cells appears constituted in bundles twisted at 90° but with bizarre trend

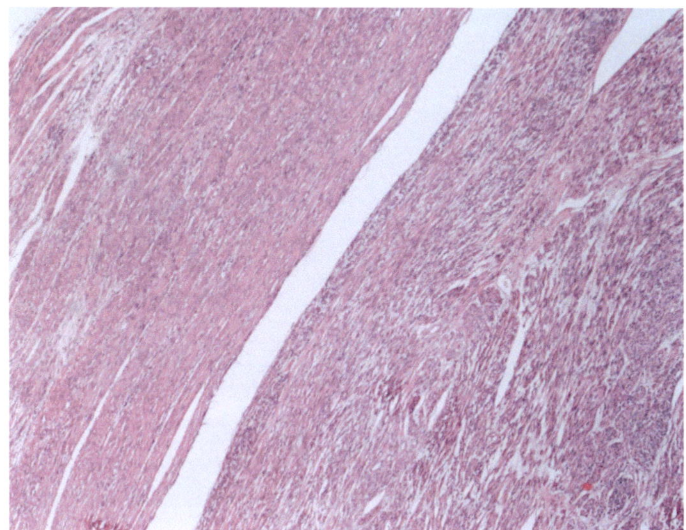

FIGURE 1.17 Another example of a comparison between the leiomyoma (*bottom right*) and pseudocapsule compressed uterine muscle tissue

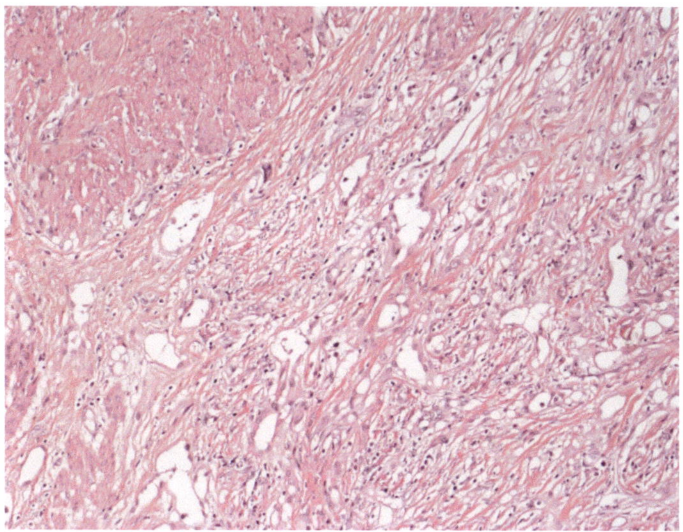

FIGURE 1.18 At higher magnification, the pseudocapsule appears rich in newly formed vessels, sometimes with minimal reactive lymphocytic infiltration

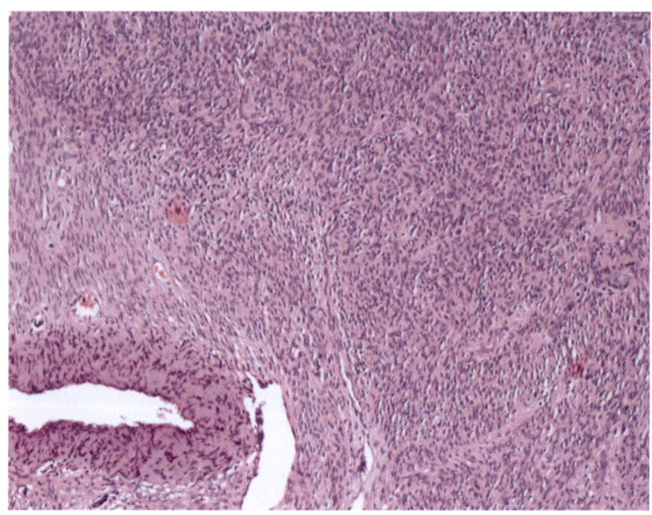

FIGURE 1.19 Leiomyoma cell. The cells appear thickly crammed with scant cytoplasm and nuclei in close contact with each other. In this case the evolution of the neoplastic cell-sorted bundles is still evident

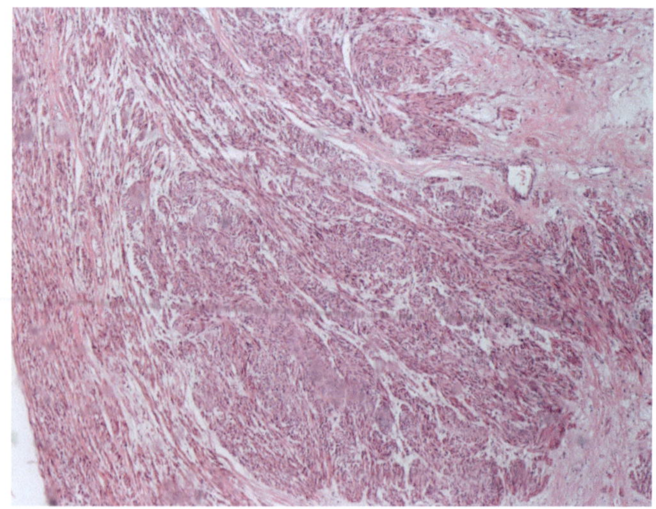

FIGURE 1.20 Leiomyoma with fibrosis. The muscle cell bundles are separated by collagen fibers (eosinophilic less), limiting the growth of the tumor. This is most common in postmenopausal women

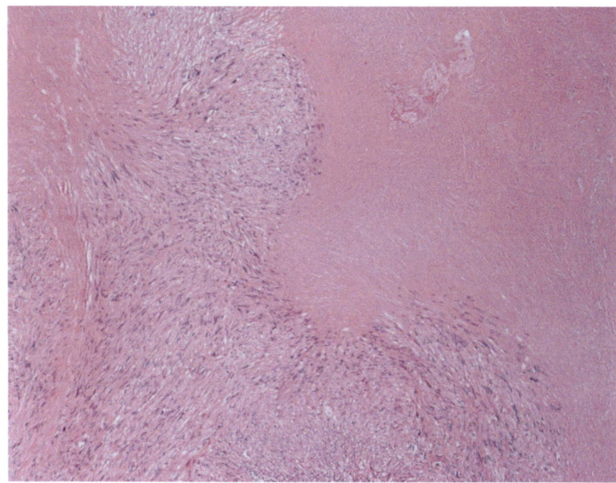

FIGURE 1.21 In some hormonal conditions (pregnancy, hormonal treatment, and suppressive therapy), leiomyoma may have more or less extensive areas of necrosis (defined improperly "hyaline"). This necrosis is differentiated from typical coagulation necrosis of leiomyosarcoma

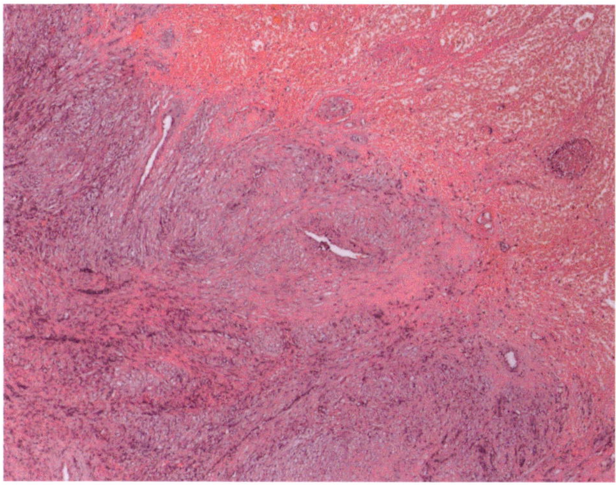

FIGURE 1.22 Also for hormonal conditions or mechanical effects, it may also exhibit large areas of hemorrhage (leiomyoma apoplexy). These factors should always be differentiated from regressive areas of leiomyosarcoma

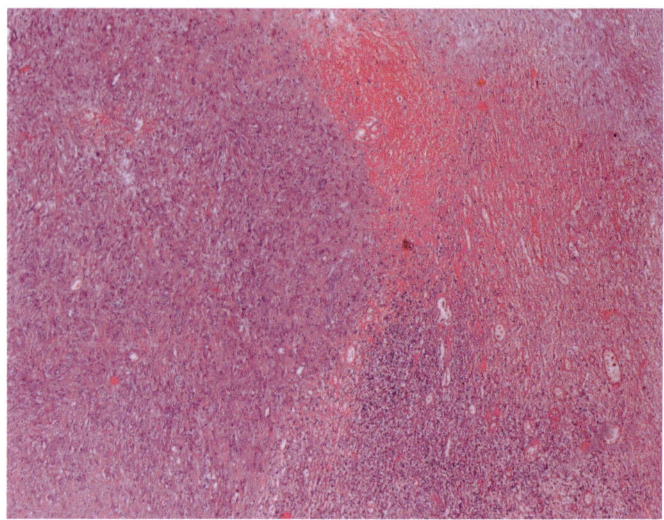

FIGURE 1.23 Another image of apoplexy

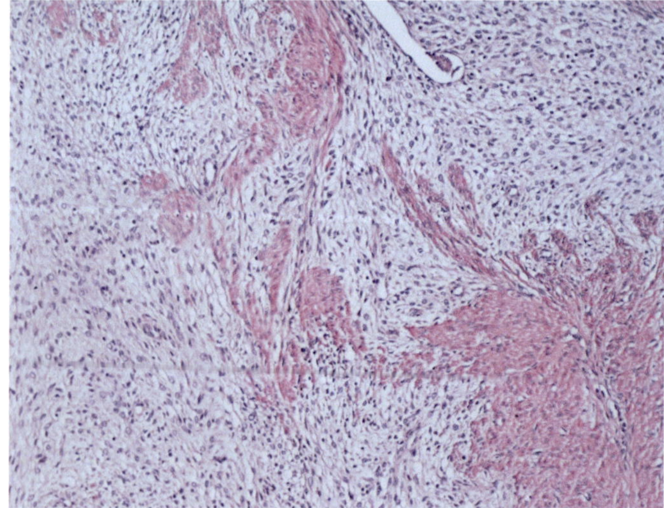

FIGURE 1.24 Myxoid leiomyoma. Vast areas of the tumor are formed by one frame basophilic stroma in which cancer cells take on a starry appearance. This cancer must be studied carefully, because even a low mitotic index is suggestive of malignancy

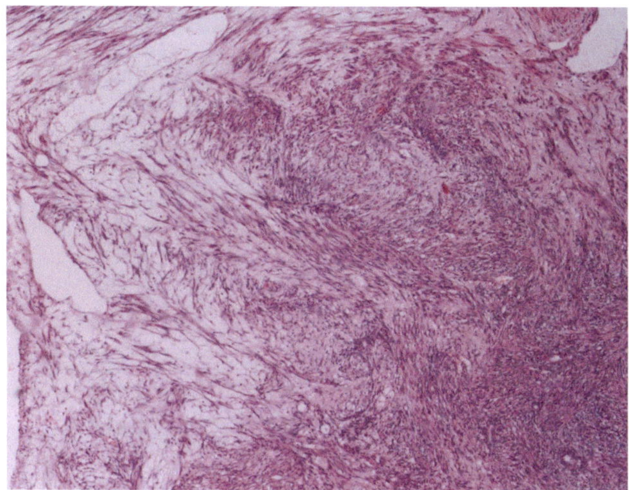

FIGURE 1.25 Unlike the myxoid leiomyoma, leiomyoma with myxoid stroma degeneration presents basophilic spindle but cancer cells and not stellate. The risk of malignant behavior in this case is exceptional

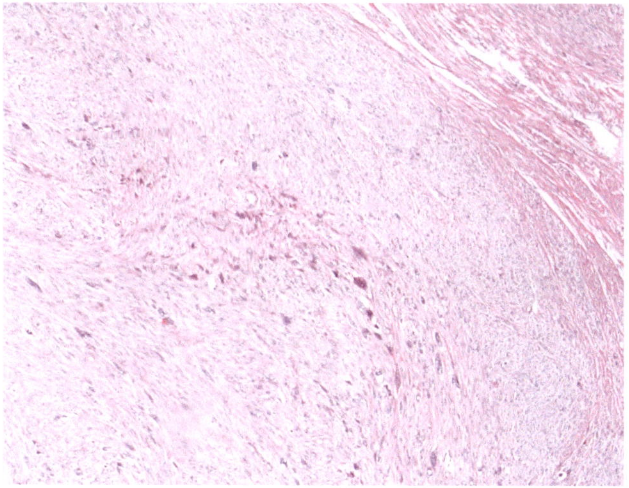

FIGURE 1.26 Leiomyoma with bizarre or atypical nuclei or symplastic leiomyoma. This cancer has voluminous cells with multiple nuclei and hyperchromatic. The absence of necrosis and low mitotic index excludes the malignant nature of the tumor

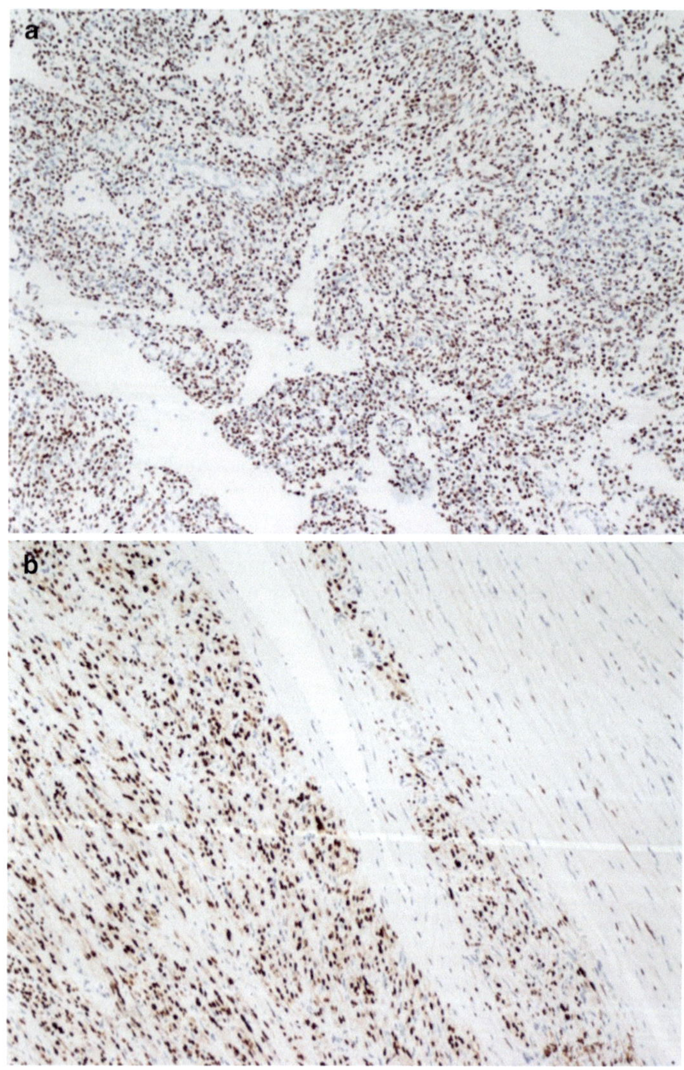

FIGURE 1.27 Expression of estrogen receptor (**a**) and for progesterone (**b**) in almost all of leiomyoma cells. Note the low expression of progesterone receptors in the normal myometrium (*right*)

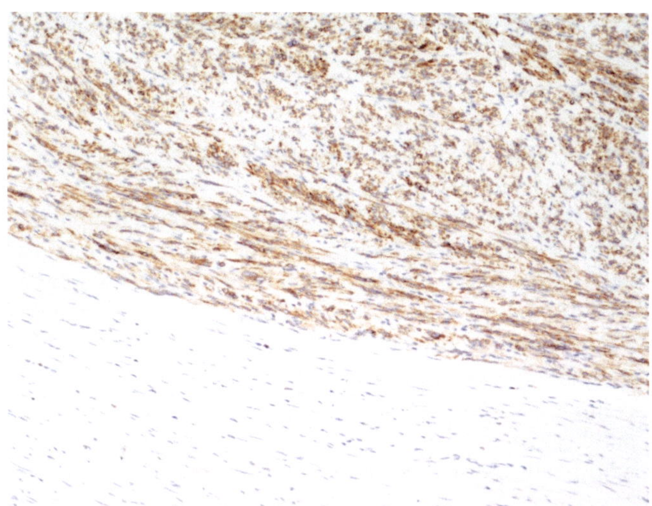

FIGURE 1.28 Expression of BCL2 (known as anti-apoptotic gene) in leiomyoma cells. The normal myometrium appears negative. The interference of BCL2 on the cell cycle ensures the persistence of the tumor

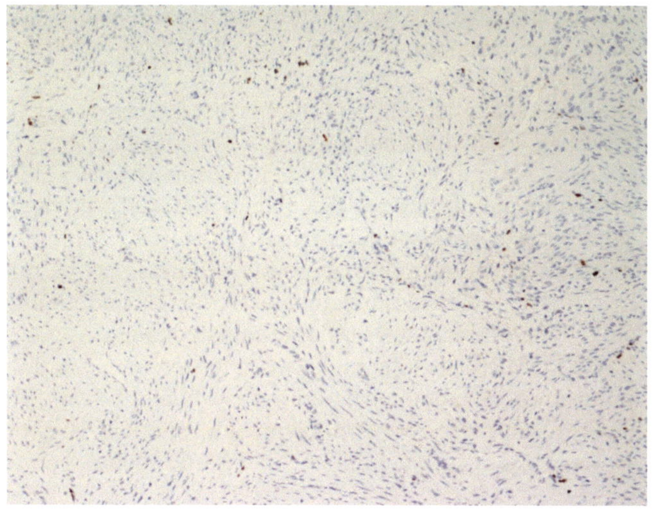

FIGURE 1.29 In a simple leiomyoma, research of proliferating cells (positive for Ki-67) is at minimum value (always below 5% of the neoplastic cells)

1. Red degeneration fibroid (characterized by coagulative necrosis, often associated with pregnancy or oral contraceptive use).
2. Fibroid with apoplexy.
3. Fibroid with hydropic degeneration (mimicking myxoid leiomyosarcoma).
4. Fibroid with lymphoid infiltration (mimicking lymphoma).
5. Fibroid with high cellularity (tumor that has an increased cellularity but not coagulative necrosis, atypia, or an excessive number of mitotic figures—the differential diagnosis includes the leiomyosarcoma).
6. Atypical, bizarre, or pleomorphic fibroid (includes atypical cellular elements but not coagulation necrosis or mitotic activity).
7. Mitotically active fibroid (tumors that have from 5 to 10xHPF mitosis but the absence of coagulative necrosis or cytologic atypia.
8. Leiomyolipoma, epithelioid fibroid, and parasite fibroid different from skeletal intravenous leiomyomatosis (with growth in the lumen of the uterine or pelvic veins, going up to the vena cava and right atrium), in which distant metastases are exceptionally rare and long-term survival is excellent.
9. Benign metastasizing fibroid (tumor that has characteristics typical of leiomyoma but the absence of coagulative necrosis, increased mitotic activity, or significant atypia), accompanied by pulmonary nodules, lymph nodes, etc. It has the same characteristics of the original and probably represents metastases. The extrauterine nodule features may be mild or show characteristics of leiomyosarcoma or smooth muscle tumors of uncertain or indeterminate malignant potential (STUMP). The interval between hysterectomy and the occurrence of pulmonary nodules is about 15 years. The clinical course is more indolent, and survival is about 10 years after excision of these "metastatic" nodules.

This neoplasm should be called also leiomyomas metastasizing or leiomyosarcomas of low grade.

Despite scientific advances, there is an unsolved problem on pathologic differentiation of fibroids in surgical pathology. Adapting the criteria of classification of Kempson, such as mitosis, atypia, coagulative necrosis, etc., to surgical pathology, these aspects alone or in combination constitute an accurate method but not infallible to predict the prognosis of these tumors. Some pathologists suggest calling fibroid as smooth muscle tumors because of the likelihood of an estimated percentage of such tumors to recur or metastasize on the basis of the mentioned parameters and on phenotypic and genotypic data assisting pathologist in terms of prognosis and recommended treatment.

Discussing on fibroid developing in the context of myometrium, it does not have a real structural continuity with the surrounding myometrium. Fibroid has a round shape made of fibers of smooth muscle tissue with concentric spiral, with fibrous connective tissue, vessels, and neurofibers forming a pseudocapsule, anchored to the myometrium by fibromuscular bridges. This structure was evaluated by several investigations [36].

Anatomy and Functionality of Myoma Pseudocapsule

Ito et al. [37] performed a histopathology evaluation of the myoma and its surrounding structure, the myoma pseudocapsule; the study of the architecture of the myometrium and the extracellular matrix in the presence of myomas demonstrated how a pseudocapsule is formed surrounding the myoma, which separates the myoma from normal tissue. The authors concluded that the fibroid is anchored to the pseudocapsule by connective bridges but lacks its own true vascular pedicle.

Dapunt [38] previously confirmed that a vascular network surrounds the myoma as in a pseudocapsule, so that if the detachment of the myoma occurs inside the pseudocapsule burning this network, it leads to less bleeding during myomectomy.

Fox and Buckley [39], using ultrastructural microscopy to study a series of enucleated myomas, founded an anatomical structure different from normal myometrium: they affirmed that leiomyomas have a well-defined regular outline and a surrounding pseudocapsule of compressed muscle fibers.

The hypothesis of the presence of a pseudocapsule was also asserted by Vizza and Motta [40], who demonstrated that, in a section of myoma with pseudocapsule, the surrounding fibers tend to bulge out from the surrounding myometrium and to have a firm, whorled, or trabeculate surface. Furthermore, ultrasonographic (US) evaluations have been recently performed on myomas and their connecting structures: the pseudocapsule appears, by transabdominal and transvaginal US, as an echogenic line around the myoma, with a 1 cm or less clear wall, and with reinforcement of distal echoes. A color Doppler investigation on fibroids by Kurjak et al. [41] demonstrated a "fire ring" surrounding the myoma, and this has led to the myoma pseudocapsule ultrasound definition.

On the basis of these reports of 20 years ago, histological investigations on the fibroid vascular pseudocapsule were performed, to better understand their role in the modern minimally invasive surgical approach in women [42].

The macroscopic evaluation of the pseudocapsule and of the adjacent myometrium showed parallel arrays of extremely dense capillaries and of larger vessels forming the capsule, separated from the myometrial vasculature by a narrow avascular cleft. The pseudocapsule vessels coming from the surrounding myometrium throw themselves in a group to the center of the vascular network, to form a sort of pedicle: the veins surrounding the myoma circulate under the pseudocapsule arranged in a plexus [43] (Fig. 1.30).

Moreover, the biochemical growth factor evaluation in pseudocapsule vessels showed intense angiogenesis in pseudocapsule, probably promoted by the same fibroid presence. The angiogenesis of the myoma pseudocapsule leads, probably, to the formation of a "protective" vascular capsule responsible for the supply of blood to the growing tumor [44].

The fibroid pseudocapsule is a structure which surrounds the uterine fibroid and separates it from the uterine tissue. At the ultrastructural level, visualized by transmission electron

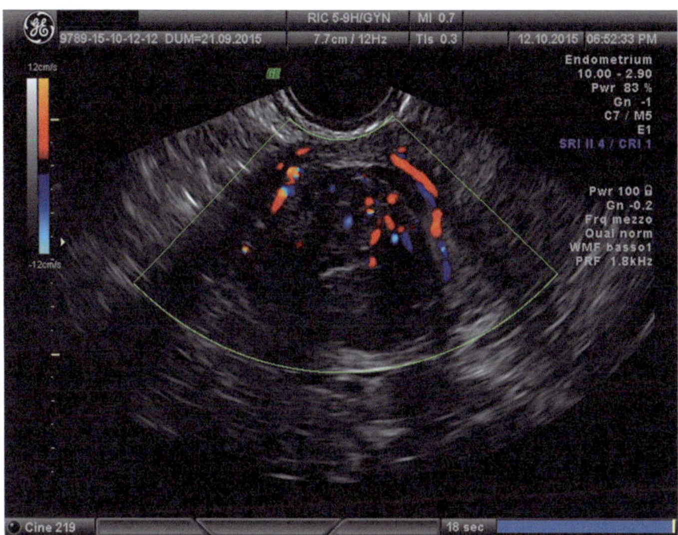

FIGURE 1.30 A transvaginal ultrasonographic scan, showing a fibroid surrounded by its pseudocapsule vessels. They, coming from the surrounding myometrium, throw themselves in a group to the center of the vascular network, to form a sort of pedicle: the veins surrounding the myoma circulate under the pseudocapsule arranged in a plexus

microscopy, the pseudocapsule cells have the features of smooth muscle cells similar to the myometrium. So, the pseudocapsules are part of the myometrium which compresses the leiomyoma [45].

This ultrastructural feature suggests that, when removing fibroids, the pseudocapsules should be always preserved, to preserve the myometrium and postsurgical uterine anatomy.

Wei et al. [46] demonstrated that in large uterine fibroids, the most biologically active zone is the region next to the periphery with a higher level of gene expression, a higher density of blood vessels, a higher proliferative rate, and a lower level of hyaline degeneration.

These studies confirm preliminary evidence that pseudocapsules contain neuropeptides together with their related fibers, as a neurovascular bundle, containing a vascular network rich in neurotransmitters like a neurovascular bundle [47].

Literature data confirm that pseudocapsules contain many neuropeptides and neurotransmitters, physiologically active. Moreover, these substances may play a significant role in wound healing and innervation repair and may be essential for reproductive and sexual function [48].

In fact, a research on gene expression analysis in uterine leiomyoma pseudocapsule revealed an angiogenic profile in the pseudocapsule. In this investigation [49], authors performed, by quantitative real-time RT-PCR method (qRT-PCR), a gene expression analysis of PC, matching it with the same analysis in UL and UM and evaluating the expression levels of IGF-2, used as tumoral marker, and COL4A2, CYR61/CCN1, CTGF/CCN2, VEGF-A, and vWF, known to be involved in angiogenic processes. The results clearly indicated that the pseudocapsule was a structure anatomically distinguishable from the myometrium and the surrounding fibroid, displaying a significant and specific gene expression profile. The pseudocapsule, as the fibroid, exhibits a significantly reduced expression of the IGF-2 gene [50], known to be a tumor growth marker, if compared to the fibroid, suggesting that it has a non-fibroid origin and that it has a structural continuity with the myometrium. The pseudocapsule also showed a statistical relevant overexpression of the endoglin/CD105 gene, when compared to the myometrium and to the fibroid. Based on these evidences, the overexpression of the endoglin gene, rather than of other angiogenic genes, seemed to indicate the presence of an active angiogenesis correlated with reparative process in the pseudocapsule. Altogether these data clearly depicted the pseudocapsule as a site of intense angiogenesis linked to the endoglin activation rather than other angiogenic factors such as VEGF-A or vWF. The presence of an active angiogenesis is concordant with the histological studies that describe a parallel array of extremely dense capillaries in the pseudocapsule and in the adjacent myometrium that are absent in fibroid. This can define the structural and functional features of the pseudocapsule that could explain its possible roles in the uterine regenerative process.

Moreover, in such regenerative process, there is also the involvement of neuropeptides and neurotransmitters extremely important in wound healing. In fact, there is evidence that the nervous system and its neurotransmitters, such as substance P (SP) and vasoactive intestinal peptide (VIP) [51], neuropeptide Y (NPY), neurotensin (NT), and PGP9.5 [52], enkephalin, and oxytocin [53], play a role in mediating inflammation and healing. Referring to uterine musculature scar physiology, this peptide sparing enhances a correct healing of a hysterotomy, as evidenced by Mettler et al. [44].

Most of these neuropeptides have been already highlighted in the pseudocapsule [17].

Clinical Symptoms

Fibroids affect the quality of life and can cause morbidity; patients submitted to hysterectomies for fibroid-related symptoms (Fig. 1.31) have significantly worse scores on SF-36 quality-of-life questionnaires than women with hypertension, heart disease, chronic lung disease, or arthritis [54].

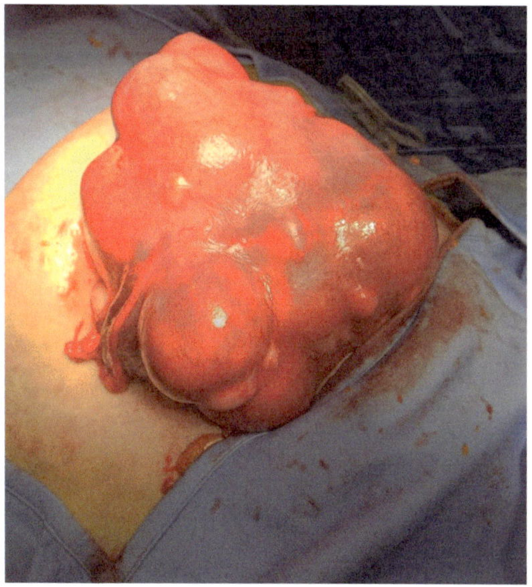

FIGURE 1.31 A laparotomic hysterectomy for a symptomatic giant multi-myomatosic uterus

The association of fibroids with heavy menstrual bleeding has not been clearly established, so it is important to consider other possible etiologies including coagulopathies such as von Willebrand's disease [55].

One study found that women with fibroids used 7.5 pads or tampons on the heaviest day of bleeding compared with 6.1 pads or tampons used by women without fibroids. Women with fibroids larger than 5 cm (Fig. 1.32) had slightly more gushing and used about three more pads or tampons on the heaviest day of bleeding than women with smaller fibroids [56].

A recent study reported that 259 women found to have submucous fibroids on hysteroscopic examination had objective measures of heavy menstrual bleeding, i.e., lower hemoglobin levels and a higher risk of anemia than women without submucous fibroids, although self-reported pictorial blood loss assessment did not differ [57]. Women with fibroids are only slightly more likely to experience pelvic pain than women without fibroids. In one study, 96 women found to have fibroids based on transvaginal sonography reported

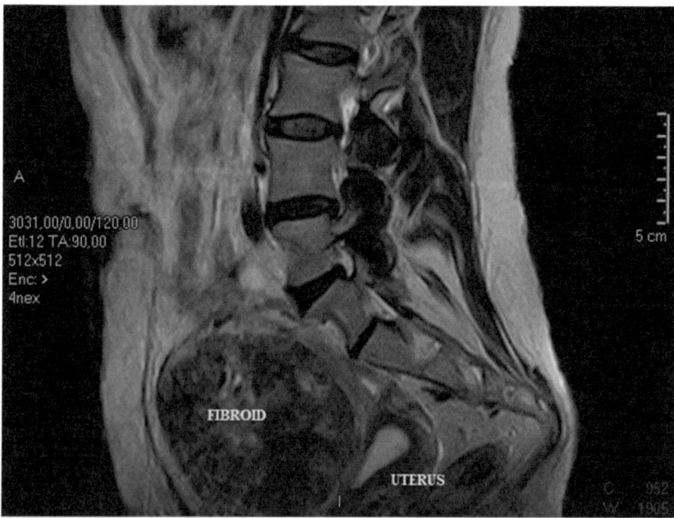

FIGURE 1.32 A magnetic resonance imaging (MRI) sagittal T2 scan showing an anterior fibroid of 11 cm in diameter

moderate or severe dyspareunia or noncyclic pelvic pain only slightly more than women without fibroids; there was no difference in moderate or severe dysmenorrhea [57]. A study of 827 women with ultrasound-detected fibroids found that deep dyspareunia was related to fibroids, and the relationship was even stronger for "severe deep dyspareunia" [57].

Patients presenting to gynecologists for evaluation with fibroid-associated pain may be different than those in the general population. As fibroids enlarge, they may outgrow their blood supply with resulting cell death and degeneration (Fig. 1.33). The type of degeneration, as hyaline, cystic, or hemorrhagic, appears to be unrelated to the clinical symptoms [58].

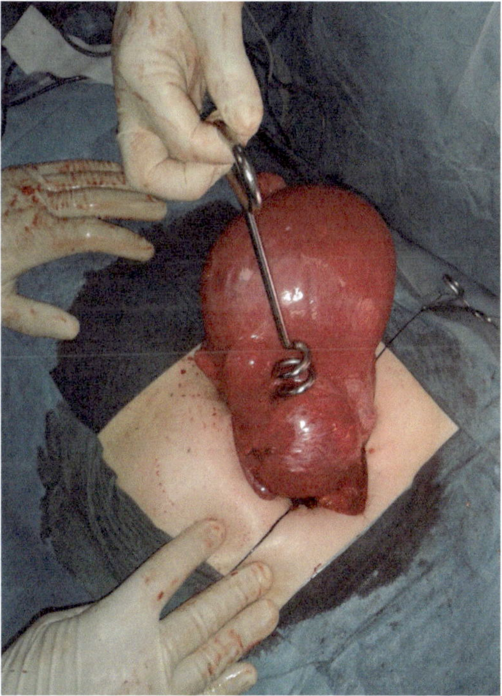

FIGURE 1.33 A laparotomic hysterectomy for a myomatosic uterus; patient referred to surgery for fibroid growth, after 2 years of absence of gynecological check. The histological analysis coagulative necrosis and no malignant degeneration

Torsion of pedunculated subserosal fibroid may, rarely, occur and produce acute pelvic pain, until the surgical intervention [20, 59].

Fibroids can cause urinary symptoms, although few studies have examined this association. Following uterine artery embolization and a 35% reduction in mean uterine volume, 68% of women had great or moderate improvement in frequency and urgency [60].

A 55% decrease in uterine volume following a 6-month treatment with GnRH-a leads to a likewise decrease in urinary frequency, nocturia, and urgency [61]. There were no changes in urge or stress incontinence as measured by symptoms or urodynamic studies. These findings may be related to decrease in uterine volume or other effects of GnRH treatment.

Unfortunately, predicting fibroid growth is not possible. Serial MRIs from 72 premenopausal women with fibroids found a median growth rate over 1 year of 9%, although 7% of fibroids got smaller over the study period. The range of growth and shrinkage was very large: −89% to +138% [62].

Fibroids with diameter <5 cm had more frequent growth spurts than did larger fibroids. Surprisingly, multiple fibroids found in the same woman showed very variable growth rates, suggesting that a woman's hormone levels do not determine the growth rate. After age 35, growth rates did not decline with age for black women but did decline in white women [1].

In premenopausal women, "rapid uterine growth" almost never indicates presence of uterine sarcoma. One study found only one sarcoma among 371 (0.26%) women operated for rapid growth of presumed fibroids [63].

No sarcomas were found in the 198 women who had a 6-week increase in uterine size over 1 year, one published definition of rapid growth. Women found to have uterine sarcoma are often clinically suspected of having a pelvic malignancy [64].

Between 1989 and 1999, the SEER database reported 2098 women with uterine sarcomas with an average age of 63 years [65].

Genetic differences between fibroids and leiomyosarcomas indicate that leiomyosarcomas do not result from malignant degeneration of fibroids, and comparative genomic hybridization did not find specific anomalies shared by fibroids and leiomyosarcomas [66].

If that fibroid growth is not predictable, women with fibroids who are mildly or moderately symptomatic may choose to defer treatment. As women approach menopause and there is limited time to develop new symptoms, "watchful waiting" may be considered. There is no evidence that not having treatment for fibroids results in harm, except for women with severe anemia from fibroid-related heavy menstrual bleeding or hydronephrosis due to obstruction of the ureter(s) from an enlarged fibroid uterus (Fig. 1.34).

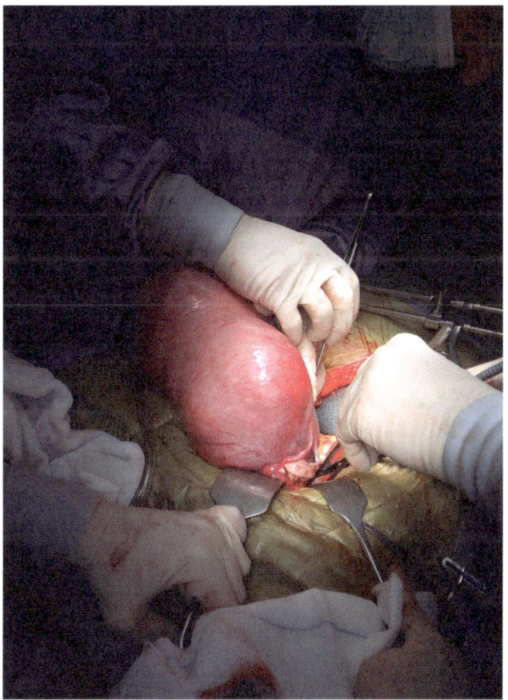

FIGURE 1.34 A laparotomic hysterectomy for a symptomatic giant myomatosic uterus causing bilateral hydronephrosis due to obstruction of the ureters

After 1 year of "watchful waiting," 77% of women with uterine size 8 weeks or greater had no significant changes in the self-reported amount of bleeding, pain, or degree of bothersome symptoms [67].

However, of the 106 women who initially chose "watchful waiting," 23% opted for hysterectomy during the course of the year [67].

The majority of symptomatic women may require surgical treatment, as most medical approaches available at present have not been completely successful, particularly in the long term [68].

References

1. Sparic R, Mirkovic L, Malvasi A, Tinelli A. Epidemiology of uterine Myomas: a review. Int J Fertil Steril. 2016;9(4):424–35.
2. Di Tommaso S, Massari S, Malvasi A, Vergara D, Maffia M, Greco M, et al. Selective genetic analysis of myoma pseudocapsule and potential biological impact on uterine fibroid medical therapy. Expert Opin Ther Targets. 2015;19(1):7–12.
3. Reis FM, Bloise E, Ortiga-Carvalho TM. Hormones and pathogenesis of uterine fibroids. Best Pract Res Clin Obstet Gynaecol. 2016;34:13–24. pii: S1521-6934(15)00229-1.
4. Puchar A, Luton D, Koskas M. Ulipristal acetate for uterine fibroid-related symptoms. Drugs Today (Barc). 2015;51(11):661–7.
5. Sparic R, Hudelist G, Berisava M, Gudovic A, Buzadzic S. Hysterectomy throughout history. Acta Chir Iugosl. 2011;58(4):9–14.
6. Styer AK, Rueda BR. The epidemiology and genetics of uterine leiomyoma. Best Pract Res Clin Obstet Gynaecol. 2016;34:3–12. pii: S1521-6934(15)00232-1.
7. Wise LA, Laughlin-Tommaso SK. Epidemology of uterine fibroids: from menarche to menopause. Clin Obstet Gynecol. 2015;59(1):2–24.
8. Laughlin S, Baird DD, Savitz DA, Herring AH, Hartmann KE. Prevalence of uterine leiomyomas in the first trimester of pregnancy: an ultrasound screening study. Obstet Gynecol. 2009;113(3):630–5.
9. Wise LA, Lauglin-Tommaso SK. Uterine leiomyomata. In: Goldman MB, Troisi R, Rexrode KM, editors. Women and health. San Diego: Academic; 2013. p. 285–306.

10. Parazzini F, Di Martino M, Candiani M, Vigano P. Dietary components and uterine leiomyomas: a review of the publishe data. Nutr Cancer. 2015;67(4):569–79.
11. Brakta S, Diamond AS, Al-Hendy A, Diamond MP, Halder SK. Role of vitamin D in uterine fibroid biology. Fertil Steril. 2015;104(3):698–706.
12. Haan YC, Oudman I, de Lange ME, Timmermans A, Ankum WM, van Montfrans GA, et al. Hypertension risk in Dutch women with symptomatic uterine fibroids. Am J Hypertens. 2015;28(4):487–92.
13. Hashimoto K, Azuma C, Kamiura S, Kimura T, Nobunaga T, Kanai T, et al. Clonal determination of uterine leiomyomas by analyzing differential inactivation of the X-chromosome-linked phosphoglycerokinase gene. Gynecol Obstet Invest. 1995;40(3):204–8.
14. Ono M, Qiang W, Serna VA, Yin P, Coon JS 5th, Navaro A, et al. Role of stem cells in human uterine leiomyoma growth. PLoS One. 2012;7(5):e36935.
15. Sozen I, Arici A. Interactions of cytokines, growth factors, and the extracellular matrix in the cellular biology of uterine leiomyomata. Fertil Steril. 2002;78(1):1–12.
16. Bogusiewicz M, Stryjecka-Zimmer M, Postawski K, Jakimiuk AJ, Rechberger T. Activity of matrix metalloproteinase-2 and -9 and contents of their tissue inhibitors in uterine leiomyoma and corresponding myometrium. Gynecol Endocrinol. 2007;23(9):541–6.
17. Tinelli A, Malvasi A. Uterine fibroid pseudocapsule. In: Tinelli A, Malvasi A, editors. Uterine myoma, myomectomy and minimally invasive treatments. Cham: Springer Publisher; 2015. p. 73–93.
18. Grings AO, Lora V, Dias Ferreira G, Brum IS, Corleta HV, Capp E. Protein expression of estrogen receptors α and β and aromatase in myometrium and uterine leiomyoma. Gynecol Obstet Invest. 2012;73(2):113–7.
19. Maruo T, Matsuo H, Shimomura Y, Kurachi O, Nikago S, Yamada T, et al. Effects of progesterone on growth factor expression in human uterine leiomyoma. Steroids. 2003;68(10–13):817–24.
20. Sparic R, Terzic M, Malvasi A, Tinelli A. Uterine fibroids-clinical presentation and complications. Acta Chir Iugosl. 2014;61(3):41–8.
21. Lora V, Grings AO, Capp E, von Eye CH, Brum IS. Gene and protein expression of progesterone receptor isoforms a and B,

p53 and p21 in myometrium and uterine leiomyoma. Arch Gynecol Obstet. 2012;286(1):119–24.

22. Matsuo H, Kurachi O, Shimomura Y, Samoto T, Maruo T. Molecular bases for the actions of ovarian sex steroids in the regulation of proliferation and apoptosis of human uterine leiomyoma. Oncology. 1999;57(Suppl 2):49–58.

23. Wang L, Mou X, Xiao L, Tang L. T-cadherin expression in uterine leiomyoma. Arch Gynecol Obstet. 2013;288(3):607–14.

24. Mäkinen N, Mehine M, Tolvanen J, Kaasinen E, Li Y, Lehtonen HJ, et al. MED12, the mediator complex subunit 12 gene, is mutated at high frequency in uterine leiomyomas. Science. 2011;334(6053):252–5.

25. Mittal P, Shin YH, Yatsenko SA, Castro CA, Surti U, Rajkovic A. Med12 gain-of-function mutation causes leiomyomas and genomic instability. J Clin Invest. 2015;125(8):3280–4.

26. Croce S, Chibon F. MED12 and uterine smooth muscle oncogenesis: state of the art and perspectives. Eur J Cancer. 2015;51(12):1603–10.

27. Vergara D, Greco M. Genetics and genomics of uterine myomas. In: Tinelli A, Malvasi A, editors. Uterine myoma, myomectomy and minimally invasive treatments. Cham: Springer Publisher; 2015. p. 12–25.

28. Mäkinen N, Vahteristo P, Bützow R, Sjoberg J, Aaltonen LA. Exomic landscape of MED12 mutation-negative and -positive uterine leiomyomas. Int J Cancer. 2014;134(4):1008–12.

29. Ono M, Yin P, Navarro A, Moravek MB, Coon JS 5th, Druschitz SA, et al. Paracrine activation of WNT/β-catenin pathway in uterine leiomyoma stem cells promotes tumor growth. Proc Natl Acad Sci U S A. 2013;110(42):17053–8.

30. Karra L, Shushan A, Ben-Meir A, Rojansky N, Klein BY, Shiveiky D, et al. Changes related to phosphatidylinositol 3-kinase/Akt signaling in leiomyomas: possible involvement of glycogen synthase kinase 3alpha and cyclin D2 in the pathophysiology. Fertil Steril. 2010;93(8):2646–51.

31. Munro MG, Critchley HO, Broder MS, Fraser IS. FIGO working group on menstrual disorders. FIGO classification system (PALM-COEIN) for causes of abnormal uterine bleeding in nongravid women of reproductive age. Int J Gynaecol Obstet. 2011;113(1):3–13.

32. Worhunsky DJ, Gupta M, Gholami S, Tran TB, Ganjoo KN, van de Rijn M, et al. Leiomyosarcoma: one disease or distinct biologic entities based on site of origin? J Surg Oncol. 2015;111(7):808–12.

33. Hodge JC, Morton CC. Genetic heterogeneity among uterine leiomyomata: insights into malignant progression. Hum Mol Genet. 2007. 16 Spec No 1:R7-13.
34. Robboy SJ, Bentley RC, Butnor K, Anderson MC. Pathology and pathophysiology of uterine smooth-muscle tumors. Environ Health Perspect. 2000;108(Suppl 5):779–84.
35. Clement PB, Young RH. Atlas of gynecologic surgical pathology. 3rd ed. Philadelphia: Saunders; 2013.
36. Tinelli A, Sparic R, Kadija S, Babovic I, Tinelli R, Mynbaev OA, et al. Myomas: anatomy and related issues. Minerva Ginecol. 2016;68(3):261–73.
37. Ito F, Kawamura N, Ishimura T, Tsujimura A, Ishiko O, Ogita S. Ultrastructural comparison of uterine leiomyoma cells from the same myoma nodule before and after gonadotropin-releasing hormone agonist treatment. Fertil Steril. 2001;75(1):l25–30.
38. Dapunt O. Studies on the structure of the myoma capsule. Arch Gynakol. 1965;202:492–4.
39. Fox H, Buckley CH. Benign neoplasms of the female genital tract. In: Pathology for gynaecologists. London: Arnold Edts; 1982. p. 91–7.
40. Vizza E, Motta PM. The skeleton fibrous and muscolar of the uterus. In: Atti LXXVII Congresso SIGO. Rome: CIC Edit Int; 2001. p. 47–9.
41. Kurjak A, Jurkovic D, Alfirevic Z, Zalud I. Transvaginal color Doppler imaging. J Clin Ultrasound. 1990;18(4):227–34.
42. Tinelli A, Malvasi A, Rahimi S, Negro R, Cavallotti C, Vergara D, et al. Myoma pseudocapsule: a distinct endocrino-anatomical entity in gynecological surgery. Gynecol Endocrinol. 2009;25(10):661–7.
43. Malvasi A, Tinelli A, Rahimi S, D'Agnese G, Rotoni C, Dell'Edera D, et al. A three-dimensional morphological reconstruction of uterine leiomyoma pseudocapsule vasculature by the Allen-Cahn mathematical model. Biomed Pharmacother. 2011;65(5):359–63.
44. Mettler L, Tinelli A, Hurst BS, Teigland CM, Sammur W, Dell'Edera D, et al. Neurovascular bundle in fibroid pseudocapsule and its neuroendocrinologic implications. Expert Rev Endocrinol Metab. 2011;6(5):715–22.
45. Malvasi A, Cavallotti C, Morroni M, Lorenzi T, Dell'Edera D, Nicolardi G, et al. Uterine fibroid pseudocapsule studied by transmission electron microscopy. Eur J Obstet Gynecol Reprod Biol. 2012;162(2):187–91.

46. Wei JJ, Zhang XM, Chiriboga L, Yee H, Perle MA, Mittal K. Spatial differences in biologic activity of large uterine leiomyomata. Fertil Steril. 2006;85(1):179–87.
47. Tinelli A, Malvasi A, Hurst BS, Tsin DA, Davila F, Dominguez G, et al. Surgical management of neurovascular bundle of uterine fibroid pseudocapsule during myomectomy. JSLS. 2012;16(1):119–29.
48. Tinelli A, Hurst BS, Mettler L, Tsin DA, Pellegrino M, Nicolardi G, et al. Ultrasound evaluation of uterine healing after laparoscopic intracapsular myomectomy: an observational study. Hum Reprod. 2012;27(9):2664–70.
49. Di Tommaso S, Massari S, Malvasi A, Bozzetti MP, Tinelli A. Gene expression analysis reveals an angiogenic profile in uterine leiomyoma pseudocapsule. Mol Hum Reprod. 2013;19(6):380–7.
50. Di Tommaso S, Tinelli A, Malvasi A, Massari S. Missense mutations in exon 2 of the MED12 gene are involved in IGF-2 overexpression in uterine leiomyoma. Mol Hum Reprod. 2014;20(10):1009–15.
51. Malvasi A, Tinelli A, Cavallotti C, Morroni M, Tsin DA, Nezhat C, et al. Distribution of substance P (SP) and vasoactive intestinal peptide (VIP) neuropeptides in pseudocapsules of uterine fibroids. Peptides. 2011;32(2):327–32.
52. Malvasi A, Cavallotti C, Nicolardi G, Pellegrino M, Dell'Edera D, Vergara D, et al. NT, NPY and PGP 9.5 presence in myomeytrium and in fibroid pseudocapsule and their possible impact on muscular physiology. Gynecol Endocrinol. 2013;29(2):177–81.
53. Malvasi A, Cavallotti C, Nicolardi G, Pellegrino M, Vergara D, Greco M, et al. The opioid neuropeptides in uterine fibroid pseudocapsules: a putative association with cervical integrity in human reproduction. Gynecol Endocrinol. 2013;29(11):982–8.
54. Rowe MK, Kanouse DE, Mittman BS, Bernstein SJ. Quality of life among women undergoing hysterectomies. Obstet Gynecol. 1999;93:915–21.
55. Munro MG, Lukes AS, Abnormal Uterine Bleeding and Underlying Hemostatic Disorders Consensus Group. Abnormal uterine bleeding and underlying hemostatic disorders: report of a consensus process. Fertil Steril. 2005;84(5):1335–7.
56. Wegienka G, Baird DD, Hertz-Picciotto I, Harlow SD, Steege JF, Hill MC, et al. Self-reported heavy bleeding associated with uterine leiomyomata. Obstet Gynecol. 2003;101(3):431–7.

57. Parker WH. Uterine fibroids: clinical features. In: Tinelli A, Malvasi A, editors. Uterine myoma, myomectomy and minimally invasive treatments. Cham: Springer Publisher; 2015. p. 39–52.
58. Murase E, Siegelman ES, Outwater EK, Perez-Jaffe LA, Tureck RW. Uterine leiomyomas: histopathologic features, MR imaging findings, differential diagnosis, and treatment. Radiographics. 1999;19(5):1179–97.
59. Gaym A, Tilahun S. Torsion of pedunculated subserous myoma—a rare cause of acute abdomen. Ethiop Med J. 2007;45(2):203–7.
60. Olive DL. Review of the evidence for treatment of leiomyomata. Environ Health Perspect. 2000;108(Suppl 5):841–3.
61. Langer R, Golan A, Neuman M, Schneider D, Bukovsky I, Caspi E. The effect of large uterine fibroids on urinary bladder function and symptoms. Am J Obstet Gynecol. 1990;163(4 Pt 1):1139–41.
62. Peddada SD, Laughlin SK, Miner K, Guyon JP, Haneke K, Vahdat HL, et al. Growth of uterine leiomyomata among pre-menopausal black and white women. Proc Natl Acad Sci U S A. 2008;105(50):19887–92.
63. Parker W, Fu Y, Berek J. Uterine sarcoma in patients operated on for presumed leiomyoma and rapidly growing leiomyoma. Obstet Gynecol. 1994;83(3):414–8.
64. Boutselis J, Ullery J. Sarcoma of the uterus. Obstet Gynecol. 1962;20:23–35.
65. Brooks SE, Zhan M, Cote T, Baquet CR. Surveillance, epidemiology, and end results analysis of 2677 cases of uterine sarcoma 1989–1999. Gynecol Oncol. 2004;93(1):204–8.
66. Quade BJ, Wang TY, Sornberger K, Dal Cin P, Mutter GL, Morton CC. Molecular pathogenesis of uterine smooth muscle tumors from transcriptional profiling. Genes Chromosomes Cancer. 2004;40(2):97–108.
67. Carlson KJ, Miller BA, Fowler FJ Jr. The Maine Women's Health Study: II. Outcomes of nonsurgical management of leiomyomas, abnormal bleeding, and chronic pelvic pain. Obstet Gynecol. 1994;83(4):566–72.
68. Sparic R, Nejkovic L, Mutavdzic D, Tinelli A. Conservative surgical treatment of uterine fibroids. Acta Chir Iugosl. 2014;61(4):11–6.

Chapter 2
Uterine Fibroids and Effect on Fertility

Liselotte Mettler, Anupama Deenadayal Mettler, and Ibrahim Alkatout

Introduction

Uterine myomas are benign noninvasive but proliferative swellings of the uterine muscle located either under the endometrium, intramurally, or under the peritoneal surface. They can be symptomatic provoking pain or can just be asymptomatic.

Arising from the smooth muscle cells of the uterus, fibroids may be single or multiple. Many times they cause symptoms such as meno- and metrorrhagias.

Big fibroids, due to their size, can compress any of the neighboring organs leading to urinary, digestive, or sexual problems and seem to have a fertility-diminishing effect. Especially when large fibroids are present or when the cavity of the uterus is distorted. Here, in fact, we have to put forward one major question—If women with myomas really suffer from decreased fertility? If we find a myoma or myomas in a woman seeking fertility treatment, can we

L. Mettler, MD, PhD (✉) • A.D. Mettler, MD, PhD
I. Alkatout, MD, PhD
Department Obstetrics and Gynecology, University Clinics Schleswig-Holstein, Campus Kiel, Arnold-Heller-Str. 3, House 24, 24105 Kiel, Germany
e-mail: lmettler@email.uni-kiel.de

N.S. Moawad (ed.), *Uterine Fibroids*,
https://doi.org/10.1007/978-3-319-58780-6_2,
© Springer International Publishing AG 2018

conclude that there is a direct link between the myoma and the infertility and can we hope to improve fertility by removing the myoma?

Etiology and Microscopy

The etiology of fibroids shows a panorama of theories. Fibroids are composed primarily of smooth muscle cells. The uterus, stomach, and bladder are all organs made of smooth muscle. Smooth muscle cells are arranged so that the organ can stretch instead of being arranged in rigid units like the cells in the skeletal muscles in arms and legs that are designed to "pull" in a particular direction.

In women with fibroids, tissue from the endometrium typically looks normal under the microscope. Sometimes, however, over submucosal fibroids, there is an unusual type of uterine lining that does not have the normal glandular structures. The presence of this abnormality called aglandular functionalis (functional endometrium with no glands) in women having menstrual symptoms is sometimes a clinical clue for their doctors to look more closely for a submucosal fibroid [1]. A second pattern of endometrium termed chronic endometritis can also suggest that there may be a submucosal fibroid, although this pattern can also be associated with other problems such as retained products of conception and various infections of the uterus.

Pathophysiology

Myomas arise from genetic alternations in a single myometrial cell and thus often are described as clonal. Although estrogen may stimulate myoma development and growth, myomas also may grow when circulating estrogen levels are low, possibly because ovarian and adrenal androgens may be converted to estrogens by aromatase activity within myoma cells. Growth of myomas is clearly also regulated by progesterone and a number of local growth factors. The genetic basis for myoma growth may relate primarily to these factors and their receptors.

Although most women with uterine myomas are asymptomatic, many may have significant symptoms including pelvic and abdominal pressure or pain and menstrual irregularities. Other symptoms of myomas may result from their pressure on adjacent organs such as the bladder (urinary frequency) or rectum (tenesmus). Once we move beyond hysterectomy as a one-size-fits-all solution to fibroids, distinctions in size, position, and appearance will likely be important for treating fibroids. After understanding these issues, we may be able to tell why some women have severe bleeding and other women with a similarly sized fibroid have no problem.

Genetic Origin

It is important to us as clinicians to be up to date with the genetic advances in regard to fibroids, as it will eventually guide the best methods of treatment in women desiring fertility. The genotype is the pattern of genes that you inherit, while the phenotype is the physical manifestation or end result of the genotype. For example, with eye color, brown is a dominant color and is represented by a "B." Blue is a recessive trait and represented by a "b." Therefore, a person can have "BB," "bb," or "Bb" as genotypes for eye color. Each person gets two copies of the gene, one originally from his or her mother and the other from his or her father. The dominant gene will always dominate. It has the power to trump a recessive trait. Although there are three different genotypes (BB, bb, or Bb), there are only two phenotypes: brown eyes and blue eyes. People with the "BB" or the "Bb" genotype have brown eyes because brown is the dominant trait. Only the people with the "bb" genotype have blue eyes.

We believe that fibroids are a common phenotype that represents many different underlying genotypes. In other words, in my view fibroids can arise through multiple different pathways. In this case, "Bb" might represent two different genes that code for the estrogen receptor beta, which influences the action of estrogen on fibroid tissue. A "B" may make the fibroid more sensitive to this hormone and therefore more likely to grow. In addition, probably multiple genes influence fibroids, so that, in addition to "Bb," we may also have "Pp" for progesterone receptors, "Ff" for fibrotic factors, and so on. This information would be most helpful in advance of treatment, so that the woman who carried a high risk of recurrent fibroids and have completed their family might even choose to have a hysterectomy because their chance of having an additional surgery was so high. We currently have some clinical information (based on physicians' clinical experience with many patients) to predict prognosis for recurrence after abdominal myomectomy, but our clinical information for any other kind of treatment options is limited.

Finally, understanding the underlying genotype would open up important possibilities for the future. It may, for example, point to ways in which women can modify their risk of disease and lead to prevention of disease. If, for example, a major protein involved in body fat metabolism was found to be abnormally sensitive in women with fibroids, weight loss or preventing weight gain might be an effective strategy for decreasing the risk of fibroids. In this day and age, new therapies can be developed that are targeted to specific abnormalities. This is what happened with chronic myelogenous leukemia (CML) and Gleevec which combats this disease with minimal side effects.

Understanding which genes are involved in fibroids doesn't automatically tell us why fibroids develop or how to control them. From our understanding of fibroid behavior, we could guess that genes involved in estrogen or progesterone production, metabolism, or action would be involved. Unfortunately, science is seldom that straightforward. Most guesses regarding these "candidate genes" turn out to be wrong, and many studies are usually required to find out how these genes lead to disease.

There are also small variations called polymorphisms in genes that may play a role in influencing the risk of fibroids. Both polymorphisms and mutations are changes in the sequence of genes, but the difference is in the degree of change. A mutation makes a major change in the gene that leads to a change in the protein the gene is coding for. It changes the amino acid from alanine to glycine, for example, or causes the protein to be prematurely cut off.

Finally, in the age of molecular genetics, we can look for genes involved in a disease, which is effectively looking for a needle in a haystack. This process is called a genome-wide scan. This is a common approach to finding genes in complex diseases such as diabetes, asthma, and heart disease. With a genome-wide scan, women who are sisters and both have fibroids (an affected sibling pair) are recruited to participate in the study. Their DNA is studied for common genes. If hundreds of women are studied, each region of every chromosome can be examined, and it can be determined which genes are shared by the sisters who share the fibroid phenotype but are different in many other respects. This approach often produces novel genes that were not previously thought to be involved in the disease process [2–5].

Philosophy of Myomas in Infertility

Ideally, to prove a relationship between fibroids and infertility, prospective randomized studies should be performed comparing women desiring pregnancy with and without myomas in order to compare pregnancy rates and possibly the time needed to achieve pregnancy. These studies are lacking. A comparison between pregnancy rates and undisturbed pregnancy outcomes of infertile women with and without myomas in whom other infertility factors have been excluded however clearly speaks for the benefit of myomectomies [6–8].

A publication of the Italian team that compares spontaneous conception in infertile women with and without myomas in whom andrological and tubal infertility factors have been excluded [9], the authors found a significant difference ($P < 0.002$) in pregnancy rates between infertile women with and without myomas (11% vs. 25%). It is the only randomized prospective study to date, and if it is to be believed, infertile women with myomas have better pregnancy rates after myomectomy (42%) than infertile women without myomas (25%), who in turn have better pregnancy rates than infertile women with untreated myomas (11%).

Different theories have been proposed to explain the effects of myomas on fertility. What are the mechanisms involved? It is generally accepted that the anatomical location of a fibroid as a submucous fibroid may impair fertility, but about the influence of intramural and subserosal fibroids in causing infertility, no consensus has ever been achieved. Myomas may distort the uterine cavity making it enlarged and elongated and altering its contour and surface area. Myomas may cause dysfunctional uterine contractility which may interfere with sperm migration, ovum transport, or nidation [10–12]. Myomas may also be associated with implantation failure or gestation discontinuation due to focal endometrial vascular disturbance, endometrial inflammation, secretion of vasoactive substances, or an enhanced endometrial androgen environment [11, 13].

In an era of evidence-based medicine, we need a clear analysis of the literature. Can we draw any conclusions from what has been published or do we need to consider new studies? Well, the following discussion gives a good overview of this situation.

Myomas and Fertility Outcome?

Let us first ask the essential question if myomas do affect implantation rates of the embryo and then ask, if these surgeries may be crucial for achieving pregnancy and for avoiding problems during pregnancy. Leiomyomas of the uterus are the most common solid pelvic tumors found in women and are estimated to occur in 20–50% of women with increased frequency during the late reproductive years [14]. The incidence of myomas in infertile women without any obvious cause of infertility is estimated to be between 1 and 2.4% [11, 14, 15]. The relationship between leiomyomas and infertility remains a subject of debate. To address this issue, we have tried to evaluate the impact of myomas on fertility and pregnancy outcome in different conditions where myomas are implicated.

Implantation Rates

The Practice Committee of the American Society for Reproductive Medicine in collaboration with The Society of Reproductive Surgeons and American Society for Reproductive Medicine, Birmingham, Alabama, established some facts. The purpose of this educational bulletin is to examine the relationship between myomas and reproductive function and to review current methods for their management. Overall, evidence suggests that myomas are the primary cause of infertility in a relatively small proportion of women. Myomas that distort the uterine cavity and larger intramural myomas may have adverse effects on fertility.

It was established by J. Ben-Nagi et al. that women with submucous fibroids had significantly lower concentrations of glycodelin and IL-10 in mid-luteal phase uterine flushings [16]. It was seen that the uterine cavities of women with submucous fibroids were producing decreasing amount of substances favorable to early pregnancy development hence explaining adverse reproductive outcomes [16]. While submucous myomas may certainly impair implantation rates, the question whether intramural or subserous myomas interfere with implantation remains unanswered.

While it is accepted that it is always better to operate on myomas that distort the endometrial cavity, the controversy arises in non-cavity-distorting myomas. When the implantation rates and pregnancy outcomes were compared between women with and without non-cavity-distorting myomas, in

2007 V.Y. Fujimoto et al. did not support myomectomy before ART in patients with asymptomatic fibroids that do not significantly distort the endometrial cavity [17]. We found that live birth rates were not affected by the presence of intramural myomas in IVF patients with a hysteroscopically normal uterine cavity. However, in 2010, a meta-analysis of 6087 IVF cycles by Sunkara et al. showed a significant decrease in the live birth and clinical pregnancy rates in women with non-cavity-distorting intramural fibroids compared with those without fibroids, following IVF treatment [18]. Concluding that the presence of non-cavity-distorting intramural fibroids is associated with adverse pregnancy outcomes in women undergoing IVF treatment.

In 2004 a case-control study revealed that patients with intramural fibroids >4.0 cm had lower pregnancy rates than patients with intramural fibroids ≤4.0 cm. Patients with sub-serosal or intramural fibroids <4 cm had IVF-ICSI outcomes (pregnancy, implantation, and abortion rates) similar to those of controls [19].

In 2002 Check et al. did a prospective case-control study comparing women with and without non-cavity-distorting fibroids and found that myomas smaller than 5 cm had lower implantation rates (13.6% vs. 20.2%), lower pregnancy rates (34.4% vs. 47.5%), and lower delivery rates (22.9% vs. 37.7%) [20]. Hart and colleagues studied a similar cohort of women undergoing IVF and found that pregnancy, implantation, and ongoing pregnancy rates were reduced significantly to 23.3, 11.9, and 15% compared with 34.1, 20.2., and 28.3%, respectively, in control groups. A higher frequency of uterine peristalsis during the mid-luteal phase was thought to be one of the causes of infertility associated with intramural-type fibroids.

Yan L et al. in 2014 in the study of one of the largest reported sample sizes—245 patients after ROC analysis—identified 2.85 cm as the cutoff value for largest single fibroid diameter (SFD) [21]. Patients with fibroids with SFD >2.85 cm tended to have significantly lower delivery rate (DR) compared with patients with lower diameter. These results are in part consistent [22–24]. When comparing patients with fibroids with non-fibroid matched controls, only SFD larger than 2.85 cm showed a significant reduction in DR. The study does not claim that there is definitely a fertility benefit of myomectomy in patients whose fibroids meet the above criteria. It states that perhaps we may ignore the effect on IVF/ICSI outcomes of single IM fibroids smaller than 2.85 cm. Currently, it is impossible to achieve a consensus regarding the surgical treatment of IM fibroids that do not cause mass effect on the uterine cavity [25]. Removing IM fibroids between 2.85 and 5 cm to improve fertility remains a controversial area, but this study gives strength to the clinical consultation of infertile patients with fibroids regarding the need for surgical intervention.

In conclusion, there are various cutoff sizes of fibroids to guide the need for a myomectomy for reproductive enhancement ranging from 2.5 to 5 cm. Fibroid location, followed by size, is the most important factor determining the impact of fibroids on fertility. Surgery is indicated in cases of distortion of the endometrial cavity. Myomectomy should also be considered for patients with non-cavity-distorting fibroids based on the studies presented and for patients with unexplained unsuccessful IVF cycles after thorough evaluation of the patient and weighing the role of the fibroid as the cause for infertility.

Recurrent Pregnancy Loss

The data on association of RPL and myomas is controversial. In one study, the abortion rates in patients with and without fibroma were 71.4% and 34.9%, respectively, that indicates abortion rate is significantly higher in the presence of fibroids even after elimination of other factors ($P = 0.024$). In another large series, a miscarriage rate of 19% was reported in women following myomectomy compared to 41% for the same group of women prior to myomectomy. A review states that both submucosal and intramural fibroids were associated with an increased risk of spontaneous miscarriage [26].

While the Cochrane database review 2012 stated that there was no evidence of a significant effect of myomectomy on the miscarriage rate, the Practice Committee of the American Society for Reproductive Medicine in collaboration with the Society of Reproductive Surgeons came to the conclusion—"In infertile women and those with recurrent pregnancy loss myomectomy should be considered only after a thorough evaluation has been completed."

Myomas During Pregnancy

The question is if intracapsular myomectomies with a correct adaption of wound edges by sutures and their resulting scars impair pregnancy outcome whether performed by laparotomy, laparoscopy, or hysteroscopy.

According to Li et al. and Vercellini et al., miscarriage rates are significantly reduced after myomectomy [27, 28]. Uterine scars are associated with a risk of vicious placental implantation (accreta, increta, percreta, praevia) and a risk of uterine rupture. In our different evaluations of abdominal and laparoscopic myomectomies in more than 2000 cases over 20 years as well as over 500 hysteroscopic myomectomies, only one uterine rupture occurred during labor which was well taken care of by the attending obstetrician [6]. In Seracchioli's randomized study comparing laparoscopic and abdominal myomectomies, no uterine rupture occurred [29]. There were no significant differences between the percentages of vaginal births (35% vs. 22%) and cesarean sections (65% vs. 78%).

Of the 145 pregnancies in Dubuisson's follow-up after laparoscopic myomectomy, 38 (26.2%) resulted in miscarriage, 58 in vaginal deliveries, and 42 in cesarean sections [30]. Dubuisson describes three uterine ruptures, all occurring before labor and one attributed to the laparoscopic myomectomy. A few case reports were found in the literature on uterine rupture after laparoscopic myomectomy [30–36].

However, they do not allow us to draw any conclusions on the relative risk compared with abdominal myomectomy. Moreover, we found no recent reports on the risk of uterine rupture after abdominal myomectomy.

Some obstetricians consider the presence of a uterine scar as an indication for cesarean section [33, 37], while other authors have never expressed the need [30, 38, 39].

Treatment Possibilities

Today, in general, broad spectrums of treatment possibilities are available and are best depicted in Fig. 2.1. In our estimation, particularly for infertile patients, hysteroscopic excision and the laparoscopic enucleation are still the leading technologies.

A recent study showed that the median serum AMH levels and median AFC per ovary were significantly lowered after uterine arterial embolization (UAE) compared to women

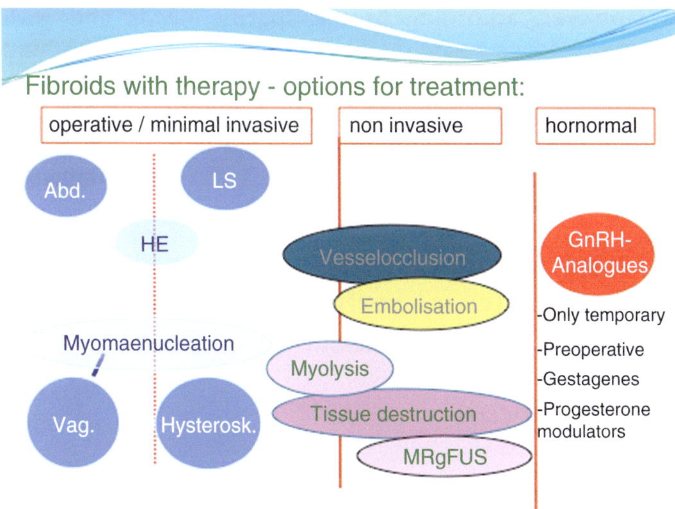

FIGURE 2.1 Treatment options for uterine fibroids

who had undergone laparoscopic myomectomy (LM) concluding that this could have an adverse impact on future response to fertility treatment and/or fecundity [40]. As the safety and effectiveness of UAE has not been established for women with myomas seeking to maintain or improve their fertility, it should not be recommended till further evidence is available.

Although studies claim that treatment of symptomatic uterine myomas with magnetic resonance-guided focused ultrasound (MgRfUS) improves both QOL and subsequent fertility, further evidence should be explored before its application in women of reproductive age [41].

Medical treatment for myomas does not improve infertility. Preoperative medical treatment with a GnRH agonist should be considered for women who are anemic and those who might be candidates for a less invasive procedure if the volume of their myoma(s) was moderately smaller the Practice Committee of the American Society for Reproductive Medicine in collaboration with the Society of Reproductive Surgeons).

However, according to the specific needs and with future evidence-based medicine UAE, focused ultrasound applied under MRI and the medical treatment with the progesterone modulator ulipristal acetate (5 mg) might be considered [42]. It has recently gained importance in the treatment of menstrual disturbances due to submucosal and intramural fibroids.

Myomectomy and Fertility: Laparoscopic and Hysteroscopic Resection of Fibroids

General Aspects

Based on immunohistochemical findings, it is proposed to remove fibroids in women seeking pregnancy while respecting the pseudocapsule by neurofiber sparing in the incision site. We published that this is of utmost importance for optimal muscular healing and myometrial function in future pregnancies. In fibroids detected under a size of 5–6 cm in diameter especially in young women wanting to achieve pregnancies, the myomectomy should be performed before the myoma reaches a size causing compression of the surrounding tissues and uterine distortion, which may result in the loss of regenerative potential [43].

It is good surgical and clinical practice to perform a hysteroscopy before advancing to the laparoscopic myomectomy. The advantage of the hysteroscopy is that, as this is a patient seeking fertility, endometrial pathology can be identified and corrected, and intracavity extension of the fibroid can be noted. A chromopertubation should be performed before proceeding to the myomectomy. It is advisable to use a uterine manipulator to stabilize the mobile uterus during a myomectomy.

A longitudinal incision is usually preferred on the uterus for a myomectomy, but if the myoma extends laterally, a horizontal incision is also acceptable. If the uterine cavity is entered during the procedure, it just has to be sutured additionally in a special layer. If the fibroid is posterior, there might be an increased risk of adhesion formation, and an anti-adhesive strategy needs to be adopted. The patient should always be informed that there might be a rare possibility to convert the surgery to a laparotomy.

The Practice Committee of the American Society for Reproductive Medicine in collaboration with The Society of Reproductive Surgeons concluded that myomectomy is a relatively safe surgical procedure associated with few serious complications. However, postoperative adhesions are common after abdominal myomectomy and pose a significant potential threat to subsequent fertility. Hence, a laparoscopic and/or hysteroscopic myomectomy should be preferred to an abdominal. However, each surgeon should determine his or her own criteria for laparoscopic myomectomy.

Post-surgery, the patient is usually advised to attempt pregnancy after 3 months to give adequate time for the uterine scar to heal.

Laparoscopic Stepwise Enucleation of an Intramural Fibroid and Uterine Reconstruction

Figures 2.2, 2.3, 2.4, 2.5, 2.6, 2.7, and 2.8 give a detailed diagnostic and surgical description of myomectomy and surgical reconstruction of the uterine wall.

This stepwise description of laparoscopic myoma enucleation as an intracapsular approach with an adequate reconstruction of the uterine wall gives the patients a good start for further fertility results. The adaption of wound edges may be in 1, 2, or 3 layers depending of the situation. If the uterine cavity has been opened, an extra layer of sutures has to be applied. Conventional or barbed sutures are acceptable.

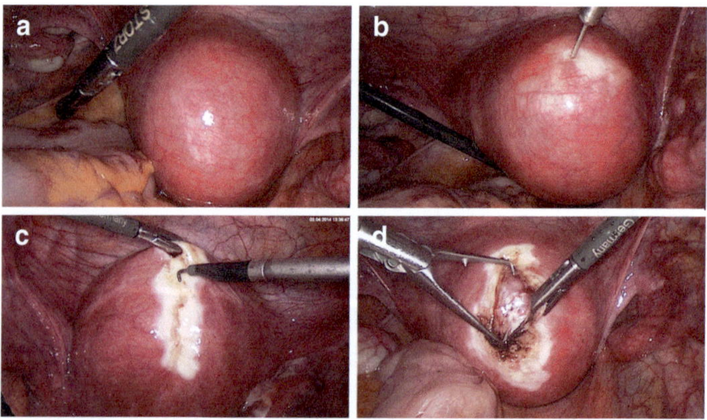

FIGURE 2.2 Laparoscopic myoma enucleation. (**a**) Situs of a fundal/anterior wall fibroid. (**b**) Prophylactic hemostasis with 1:100 diluted vasopressin solution (Gylpressin) in separate wells. The injection intends to separate the pseudocapsule from the fibroid and reduces bleedings. (**c**) Bipolar superficial coagulation of the longitudinal incision strip and opening of the uterine wall with the monopolar hook or needle till the fibroid surface. (**d**) Grasping of the fibroid and beginning of the enucleation. The pseudocapsule remains within the uterine wall and is pushed off bluntly

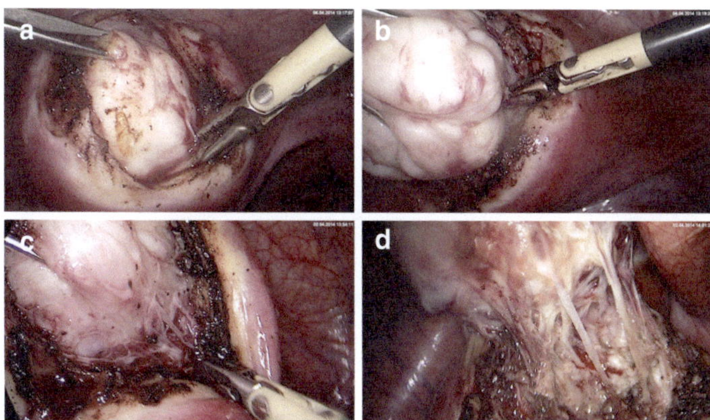

FIGURE 2.3 Laparoscopic myoma enucleation. (**a**) Traction of the fibroid with a tenaculum and blunt delineation from the capsule. (**b**) Focal bipolar coagulation of basic vessels. (**c**) Continuous enucleation of the fibroid under traction and specific coagulation of capsule fibers containing vessels. (**d**) Magnification of remaining capsule fibers to be coagulated and cut

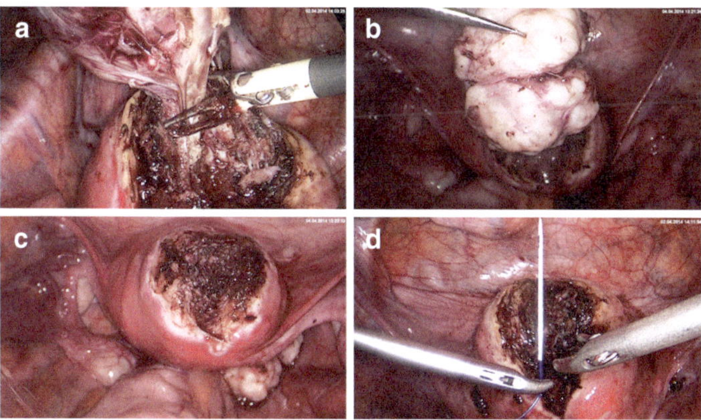

FIGURE 2.4 Laparoscopic myoma enucleation. (**a**) Final coagulation of the capsule vessels. (**b**) Double belly fibroid after complete enucleation. (**c**) Minimal coagulation of bleeding vessels under suction and irrigation. (**d**) Approximation of wound edges with either straight or round sharp needle and a monofilar late resorbable suture

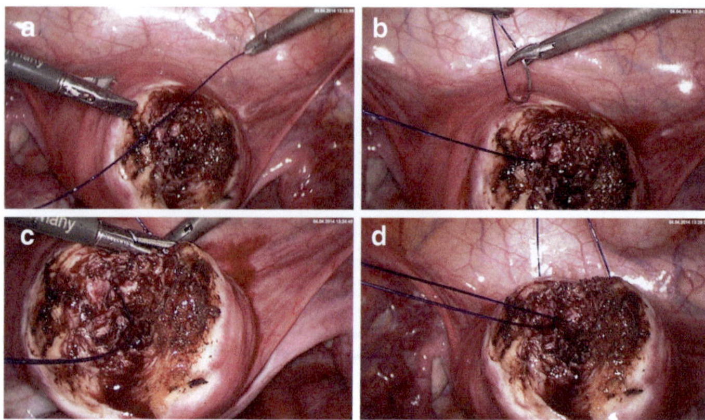

FIGURE 2.5 Laparoscopic myoma enucleation. (**a**) Advantage of round needle stitch. The wound angle is elevated safely and completely by elevating it with a Manhes forceps. Deeper layers of the myometrium can be grasped more easily using a round needle. (**b**) Needle exit and simplified regrasping with the right needle holder. (**c**) Final stich to invert the knot. (**d**) Extirpation of the needle and completing the extracorporeal knot and preparing to push down the extracorporeal knot

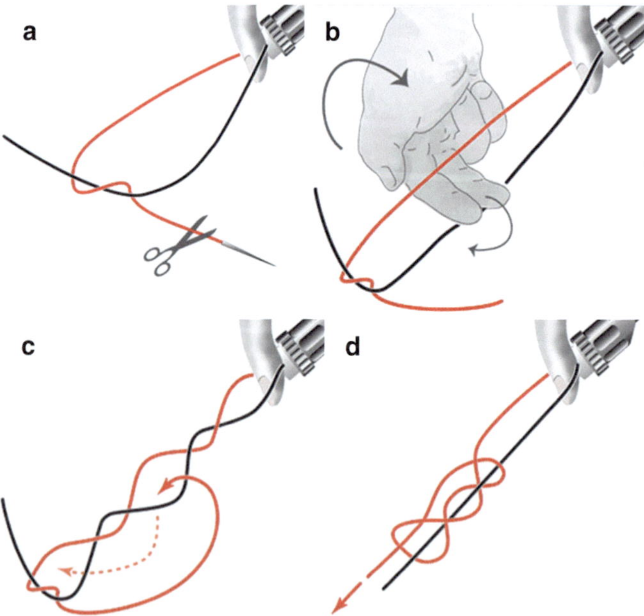

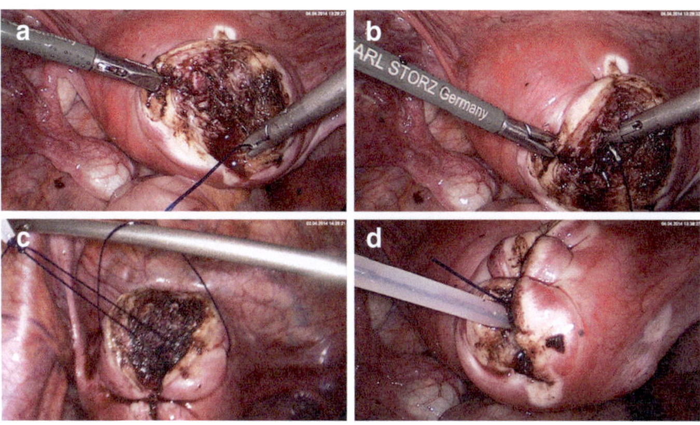

FIGURE 2.7 Laparoscopic myoma enucleation. (**a**) Second single stich starting as deep as possible in the uterine wound. (**b**) Exiting of the needle on the left wound margin (just next to the Manhes forceps). (**c**) Completing of the stich and preparation of the extracorporeal von Leffern knot. The needle holder elevates the thread to avoid tearing of the uterine wall while pulling through the monofilar thread (PDS). (**d**) Pushing down the extracorporeal performed knot with a plastic pushrod in the depth of the wound to dump the knot minimizing the external suture part

FIGURE 2.6 Performance of the extracorporeal "von Leffern" knot. (**a**) Pulling out the suture, removing the needle, half hitch. (**b**) Holding the knot with the left hand and reaching over with the right hand. (**c**) Grasping the short end from below and leading it back, exiting before the half hitch. (**d**) Turning back the knot. Holding the straight suture and tightening the knot

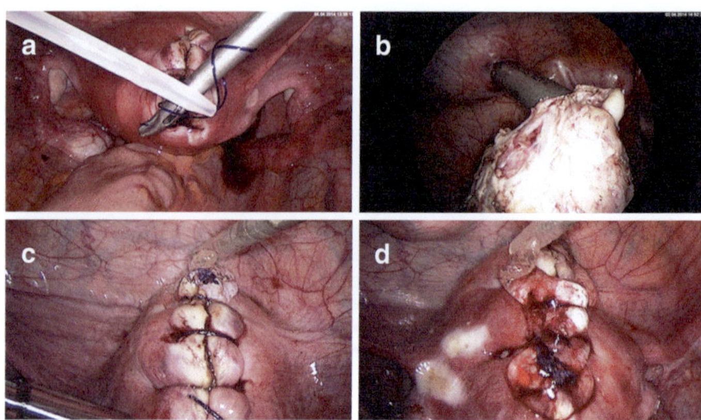

FIGURE 2.8 Laparoscopic myoma enucleation. (**a**) Intracorporeal safety knot of the performed extracorporeal knot. (**b**) Morcellation of the fibroid with the Rotocut morcellator (Storz) in an apple peeling manner. (**c**) Final situs showing the extracorporeal sutures to adapt the uterine wound edges. (**d**) Application of Hyalobarrier (Nordic Pharma) for adhesion prevention

Hysteroscopic Myoma Enucleation Has to Be Performed According to the Depth of Infiltration into the Myometrium

Submucous myomas may cause serious implantation problems and raise the frequency of abortions. The best time of surgery is the early phase in the cycle without bleeding. Saline infusion sonography best reveals the fibroid enucleation level and helps to plan the correct surgery which sometimes needs to be combined with a laparoscopic approach [8].

Differentiation of Fibroids and Focal Endometriosis to Adenomatoid Tumors

Focal adenomyosis may create a lot of pain and has to be resected if the patient is below the childbearing age or wants to conceive sooner or later, although hysterectomy best solves the dysmenorrhea of these patients. But, this is of course not an option in infertile women. Focal adenomyosis is of mesothelial origin and affects the epididymis, testis, tunica albuginea, ejaculatory duct, prostate, and spermatic cord in men and uterus, ovary, and fallopian tubes in women. Cases have been reported of adenomatoid tumors located in the heart, pleura, liver, and adrenals [44–47]. Multifocal or multicentric appearance is exceptional [48, 49].

The excision of these lesions is much more difficult than any myomectomy as there is no myoma capsule. Adenomatoid tumors also resemble fibroids without a capsule, sometimes after GnRH analogue treatments. They can also be mistaken for lymphangiomas, metastatic adenocarcinoma, and metastasis of other origin.

These tumors form circumscribed tubercular solid masses. A recognizable separating layer or capsule enclosing the lesion is missing, as the tumors are densely adherent to the surrounding tissue. These circumstances make intraoperative preparation difficult and inhibit the definite macroscopic exclusion of a malignant event. Sixty percent of the uterine adenomatoid tumors are subserosal or at least in the external region of the myometrium. As described in our cases, most frequently they are situated in the fundus or in the posterior wall of the uterus [44–46, 50, 51]. The following two case reports reflect the complexity of the problem.

Case 1

A 26-year-old Caucasian woman, nulliparous, was transferred for surgery with a recurring symptomatic ovarian cyst. During the gynecological examination, in addition to an unsuspicious-looking cyst on the left ovary, a 2.1 cm diameter well-circumscribed uterine mass located in the posterior wall of the fundus, 1.2 cm from the serosal surface, was recorded as a fibroid (Fig. 2.9). This known tumor had been seen by an ultrasound scan 1 year earlier measuring 1 cm in diameter. The patient had a medical history of three laparoscopic surgeries for the enucleation of relapsing functional ovarian cysts with no evidence of endometriosis.

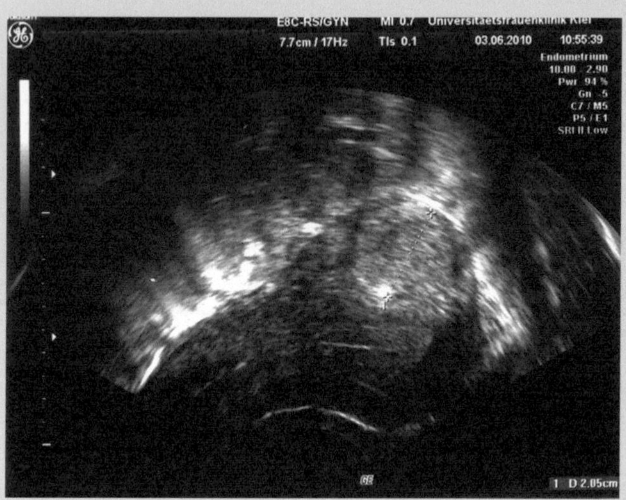

FIGURE 2.9 Preoperative transvaginal ultrasound scan showing the typical misleading sonographic picture of a fibroid (Case 1)

The patient required a fourth laparoscopy to treat the symptomatic ovarian cyst. Because of the growth of the tumor on the posterior wall, the age of the patient, and possible problems in future family planning, it was decided to simultaneously excise the suspected myoma. At laparoscopy, the ovarian cyst was enucleated, and the presumed fibroid was resected. Excision of the tumor was difficult as it was smoother than a typical myoma and more difficult to grasp with forceps. The tumor was enucleated with a special instrument which we also use to remove myomas. The usual enucleation performed in fibroid surgery was not possible as there was no capsule separating nodule from the myometrium, and the tumor seemed to grow into the orthotope myometric tissue (Fig. 2.10a). After removal of the nodule and the surrounding myometrial layer, the uterine wall was reconstructed in a

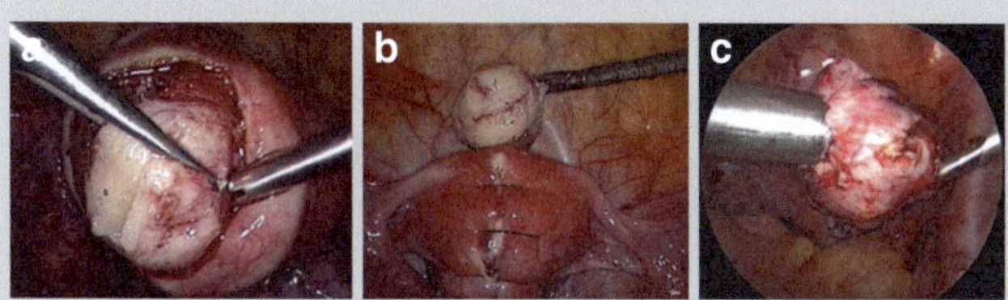

FIGURE 2.10 (**a**) Intraoperative sight of the adenomatoid tumor connected to the surrounding myometrium (Case 1). (**b**) Reconstruction of the uterine wall after excision of the tumor (Case 1). (**c**) Removing the adenomatoid tumor by morcellation (Case 2)

single layer with reversed and inverted single stitches (Fig. 2.10b). The tumor was removed after intra-abdominal morcellation (Fig. 2.10c).

Case 2

A 19-year-old *nulligravida* presented with pain in the lower abdomen for the last 6 months, dyspareunia and pain in the back. Transvaginal ultrasound revealed a well-circum-scribed 5 cm mass in the fundus of the uterus. No additional lesions were noted in the pelvis. The patient underwent an uneventful laparoscopic procedure with excision of the tumor and reconstruction of the uterus wall.

The postoperative recovery was in each case unre-markable, and the patients were discharged 2 days after surgery free of pain. The follow-up period was without pathological findings.

Histological tissue was available from both original tumor specimens. Routine histological studies were performed according to the usual procedures: 4 μm thick sections of formaldehyde-fixed, paraffin-embed-ded tissue were stained with hematoxylin and eosin (H&E) for the light microscopic histological examina-tion. Immunohistochemistry was performed using the following antibodies: calretinin for staining cells of mesothelial origin and CD34 for marking endothelial cells; KI-67 was used as a proliferation marker [47, 52].

Macroscopically, both tumors showed a white-gray, nodular, non-capsulated surface. The histological examination showed smooth muscle cells of normal myometrium and in between the myometrium tumor elements consisted of slit-like, tubular, cystic, or cribriform anastomosing gland-like spaces reminiscent of vascular structures (Fig. 2.11a, b). The lining cells were columnar, cuboidal to flat with bland cytologic features and mitotic activity. The angiomatoid spaces were lined by a single layer of flattened cells with oval or round nuclei, divided by fine connective tissue septa rich in blood vessels with a slight lymphocytic infiltration. The spaces contained cells with slightly eosinophilic cytoplasm and prominent cytoplasmic vacuoles that mimic signet ring cells. The pseudoglandular spaces were surrounded by hyperplastic smooth muscle with a sprinkling of stromal lymphocytes. Nuclei were usually small with inconspicuous nucleoli. Neither atypical nuclei, mitoses, nor necrosis was found.

Immunohistochemical techniques showed a strong staining of tumor cells with calretinin but no staining with CD34 (Fig. 2.11c, d). However, CD34 marked the endothelial cells and the surrounding orthotopic lymphovascular vessels (Fig. 2.11e, f). The Ki-67 index of the tumor cells was <1% (Fig. 2.11g).

Adenomatoid tumors occur most commonly during the reproductive years. Nevertheless, they are rare, benign neoplasms, occurring in about 1% of pathologically examined hysterectomies and are mostly incidental findings [45, 53]. In the majority of the known case reports, the diagnosis is made only after pathological examination of other suspected tumor origins. As in our case, most of the adenomatoid tumors remain asymptomatic. Adenomatoid tumors of the uterus can be either subserosal or intramural and can involve the subendometrial myometrium. Due to their anatomical

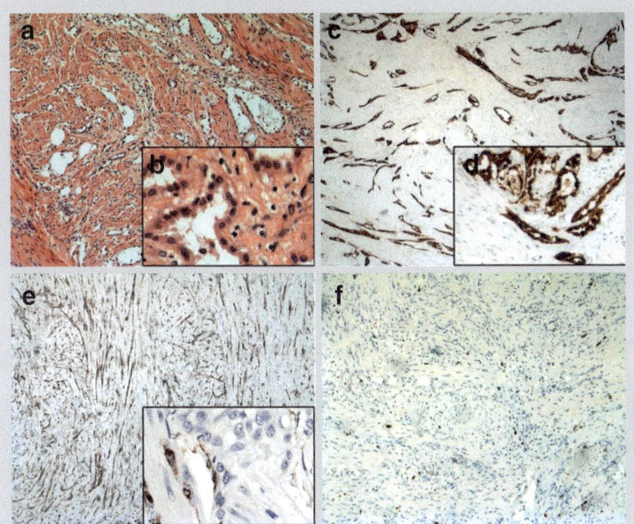

FIGURE 2.11 (**H&E**) (**a**) low magnification (×25) of the uterine adenomatoid tumor showing the typical tubular-glandular growth pattern and surrounding small muscle cells. (**b**) The lining cells in typical cuboidal growth pattern with unsuspicious nuclei at high magnification (×400). (**Calretinin**) (**c**), showing the strongly positive immunohistochemical calretinin staining of the tumor tissue (×25). (**d**) positive-stained tumor cells at high magnification (×400). (**CD34**) immunohistochemical CD34 staining (**e, f**) showing no positive staining of the tumor cells but the surrounding lymphovascular endothelial cells in low and high magnification (×25 and ×400). (**Ki-67**) immunohistochemical Ki-67 staining (×10) showing no enhanced mitotic activity of the tumor tissue (**g**)

localization, the most common symptoms are pain and menorrhagia or symptoms associated with adenomyosis uteri. Many cases of incidental diagnosis do not show any clinical symptoms at all [45, 46, 52, 54–56]. In females, adenomatoid tumors are mostly situated in the fallopian tubes and the uterus and less frequently in the ovaries or the periovarial tissue. In males, they occur in the epididymitis, tunica albuginea, and testicular parenchyma. Very seldom, adenomatoid tumors are seen in extragenital regions, e.g., the adrenal gland, omentum majus, or liver. Accordingly, the clinical symptoms are similar to those caused by other benign space-consuming lesions in these regions. There is no evidence of recurrence, malignant transformation, or metastasis [46].

In the majority of cases, preoperative detailed differential diagnostics are the exception as adenomatoid tumors are found incidentally. Despite the well-established microscopic features that distinguish adenomatoid tumors from all other entities, preliminary clinical examination, ultrasound, or MRI cannot differentiate adenomatoid tumors from their differential diagnosis [52, 56, 57].

The dissimilarity to uterine fibroids, the most frequent misdiagnosis of uterine adenomatoid tumors, is seen in the intraoperative complexity of the separation between tumor and myometrium. Mitsumori et al. report two cases of adenomatoid tumors of the uterus that also imitated leiomyoma and were only diagnosed postoperatively [57]. Histologically, fibroids have their own capsule of connective tissue. This is missing in adenomatoid tumors [49], and it is, therefore, necessary to include a layer of unaffected myometrium when operating adenomatoid tumors. Nevertheless, laparoscopic surgery for the treatment of adenomatoid tumors is feasible and recommended. In contrast to adenomyosis uteri, there is no histological infiltration of endometrial glands and stroma into the myometrial tissue. Adenomyosis uteri in its primary and disseminated forms infiltrate the entire myometrial wall. A more disseminated spreading of adenomatoid tumor has been reported in women with immunosuppression [58].

The term adenomatoid tumor was first presented by Golden and Ash in 1945 based on its histological appearance [48–50]. Mesonephric, mullerian, endothelial, and mesothelial origins have been discussed. Extensive research has been needed to prove that adenomatoid tumors have their origin in the uterine wall and are of mesothelial origin [44–46, 54, 59, 60]. All affected organs have a common embryological origin, that is, a celomic thickening, and are influenced by different steroid hormones, which support the mesothelian concept. Nevertheless, the pathogenesis remains uncertain, as the superficial location suggests a peritoneal origin, whereas the mesothelian part could in the same way originate from the muscle. In contrast, fibroids are of mesenchymal origin. These results have however led to an immunohistological differentiation distinguishing adenomatoid tumors from other morphological entities. The corresponding immunohistological markers are CD34, calretinin, and Ki-67. Other markers are HMBE1, other cytokeratins, EMA, WT1, and vimentin [48, 60].

There have been different attempts to classify adenomatoid tumors. They can be macroscopically separated into *small solid* tumors measuring 0.2–3.5 cm and *large cystic* tumors measuring 7–10 cm [46]. The small solid tumors, if recognized preoperatively by ultrasound or MRI, are similar to fibroids. However, the large cystic tumors resemble cystic-degenerated fibroids, cystic adenomyosis, congenital uterine cysts such as mesonephric or paramesonephric cysts, lymphangiomas, cervical ovula nabothi, or echinococcus cysts. Lee et al. described three different histological growth patterns of adenomatoid tumors: (a) *plexiform*, (b) *tubular*, and (c) *canalicular* although most tumors show more than one pattern [51]. Quigley and Hart differentiated adenomatoid tumors of the uterus into four different types according to their microscopic features: (a) *angiomatoid*, (b) *adenoid*, (c) *solid*, and (d) *cystic*. Many of the tumors show two or more patterns, with one pattern predominating [61].

Even though adenomatoid tumors are benign, nonmetastasizing, and nonrecurring, the preoperative and intraoperative differential diagnosis has to consider more threatening possibilities: lymphangioma, metastatic adenocarcinoma, and metastasis of other origins. For this reason, all specimens need to be analyzed histologically.

Intraoperative frozen section could be of use in protecting women of reproductive age from an unnecessary hysterectomy due to the misleading picture an adenomatoid tumor can present. Nevertheless, as adenomatoid tumors are usually encountered during the reproductive age and can be treated by similar surgical techniques used for the enucleation of fibroids, laparoscopic surgery is the gold standard.

Morcellation of Fibroids and the Threat of Sarcomas

This topic has only minor concern for myomectomy and infertility. However, **endometrial stromal sarcoma (ESS)** accounts for approximately 20% of all uterine sarcomas and commonly affects premenopausal age women. All other sarcomas appear beyond the reproductive age and are not an issue within this chapter. Nucci [62] describes that on macroscopic examination, LG-ESS generally forms multiple soft, poorly defined, attached nodules within the endometrium and myometrium which tend to have a tan to yellow color. It is difficult to make reliable preoperative diagnoses by way of imaging modalities and endometrial sampling. Consequently, surgical procedures are often incorrectly carried out for a presumed fibroid, polyp, or adenomyosis. The hysterectomy with bilateral oophorectomy is the initial surgical procedure for early stages of LG-ESS; however in young women ovarian preservation may be a possibility. Clinical course of LG-ESS is favorable due to its high response to progesterone therapy .Patients with low-grade ESS have a 90% 5-year disease-free survival (DFS) rate for stage (I/II); this 5-year outlook drops to 50% if high stage (III/IV), and recurrence is possible 10–20 years after the primary diagnosis [63]. However, morcellation of ESS can cause negative consequences. Park et al. [64] analyzed the surgical outcomes of 50 women with (Low Grade Endometrial Stromal Sarcoma) LG-ESS diagnosis (27 cases without morcellation and 23 cases with morcellation). The results showed that abdominopelvic recurrence was significantly higher in the group where morcellation was applied than in the group without morcellation. In addition, the 5-year DFS rates were 84% in the group where morcellation was not used and 55% for the group where morcellation was used. [64].

In a study over a period of 12 years in our department, seven uterine sarcomas within 2297 patients with fibroid surgery were detected. In six patients the preoperative evaluation clarified the possibility of malignancy, and the patient was operated by open abdominal surgery in the usual radical way. Only one patient with low-grade endometrial stromal sarcoma (LG-ESS) was preoperatively diagnosed by ultrasound (US) and endometrial sampling as having symptomatic uterine fibroids; however, when this patient underwent laparoscopic supracervical hysterectomy, postoperative histopathological examination detected ESS. Thus, the incident of ESS among women who underwent benign uterine fibroid surgery is 1/2297 (0.043%). Other publications results: Graebe et al. (2005) identified three ESS cases among 1361 patients who had uterine fibroids surgery (0.22%); Bojar et al. (2015) reported four ESS cases of ESS among 10,119 LASH procedures (0.037%); and Kto et al. (2016) reported two cases of ESS among 10,119 hysterectomies (0.019%) [65–67]. The risk of ESS seems to be low, but morcellation can negatively impact the patient's prospects. The risk of morcellation of uterine sarcoma is low; however, it has negative affect on recurrence and survival rate of the disease and should be avoided if there is any risk of malignancy especially in infertility surgery.

Discussion

Recurrence Rates

Even with the best, at this moment, surgical intracapsular excision of fibroids gives no guarantee of a nonrecurrence at another sight. Myomas do reoccur and we do not yet know the causing factors. One of our patients had five laparoscopic myomectomies in a span of 16 years. She then conceived and delivered two healthy children; finally, by the age of 43, she had reoccurring symptomatic fibroids. We performed a subtotal laparoscopic hysterectomy (SLH). At this occasion we even found some small retrocervical implants that histologically proved to be myomatosis. Hence, it is always safe to explain this to the patient preoperatively. It was observed that women with a single fibroid tended to experience a lower rate of cumulative recurrence after myomectomy.

Fertility Outcome: Our Experience

Of the 392 patients who underwent laparoscopic surgery for fertility in our department, in 129 cases (32%) the indication for surgery was myomas. Of these 129 patients, in 56 cases (14.3%) myomas were the only indication with infertility lasting more than 3 years. In 44 cases (11.2%), myomas appeared along with other factors: in 20 cases (5.1%) with other genital abnormalities, in 18 cases (4.6%) with tubal pathology, in 3 cases (0.8%) with endometriosis, and in 3 cases (0.8%) with ovarian cysts [68].

Location of Myoma

The different locations of myomas are clearly visible in (Fig. 2.12). The location of fibroids was evaluated as diffuse (this group comprised of all partly intramurally and partly subserously located myomas), submucous, intramural, and subserous. Primarily a deep, diffuse myomatosis with partly subserous and partly intramural location of fibroids was found in 60% of patients, submucous fibroids in 16%, and subserous fibroids in 13%.

In 122 patients a laparoscopic myoma enucleation was performed. In 61% of patients, the myomas were situated subserous-intramural, in 18% submucous, in 13% subserous,

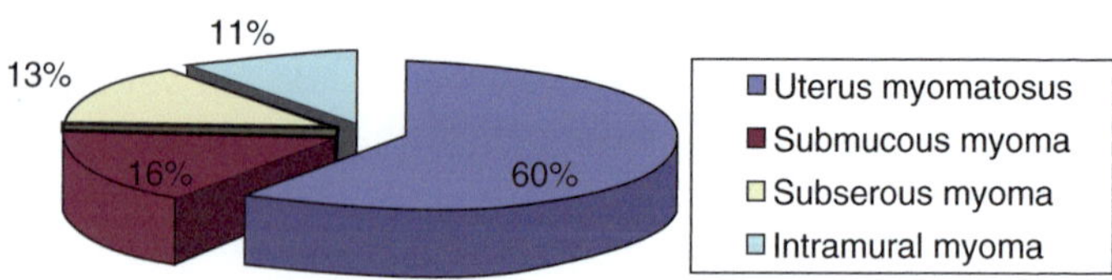

FIGURE 2.12 Localization of myomas in the 392 patients

and in 8% intramural. In 33 patients adhesiolysis was necessary prior to the myomectomy.

Figure 2.13 shows the additional surgical procedures performed on the 392 patients who underwent laparoscopic surgery for infertility in 2008/2009. Pregnancy rates clearly increased after surgery (Fig. 2.14).

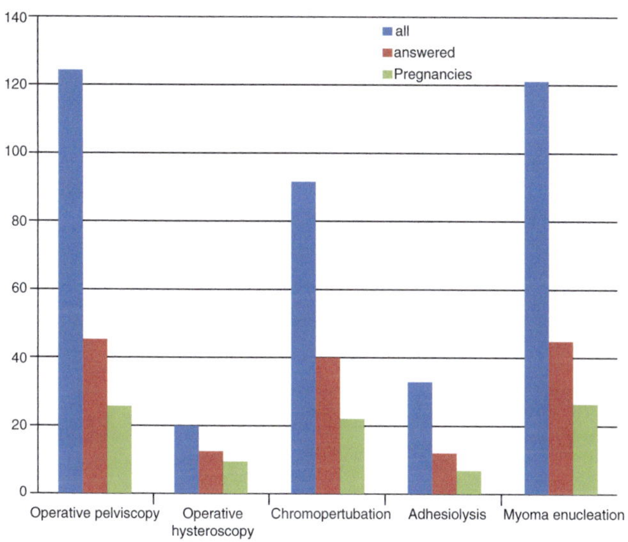

FIGURE 2.13 Laparoscopic surgical procedures performed for infertility according to groups A, B, and C

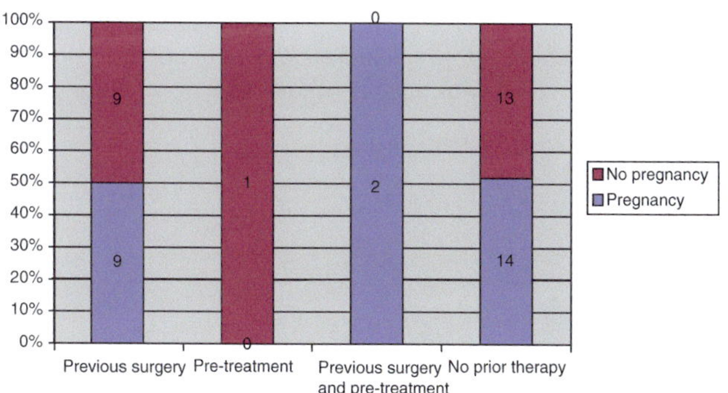

FIGURE 2.14 Influence of surgery and pretreatment on pregnancy rates of patients with myomas

Pregnancies and Deliveries

The average age of the evaluated patients was 34.6 years. Different pregnancy rates resulted depending on the localization of the fibroids. The resection of intramural-subserous fibroids resulted in a good pregnancy and delivery rate, and the highest pregnancy rate was achieved after submucous fibroid resection (Figs. 2.15 and 2.16). The lowest pregnancy rate was achieved after intramural fibroid resection.

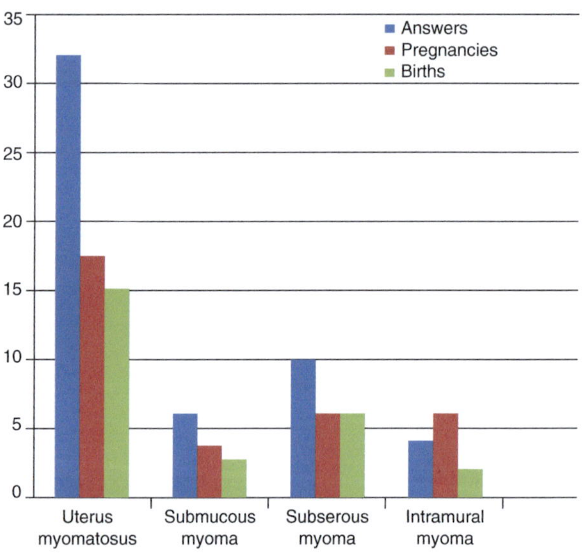

FIGURE 2.15 Number of pregnancies and deliveries according to localization of myoma with display of answers

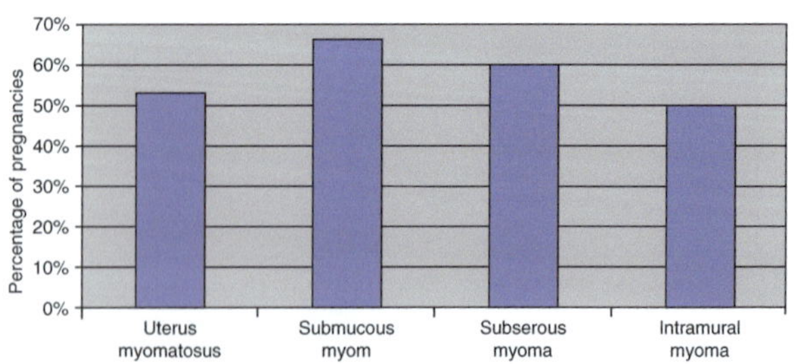

FIGURE 2.16 Number of pregnancies according to myoma localization

Mode of Delivery

Eleven of the 129 myomectomy patients underwent a cesarean section. Of these 129 patients, only 25 suffered from myomas alone; all others had multiple morbidities. The 14 pregnancies (56%) which resulted in this group of 25 led to 12 deliveries (48%), 5 (42%) of which were spontaneous and 7 (58%) cesarean sections. In the group of patients who underwent myomectomy for infertility, we had a pregnancy rate of 53% ($n = 17$) and a delivery rate of 47% ($n = 15$).

Complications

Four complications occurred in the group of myomectomy patients at or after delivery: genital descent after delivery, placenta accreta, one uterine rupture with cesarean section, and one emergency cesarean section due to imminent asphyxia of the baby.

Two of these appear to be normal intrapartum complication, while the placenta accreta and the uterine rupture may be seen in connection with the myomectomy. The size of the enucleated fibroid was 12 cm, but it could have occurred after a laparotomy myomectomy as well.

Conclusions

The role of uterine fibroids in infertility remains unknown. A causal relationship between fibroids and infertility has not been definitively demonstrated. Ideally, a comparison of pregnancy rates should be made between women with known fibroids and women post myomectomy. Such prospective studies have not been conducted, so our knowledge of the relationship between infertility and myomas results from indirect studies. The IVF/ET evaluations indicate that pregnancy rates only decrease when myomas are submucosal. However, only study comparing infertile women without tubal and andrological infertility factors, with and without myomas before and after myomectomy, seems to suggest that the presence of myomas decreases pregnancy rates, while their removal increases pregnancy rates.

The favorable pregnancy rates obtained after myomectomy lead us to believe that myomas influence fertility. Surprisingly, the global pregnancy rates are the same after hysteroscopic, laparoscopic, and abdominal myomectomy. However, we have no control groups of women who did not undergo surgery.

So the question remains: do myomas influence fertility? Every situation has to be judged separately, and efforts must be made to develop the best technique, that is, to say, the technique with the least risk of impairing fertility or causing complications during pregnancy. Although more fundamental research should be carried out to detect the mechanisms of infertility and understand the genetic basis for fibroid development and the molecular and hormonal mechanisms of myometrial proliferation, it is clear that intramural myomas may complicate pregnancies and healthy child delivery [69]. Myomectomies at cesarean sections have led to dramatic complications, and it is not advisable to be performed at that time [70].

A better understanding of the genetic basis of fibroid development in the future may show possibilities for the development of an effective prevention strategy in genetically predisposed individuals and provide strategies to slow the growth of myomas.

References

1. Patterson-Keels LM, Selvaggi SM, Haefner HK, Randolph JF Jr. Morphologic assessment of endometrium overlying submucosal leiomyomas. J Reprod Med. 1994;39(8):579–84.
2. Al-Hendy A, Salama SA. Catechol-O-methyltransferase polymorphism is associated with increased uterine leiomyoma risk in different ethnic groups. J Soc Gynecol Investig. 2006;13(2):136–44.
3. Tsibris JC, Segars J, Coppola D, Mane S, Wilbanks GD, O'Brien WF, et al. Insights from gene arrays on the development and

growth regulation of uterine leiomyomata. Fertil Steril. 2002;78(1):114–21.

4. Wang H, Mahadevappa M, Yamamoto K, Wen Y, Chen B, Warrington JA, et al. Distinctive proliferative phase differences in gene expression in human myometrium and leiomyomata. Fertil Steril. 2003;80(2):266–76.

5. Gross K, Morton C, Stewart E. Finding genes for uterine fibroids. Obstet Gynecol. 2000;95(4 Suppl 1):60.

6. Mettler L, Semm K, Gebhardt IH, Schollmeyer TH, Schollmeyer M, Meyer P, et al., editors. Endoskopische Abdominalchirurgie in der Gynäkologie. Stuttgart: Schattauer; 2002.

7. Mettler L, Semm K, Schollmeyer TH, Schollmeyer M, Meyer P, Ternamian A, editors. Manual for laparoscopic and hystero-scopic gynecological surgery. New Delhi: Jaypee Brothers Medical Publishers LTD; 2006.

8. Schollmeyer TH, Mettler L, Rüther D, Alkatout I, editors. Practical manual for laparoscopic & hysteroscopic gynecological surgery. New Delhi: Jaypee Brothers Medical Publishers; 2013.

9. Bulletti C, De Ziegler D, Polli V, Flamigni C. The role of leio-myomas in infertility. J Am Assoc Gynecol Laparosc. 1999;6(4):441–5.

10. Hunt JE, Wallach EE. Uterine factors in infertility—an over-view. Clin Obstet Gynecol. 1974;17(4):44–64.

11. Buttram VC Jr, Reiter RC. Uterine leiomyomata: etiology, symptomatology, and management. Fertil Steril. 1981;36(4):433–45.

12. Vollen-Hoven BJ. Uterine fibroids: a clinical review. Br J Obstet Gynaecol. 1990;97:285–8.

13. Deligdish L, Loewenthal M. Endometrial changes associated with myomata of the uterus. J Clin Pathol. 1970;23(8):676–80.

14. Verkauf BS. Myomectomy for fertility enhancement and preser-vation. Fertil Steril. 1992;58(1):1–15.

15. Robert HG. Prècis de gynecologie. Paris: Masson; 1974.

16. Ben-Nagi J, Miell J, Mavrelos D, Naftalin J, Lee C, Jurkovic D. Endometrial implantation factors in women with submucous uterine fibroids. Reprod Biomed Online. 2010;21(5):610–5.

17. Klatsky PC, Lane DE, Ryan IP, Fujimoto VY. The effect of fibroids without cavity involvement on ART outcomes indepen-dent of ovarian age. Hum Reprod. 2007;22(2):521–6.

18. Sunkara SK, Khairy M, El-Toukhy T, Khalaf Y, Coomarasamy A. The effect of intramural fibroids without uterine cavity

involvement on the outcome of IVF treatment: a systematic review and meta-analysis. Hum Reprod. 2010;25(2):418–29.

19. Oliveira FG, Abdelmassih VG, Diamond MP, Dozortsev D, Melo NR, Abdelmassih R. Impact of subserosal and intramural uterine fibroids that do not distort the endometrial cavity on the outcome of in vitro fertilization-intracytoplasmic sperm injection. Fertil Steril. 2004;81(3):582–7.

20. Check JH, Choe JK, Lee G, Dietterich C. The effect on IVF outcome of small intramural fibroids not compressing the uterine cavity as determined by a prospective matched control study. Hum Reprod. 2002;17(5):1244–8.

21. Yan L, Ding L, Tang R. ZJ4 C, Li C, Wang Y. Effect of fibroids not distorting the endometrial cavity on the outcome of in vitro fertilization treatment: a retrospective cohort study. Fertil Steril. 2014;101(3):716–21.

22. Somigliana E, De Benedictis S, Vercellini P, Nicolosi AE, Benaglia L, Scarduelli C, et al. Fibroids not encroaching the endometrial cavity and IVF success rate: a prospective study. Hum Reprod. 2011;26(4):834–9.

23. He Y, Zeng Q, Dong S, Qin L, Li G, Wang P. Associations between uterine fibroids and lifestyles including diet, physical activity and stress: a casecontrol study in China. Asia Pac J Clin Nutr. 2013;22:109–17.

24. Dandolu V, Singh R, Lidicker J, Harmanli O. BMI and uterine size: is there any relationship? Int J Gynecol Pathol. 2010;29(6):568–71.

25. Marret H, Fritel X, Ouldamer L, Bendifallah S, Brun JL, De Jesus I, et al. Therapeutic management of uterine fibroid tumors: updated French guidelines. Eur J Obstet Gynecol Reprod Biol. 2012;165(2):156–64.

26. Ezzati M, Norian JM, Segars JH. Management of uterine fibroids in the patient pursuing assisted reproductive technologies. Womens Health (Lond Engl). 2009;5(4):413–21.

27. Li TC, Mortimer R, Cooke ID. Myomectomy: a retrospective study to examine reproductive performance before and after surgery. Hum Reprod. 1999;14(7):1735–40.

28. Vercellini P, Maddalena S, De Giorgi O, Pesole A, Ferrari L, Crosignani PG. Determinants of reproductive outcome after abdominal myomectomy for infertility. Fertil Steril. 1999;72(1):109–14.

29. Seracchioli R, Rossi S, Govoni F, Rossi E, Venturoli S, Bulletti C, et al. Fertility and obstetric outcome after laparoscopic

myomectomy of large myomata: a randomized comparison with abdominal myomectomy. Hum Reprod. 2000;15(12):2663–8.
30. Dubuisson JB, Fauconnier A, Deffarges JV, Norgaard C, Kreiker G, Chapron C. Pregnancy outcome and deliveries following laparoscopic myomectomy. Hum Reprod. 2000;15(4):869–73.
31. Harris WJ. Uterine dehiscence following laparoscopic myomectomy. Obstet Gynecol. 1992;80(3 Pt 2):545–6.
32. Mecke H, Wallas F, Brocker A, Gertz HP. Pelviscopic myoma enucleation: technique, limits, complications. Geburtshilfe Frauenheilkd. 1995;55(7):374–9.
33. Friedmann W, Maier RF, Luttkus A, Schafer AP, Dudenhausen JW. Uterine rupture after laparoscopic myomectomy. Acta Obstet Gynecol Scand. 1996;75(7):683–4.
34. Pelosi MA 3rd, Pelosi MA. Spontaneous uterine rupture at thirty-three weeks subsequent to previous superficial laparoscopic myomectomy. Am J Obstet Gynecol. 1997;177(6):1547–9.
35. Foucher F, Leveque J, Le Bouar G, Grall J. Uterine rupture during pregnancy following myomectomy via coelioscopy. Eur J Obstet Gynecol Reprod Biol. 2000;92(2):279–81.
36. Hockstein S. Spontaneous uterine rupture in the early third trimester after laparoscopically assisted myomectomy. A case report. J Reprod Med. 2000;45(2):139–41.
37. Seinera P, Arisio R, Decko A, Farina C, Crana F. Laparoscopic myomectomy: indications, surgical technique and complications. Hum Reprod. 1997;12(9):1927–30.
38. Darai E, Dechaud H, Benifla JL, Renolleau C, Panel P, Madelenat P. Fertility after laparoscopic myomectomy: preliminary results. Hum Reprod. 1997;12(9):1931–4.
39. Ribeiro SC, Reich H, Rosenberg J, Guglielminetti E, Vidali A. Laparoscopic myomectomy and pregnancy outcome in infertile patients. Fertil Steril. 1999;71(3):571–4.
40. Arthur R, Kachura J, Liu G, Chan C, Shapiro H. Laparoscopic myomectomy versus uterine artery embolization: long-term impact on markers of ovarian reserve. J Obstet Gynaecol Can. 2014;36(3):240–7.
41. Gizzo S, Saccardi C, Patrelli TS, Ancona E, Noventa M, Fagherazzi S, et al. Magnetic resonance-guided focused ultrasound myomectomy: safety, efficacy, subsequent fertility and quality-of-life improvements, a systematic review. Reprod Sci. 2014;21(4):465–76.
42. Donnez J, Tomaszewski J, Vazquez F, Bouchard P, Lemieszczuk B, Baro F, et al. Ulipristal acetate versus leuprolide acetate for uterine fibroids. N Engl J Med. 2012;366(5):421–32.

43. Tinelli A, Malvasi A, Cavallotti C, Dell'Edera D, Tsin DA, Stark M, et al. The management of fibroids based on immunohisto-chemical studies of their pseudocapsules. Expert Opin Ther Targets. 2011;15(11):1241–7.
44. Youngs LA, Taylor HB. Adenomatoid tumors of the uterus and fallopian tube. Am J Clin Pathol. 1967;48(6):537–45.
45. Tiltman AJ. Adenomatoid tumours of the uterus. Histopathology. 1980;4(4):437–43.
46. Nogales FF, Isaac MA, Hardisson D, Bosincu L, Palacios J, Ordi J, et al. Adenomatoid tumors of the uterus: an analysis of 60 cases. Int J Gynecol Pathol. 2002;21(1):34–40.
47. Hes O, Perez-Montiel DM, Alvarado Cabrero I, Zamecnik M, Podhola M, Sulc M, et al. Thread-like bridging strands: a mor-phologic feature present in all adenomatoid tumors. Ann Diagn Pathol. 2003;7(5):273–7.
48. Di Stefano D, Faticanti Scucchi L, Covello R, Martinazzoli A, Meli C, Bosman C. Uterine diffuse adenomatoid tumor. Does it represent a different biological entity? Gynecol Obstet Invest. 1998;46(1):68–72.
49. Kalidindi M, Odejinmi F. Laparoscopic excision of uterine ade-nomatoid tumour: two cases and literature review. Arch Gynecol Obstet. 2010;281(2):311–5.
50. Golden A, Ash JE. Adenomatoid tumors of the genital tract. Am J Pathol. 1945;21(1):63–79.
51. Lee MJ Jr, Dockerty MB, Thompson GJ, Waugh JM. Benign mesotheliomas (adenomatoid tumors) of the genital tract. Surg Gynecol Obstet. 1950;91(2):221–31.
52. Irikoma M, Takahashi K, Kurioka H, Miyazaki K, Kamei T. Uterine adenomatoid tumors confirmed by immunohisto-chemical staining. Arch Gynecol Obstet. 2001;265(3):151–4.
53. Tiltman A. Adenomatoid tumors of the uterus. Int J Gynecol Pathol. 2002;21(3):305; author reply
54. Agbata AI, Kovi J. Adenomatoid tumor of the uterus. Report of two cases. J Natl Med Assoc. 1975;67(6):447–9.
55. Bisset DL, Morris JA, Fox H. Giant cystic adenomatoid tumour (mesothelioma) of the uterus. Histopathology. 1988;12(5):555–8.
56. Saran M, Sanghi A, Faruqi A. Adenomatoid tumour of the uterus presenting as cyst. J Obstet Gynaecol. 2007;27(6):637–8.
57. Mitsumori A, Morimoto M, Matsubara S, Yamamoto M, Akamatsu N, Hiraki Y. MR appearance of adenomatoid tumor of the uterus. J Comput Assist Tomogr. 2000;24(4):610–3.

58. Cheng CL, Wee A. Diffuse uterine adenomatoid tumor in an immunosuppressed renal transplant recipient. Int J Gynecol Pathol. 2003;22(2):198–201.

59. Salazar H, Kanbour A, Burgess F. Ultrastructure and observations on the histogenesis of mesotheliomas, "adenomatoid tumors", of the female genital tract. Cancer. 1972;29(1):141–52.

60. Lehto VP, Miettinen M, Virtanen I. Adenomatoid tumor: immunohistological features suggesting a mesothelial origin. Virchows Arch B Cell Pathol Incl Mol Pathol. 1983;42(2):153–9.

61. Quigley JC, Hart WR. Adenomatoid tumors of the uterus. Am J Clin Pathol. 1981;76(5):627–35.

62. Nucci MR. Practical issues related to uterine pathology: endometrial stromal tumors. Mod Pathol. 2016;29(Suppl 1):S92–S103. doi:10.1038/modpathol.2015.140. PMID: 26715176.

63. Rauh-Hain JA, Goodman A, Boruta DM, et al. Endometrial stromal sarcoma: a clinicopathologic study of patients. J Reprod Med. 2014;59:547–52.

64. Park JY, Kim DY, Kim JH, Kim YM, Kim YT, Nam JH. The impact of tumor morcellation during surgery on the outcomes of patients with apparently early low-grade endometrial stromal sarcoma of the uterus. Ann Surg Oncol. 2011;18(12):3453–61. doi:10.1245/s10434-011-1751-y. Epub 2011 May 4. PMID: 21541824.

65. Graebe K, Garcia-Soto A, Aziz M, Valarezo V, Heller PB, Tchabo N, Tobias DH, Salamon C, Ramieri J, Dise C, Slomovitz BM. Incidental power morcellation of malignancy: a retrospective cohort study. Gynecol Oncol. 2015;136(2):274–7. doi:10.1016/j.ygyno.2014.11.018. Epub 2014 Nov 26. PMID: 25740603.

66. Harris JA, Swenson CW, Uppal S, Kamdar N, Mahnert N, As-Sanie S, Morgan DM. Practice patterns and postoperative complications before and after US Food and Drug Administration safety communication on power morcellation. Am J Obstet Gynecol. 2016;214(1):98.e1–98.e13. doi:10.1016/j.ajog.2015.08.047. Epub 2015 Aug 24. PMID: 26314519.

67. Hur HC, King LP, Klebanoff MJ, Hur C, Ricciotti HA. Fibroid morcellation: a shared clinical decision tool for mode of hysterectomy. Eur J Obstet Gynecol Reprod Biol. 2015;195:122–7. doi:10.1016/j.ejogrb.2015.09.044. Epub 2015 Oct 8. PMID: 26520875.

68. Genazzani AR, Brincat M, editors. Frontiers in gynecological endocrinology. Cham: Springer International Publishing; 2014.

69. Nisolle M, Gillerot S, Casanas-Roux F, Squifflet J, Berliere M, Donnez J. Immunohistochemical study of the proliferation index, oestrogen receptors and progesterone receptors A and B in leiomyomata and normal myometrium during the menstrual cycle and under gonadotrophin-releasing hormone agonist therapy. Hum Reprod. 1999;14(11):2844–50.
70. Alkatout I, Mettler L. Hysterctomy – a comprehensive surgical approach, Springer Publisher; 2017. p. 1700.

Chapter 3
Treatment Modalities for Fibroids, Indications, Risks, and Benefits

Deepika Garg and James H. Segars

Medical Management

Medical management of fibroids is usually reserved for women with the predominant symptom of heavy menstrual bleeding. It is associated with long-term failure rates. Approximately 25% of women with abnormal uterine bleeding and 50% with chronic pelvic pain experienced symptomatic improvement after 1 year of treatment [1]. Management of fibroids should be tailored to the needs of the women who display symptoms and desire future fertility.

D. Garg, MD
Department of Obstetrics and Gynecology, Maimonides Medical Center, Brooklyn, NY 11219, USA
e-mail: drgargdeepika@gmail.com

J.H. Segars, MD (✉)
Department of Gynecology and Obstetrics, Johns Hopkins School of Medicine, 720 Rutland Ave, Room 624 Ross, Baltimore, MD 21205, USA
e-mail: jsegars2@jhmi.edu

N.S. Moawad (ed.), *Uterine Fibroids*,
https://doi.org/10.1007/978-3-319-58780-6_3,
© Springer International Publishing AG 2018

Oral Contraceptives (OC)

Use of combined hormonal contraceptives was found to reduce heavy menstrual bleeding in women with fibroids but has limited efficacy in its treatment [2]. Available data on the association between fibroids and OC appears too dispersed to allow precise risk quantification [3]. Evidence suggests that use of OC is associated with decreased risk of fibroids; however, in a prospective study with 3006 cases of women with fibroids, it has been found that if OC are started before ages 13–16 years, there was an elevated risk of fibroids [4]. Some authors have suggested that OC were contraindicated in fibroids; however, data suggest that OC are associated with reduction in the risk of fibroids and alleviated fibroid-associated symptoms. Other factors such as proportion of hormones in the preparation, the timing and duration of exposure, and different route of administration may play an important role. With the use of newer delivery methods of contraceptives, further studies are required.

Progesterone Receptor Modulators

Ulipristal acetate is a progesterone receptor modulator that has been studied for fibroid treatment and has been shown to reduce the volume of fibroid and symptoms associated with fibroids [5, 6]. Ulipristal acetate inhibits ovulation and also decreases estrogen release from ovary. The compound has been approved for 3 months for preoperative management of fibroids outside the United States. Recently, a randomized controlled trial compared three different doses of ulipristal acetate (oral, 5 mg or 10 mg once daily) for 13 weeks in 242 women with fibroid-associated menorrhagia, anemia, and ≤ 16 weeks' size uterus. The authors reported significant reduction in menorrhagia, (5 mg, 91%; 10 mg, 92%; placebo, 19%), increase in hemoglobin (5 mg, 4.3 g/dL; 10 mg, 4.2 g/dL; placebo, 3.1 g/dL), and reduction in fibroid size (5 mg, −21%; 10 mg, −12%; placebo, +3%). Headache and the breast tenderness were the most common side effects noted with the use of ulipristal acetate [6]. However, effect on the endometrium after long term has spawned regimens with intermittent use. When compared with other medical treatment of fibroids, ulipristal acetate was found to be non-inferior to GnRH agonists with fewer severe side effects [7]. Oral administration and minimal side effects associated with these drugs make ulipristal acetate a suitable option. In the United States, ulipristal acetate is not currently approved for the treatment of fibroids. It is available only in a 30 mg dosage, as opposed to 5 and 10 mg that were studied for the treatment of fibroids. Also, long-term safety data after treatment with these agents are still lacking.

Mifepristone (RU-486) is an antiprogestin and has been studied for the treatment of fibroids. After treatment with 5–50 mg of mifepristone daily for 3–6 months, reduction in uterine and fibroid size was noted as 27–49% and 26–74%, respectively. This was accompanied by a reduction in severity of pressure symptoms, dysmenorrhea, and menorrhagia. Side effects were transient for transaminases in 4% of patients and endometrial hyperplasia in 28% of patients [8]. Simple endometrial hyperplasia was noted in 13.9% at 6 months and 4.8% at 12 months of its use with no patient had hyperplasia with atypia. After 5.7 months of posttreatment follow-up, most of the women had recurrence with average size of 42% less than the baseline [9]. Accumulating evidence suggests that mifepristone improves quality of life and reduces the size of the fibroid and fibroid-associated symptoms [10]. Like ulipristal acetate, mifepristone is not approved by FDA for the treatment of fibroids in the United States. Mifepristone is also available in single dose of 200 mg, not in 5–50 mg doses that have been studied for the treatment of fibroids.

Levonorgestrel-Releasing Intrauterine Device (LNG-IUS)

This device is widely used and approved by the FDA for treatment of heavy menstrual bleeding. In a prospective study, after 12 months of use in women with fibroids, heavy menstrual bleeding was decreased from 97 to 16% ($P < 0.001$), and hemoglobin and hematocrit were improved in 95% of women [11]. The LNG-IUS also acts as a contraceptive for the women. After 3 years of LNG-IUS use in women with fibroids, the mean reduction in the uterine volume was noted to be 63.6 ± 19.0 (SD) cm^3 (from 156.6 to 93 cm^3, $p = 0.014$), and for the fibroids it was 5.2 ± 3.1 (SD) cm^3 (from 12.8 to 7.6 cm^3, $P = $ NS). In addition, similar findings were noted with the reduction in menorrhagia and improvement in hematologic parameters but without any significant influence on the fibroid size [12]. Insertion of LNG-IUS is associated with an expulsion rate of 0–20% in women with fibroids, versus 0–3% in women without fibroids. However, women with submucosal fibroids were associated with a higher expulsion rate of 11% [13, 14]. The LNG-IUS is contraindicated in the presence of intracavitary fibroids that distort the uterine cavity.

Gonadotropin-Releasing Hormone (GnRH) Agonists and Antagonists

GnRH agonists are among the most effective medical therapies for fibroids. These medications work primarily by downregulation of GnRH receptors to create a hypogonadotropic state that is clinically similar to menopause. These agents are used for the short-term use as a preoperative agent to reduce the uterine bleeding and symptoms of menometrorrhagia, concomitantly to improve hematologic parameters, and to reduce the uterine and fibroid size [15, 16]. GnRH agonists are approved for 3–6 months prior to fibroid-related surgery together with iron supplementation to correct anemia and facilitate a less invasive or a minimally invasive procedure [17]. After 6 months of GnRH therapy in women with fibroids, 48.3% of women had more than 36% mean reduction in fibroid volume [18]. In a randomized double-blind study, after 24 weeks of GnRH agonist therapy in women with fibroids, there were reductions in uterine size from 601 ± 62 to 294 ± 46 cm^3 ($P < 0.01$).

GnRH agonists can result into severe hypoestrogenic symptoms, which include hot flashes, vaginal dryness, sleep disturbances, mood changes, and/or myalgias and arthralgias [19]. Osteoporosis caused by the long-term use of these drugs is the most serious side effects and limits therapy. In addition, discontinuation of GnRH agonists can lead to rapid resumption of the pretreatment uterine and/or fibroid volume. The side effects of GnRH agonists use can be reduced by "add-back" therapy with low-dose estrogen-progestin after the phase of downregulation. In a study of 51 patients with symptomatic uterine fibroids, estrogen-progestin add-back therapy for 21 months after 3 months of treatment with GnRH agonists showed no regrowth of the fibroids, thus sustaining the therapeutic role of GnRH agonists with reduction in the side effects [20]. These drugs can be used in perimenopausal women to provide short-term relief until they develop natural postmenopausal estrogen deficiency [21].

Similarly, GnRH antagonists can also be used in place of GnRH agonists to reduce the size of fibroids and associated symptoms [22]. The advantage is rapid onset of action without having the initial flare-up as observed with GnRH agonists. After a mean duration of 19 days (1–65 days) of treatment, there were maximum reductions in fibroid size. Noted was −42.7% (−77.0% to 14.1%) and −29.2% (−62.2% to 35.6%) with resolution of the hypoestrogenic side effects within 1 week after treatment [23]. Due to nonavailability of long-acting preparations, the treatment of fibroids is cumbersome with daily injections.

Selective Estrogen Receptor Modulators (Raloxifene)

The efficacy of raloxifene for the treatment of fibroids or their symptoms is uncertain. After giving raloxifene with

GnRH analog for six cycles of 28 days in premenopausal women, there was significant reduction in the size of fibroids. However, no difference was detected in fibroid-related symptoms [24]. A possible risk of venous thrombosis with high doses of raloxifene is a concern.

Aromatase Inhibitors and Androgenic Steroids (Danazol and Gestrinone)

In perimenopausal woman, aromatase inhibitors can be used to reduce the size and alleviate the symptoms associated with fibroids [25]. Limited evidence is available to determine the duration of therapy, risks, and cost-effectiveness of aromatase inhibitors [26]. Danazol and gestrinone are androgenic steroids that may be effective in the improvement of the fibroid-associated symptoms [27]. Gestrinone is not available in the United States. Danazol inhibits pituitary gonadotropin secretion, thus inhibits ovarian estrogen production. It reduces the symptoms associated with fibroids, but no effect was found on the size of fibroid. Androgenic side effects are common with the use of androgenic steroids, which include acne, hirsutism, weight gain, muscle cramps, hot flashes, mood changes, and depression.

Nonsteroidal Anti-inflammatory Drugs and Antifibrinolytic Agents (Tranexamic Acid)

Nonsteroidal anti-inflammatory drugs reduce heavy menstrual bleeding and pain associated with fibroids but less effectively in comparison with the other medical therapies [28]. Antifibrinolytic agents, such as tranexamic acid, are useful in the management of heavy menstrual bleeding. It is FDA approved, and in one trial, approximately 35% of women were from the group of fibroid-associated heavy menstrual bleeding [29, 30].

Surgical Management

Interventional Radiology

Uterine Artery Embolization (UAE)

Uterine artery embolization is an interventional radiologic technique with an excellent clinical success rate that results in similar quality of life after surgical management of fibroids [31]. By this technique, embolization of the uterine arteries causes reduction in blood supply to the fibroids and typically a 30–46% shrinkage of the fibroids [32]. There is concern about ovarian function and future pregnancies after embolization [33]. Therefore, it is most appropriately used as an effective option to treat fibroids in women who do not want future fertility but want to preserve their uterus [34].

Patients with UAE have shorter hospital stays, less pain, and quicker resumption to work after the procedure when compared with surgical management of fibroids [35]. Predictors of UAE success are size, number, and the location of the fibroids. Reduced success rates have been reported with larger fibroids or greater number of fibroids in long-term follow-up studies [36, 37]. The complications after UAE are minor and include post-procedural pain, vaginal discharge, and post-embolization syndrome which include mild fever, fatigue, nausea, vomiting, myalgia, malaise, and leukocytosis [38]. UAE is associated with a higher rate of additional surgical interventions for treatment failure [39].

Absolute contraindications to UAE include active infection, pregnancy or suspected cancer, severe vascular disease, and contrast allergy [40]. Relative contraindications are submucosal fibroids, previous internal iliac artery ligation, extensive adenomyosis, current use of GnRH agonists (decreases the size and blood flow through the uterine artery, making it difficult to catheterize the uterine artery), and future desire of pregnancy. The risk of infertility following embolization was found similar to that after myomectomy, and there were no maternal and fetal complications found during the normal course of pregnancy [41]. In contrast, another study showed 50–60% pregnancy rate following either UAE or laparoscopic myomectomy along with increased risk of preterm delivery (odds ratio 6.2; 95% CI, 1.4–27.7) and malpresentation (odds ratio 4.3; 95% CI, 1.0–20.5) in pregnancy following UAE [42].

Magnetic Resonance Imaging-Guided Focused Ultrasound Surgery (MRgFUS)

MRI-guided focused ultrasound surgery is a noninvasive method that uses ultrasound thermal ablation for the treatment of clinically significant fibroids. Magnetic resonance imaging provides better resolution of the anatomic structures and gives real-time thermal monitoring to improve tissue destruction. Limiting factors for this treatment are size, vascularity, and accessibility of fibroids. In a study of women with fibroids >10 cm in diameter, women were treated with a 3-month course of GnRH agonists followed by magnetic resonance-guided focused ultrasound treatment. Results showed a reduction in median symptoms up to 45% at 6 months; 48% at 12 months, with a 10-point reduction in symptom severity scoring 83% at 6 months; and 89% at 12 months ($P < .001$) and reduction in targeted fibroid volume of 21% at 6 months ($P < .001$), furthermore, 37% at 12 months ($P < .001$) [43]. It had shown to decrease in fibroid volume of 32.0% ($P < .001$), 3 years after the treatment [44, 45].

Usually side effects are rare and can include skin burn, fibroid expulsion, and reversible pelvic neuropathy [46]. Encouraging results for pregnancy have been reported after this treatment for the group led by Dr. Stewart. The mean time to get pregnant after this treatment was 8 months, with 41% of pregnancies resulting in live births, 28% in spontaneous abortion, and 20% in ongoing pregnancies beyond 20 weeks [47].

Minimally Invasive Approaches

Uterine Artery Occlusion (Via Laparoscopy or a Vaginally Placed Clamp)

Uterine artery occlusion either via laparoscopy or a clamp placed vaginally in treating symptomatic fibroids is a promising method [48, 49]. After 6 months of this treatment, menstrual pictogram (blood assessments) scores were reduced by 50%, and the size of dominant fibroids was reduced by 36%. In addition, reduced postoperative pain and less use of analgesics were reported when compared with embolization of uterine arteries [50]. This technique has some advantages over embolization of uterine arteries, as it provides direct laparoscopic assessment of the pelvis and abdomen and does not require introduction of foreign material. However, when compared with UAE, some of the disadvantages have less mean uterine volume reductions (33% vs. 51%) and higher recurrence of symptoms (48% vs. 17%) [51].

Myolysis

Myolysis involves ablation of fibroid tissue by laparoscopic thermal, radiofrequency, or cryoablation. A radiofrequency ablation device along with the use of intraperitoneal ultrasound to optimize detection of fibroids during surgery has been approved by the FDA [52]. Recently, a randomized trial compared radiofrequency volumetric thermal ablation (RFVTA) with laparoscopic myomectomy (LM) and found that RFVTA was associated with less hospitalization time $(10.0 \pm 5.5$ h vs. 29.9 ± 14.2 h), reduced intraoperative blood loss $(16 \pm 9$ mL vs. 51 ± 57 mL), and a greater percentage of fibroids excised (98.6% vs. 80.3%) in comparison with LM [53]. Data regarding the subsequent outcome of pregnancies after myolysis are scarce.

Endometrial Ablation

Endometrial ablation, either alone or in conjunction with hysteroscopic myomectomy, has been proposed as an alternative for the management of fibroids. It uses hot, cold, or mechanical means to ablate the endometrium and reduces the menstrual bleeding. Since this procedure does not affect intramural and subserosal fibroids, pressure symptoms associated with larger fibroids are not addressed. Endometrial ablation has been compared with hysteroscopic myomectomy, and results revealed that 8.1% in endometrial ablation group had another surgery for incomplete resolution of symptoms, in comparison with 15.9% of patients in the hysteroscopic resection group. After long-term follow-up, 91.3% of patients in endometrial ablation group did not require any surgery after 9 years in comparison with 83.9% patients in submucosal resection group after 6 years, suggesting the long-term effectiveness of endometrial ablation in fibroid treatment [54]. However, endometrial ablation does not affect the size of the fibroid [55]. Further, the presence of fibroids in the uterine cavity may interfere with the functioning of this device [56]. Subsequent pregnancies after endometrial ablation may involve the risk of ectopic pregnancy, prematurity, or abnormal placentation [16].

Hysteroscopic Myomectomy

Hysteroscopic myomectomy is the best option for the women with submucosal fibroids and fibroids extending into the uterine cavity and accessible via this route. The most common indications for this procedure are abnormal uterine bleeding, infertility, and recurrent pregnancy loss. Contraindications for hysteroscopic myomectomy are pregnancy, active pelvic infection, and genital cancers. In an observational study of 122 women, within 4 years the risk of fibroid-related surgery was significantly lower with fibroids that were ≤ 3 cm vs. 4 cm or more and mainly inside the cavity (10% vs. 60%) and uterine size ≤6 weeks [57]. The results of this study suggests that size of the uterine cavity and location and size of the fibroid play an important determinant of the long-term success of this procedure. This is an outpatient procedure associated with rapid postoperative recovery and an increased likelihood of clinical pregnancy [58]. However, the evidence showing its association with the outcome of pregnancy is limited.

Laparoscopic Myomectomy

Laparoscopic myomectomy is a minimally invasive procedure and the treatment of choice to remove intramural or subserosal fibroids in patients with abnormal uterine bleeding and/or pressure symptoms. The choice of this procedure depends upon the size, number, location of fibroids (penetration into the myometrium and position relative to uterine vessels and fallopian tubes), and the expertise of the surgeon. Contraindications of laparoscopic myomectomy are the same as laparoscopy for other medical conditions. In a prospective study of 2050 patients with symptomatic fibroids undergoing laparoscopic myomectomy, the factors that were associated with major complications, such as hemorrhaging requiring blood transfusion, visceral injury, and procedural failure, were the size of fibroids (>5 cm; OR, 6.88; $p < .001$), number of fibroids removed (>3 in number; OR, 4.46; $p < 0.001$), location of the fibroids with intramural fibroids (OR, 1.48; $p < 0.05$), and fibroids being located in the broad ligament (OR, 2.36; $p < .01$) [59]. In the same study, the pregnancy rate after 41.70 ± 23.03 months (mean $\pm$ SD) was 22.9% out of 69.8% patients who wanted to conceive, and one patient had spontaneous uterine rupture at 33 weeks.

In a meta-analysis of six randomized controlled trials including 576 women, laparoscopic myomectomy was compared with abdominal myomectomy, and results showing laparoscopic myomectomy were associated with a decrease in intraoperative bleeding (≤34 mL) and risk of complications (OR, 0.47; 95% CI, 0.26–0.85) but longer operation time (≤13 min) and no statistically significant difference in major complications such as bleeding requiring transfusion, visceral injury, and thromboembolism (OR, 0.49; 95% CI, 0.09–2.70) [60]. Interestingly, there was no difference in the recurrence of fibroids between laparoscopic or abdominal myomectomy (20% vs. 18%; OR, 1.2; 95% CI, 0.4–3.0). These results suggest that laparoscopic myomectomy is a minimally invasive approach with fewer complications and faster recovery, but the decision for this approach should be individualized based on the other factors.

Robotic-assisted Laparoscopic Myomectomy

This is an alternative to the conventional "straight stick" laparoscopic approach. In a retrospective study with 575 patients, robotic-assisted myomectomy (5.5%) was compared with abdominal myomectomy (68.3%) and traditional laparoscopic myomectomy (16.2%). The results showed that robotic-assisted myomectomy was associated with more intraoperative blood loss than conventional laparoscopic technique (150 mL vs. 100 mL), more operative time (181 min vs. 155 min), and equal duration of the hospital stay (1 day in both groups) but removal of the heaviest fibroid in robotic group (223 g) in comparison with traditional laparoscopic group (96.65 g, $P < .001$) [61].

In another study, robotic-assisted laparoscopic myomectomy was compared with abdominal myomectomy, and results showed that robotic-assisted laparoscopic myomectomy had lower intraoperative blood loss (226 mL vs. 459 mL), postoperative change in hematocrit (5.1% vs. 7.1%), length of hospital stay (0.5 day vs. 3.3 days), and postoperative febrile morbidity (1.3% vs. 38%). Nevertheless, robotic myomectomy was associated with longer intraoperative surgical times, 3.2 h vs. 2.3 h [62]. Although robotic approaches facilitate the three-dimensional view, it is not known whether robotic-assisted laparoscopic suturing technique provides secure myometrial closure, and limited data are available regarding subsequent pregnancies and their outcomes.

A recent laparoscopic advancement, myomectomy with single-port laparoscopy, or laparoendoscopic single-site surgery (LESS), has also been reported, but data are very limited regarding its limitations, risks, and benefits [63].

Abdominal Laparotomy Approaches

Myomectomy by Laparotomy

Myomectomy is the procedure of choice for the women who desire future fertility and want to retain their uterus. Abdominal myomectomy is used mostly for women with symptomatic uterine fibroids with abnormal uterine bleeding and/or pressure symptoms or if they are not a candidate for laparoscopic or hysteroscopic myomectomy. Equal efficacies have been reported for laparoscopic myomectomy and abdominal myomectomy regarding the fertility outcomes [64]. However, abdominal myomectomy is associated with higher risk of infertility due to 3–4% risk of intraoperative conversion to hysterectomy and development of postoperative adhesions [65].

Hysterectomy

Hysterectomy is often the treatment of choice for women with symptomatic fibroids who have completed childbearing. It is not current practice to advise a woman to have a hysterectomy based solely on expected blood loss and postoperative complications if she wishes to retain her uterus. A retrospective study of 394 women who had either abdominal myomectomy or hysterectomy, noted that myomectomy group had significantly lower estimated blood loss (227 mL vs. 484 mL) and less risk of hemorrhage (10% vs. 14%, defined as blood loss >500 mL), and the overall morbidity rate was comparable with 39% vs. 40% in myomectomy and hysterectomy groups [66].

Asymptomatic Fibroids

Management of asymptomatic fibroids is not recommended as these procedures are associated with postoperative morbidity, and the recurrence of the fibroids is common with at least 25% of women after myomectomy require additional treatment [58].

Conclusion

In the majority of cases, fibroids are diagnosed incidentally and may be asymptomatic. However, symptomatic fibroids may be associated with significant morbidity and impact the quality of life. Different options available for the treatment of fibroids include medical, minimally invasive methods, surgery, or a combination of either of these. Treatment of fibroids must be individualized to the clinical situation based on the symptoms, age, the size and location of fibroids, the desires for preservation of fertility, the availability of treatments, and the experience of the physician.

Acknowledgments The authors thank Kristine Massey, MBA, for assistance with manuscript preparation and proofreading the manuscript. The research was supported, in part, by the Howard and Georgeanna Seegar Jones Division of Reproductive Sciences, Department of Gynecology and Obstetrics, Johns Hopkins University School of Medicine.

References

1. Carlson KJ, Miller BA, Fowler FJ Jr. The Maine Women's Health Study: II. Outcomes of nonsurgical management of leiomyomas, abnormal bleeding, and chronic pelvic pain. Obstet Gynecol. 1994;83(4):566–72.
2. ACOG Practice Bulletin. Alternatives to hysterectomy in the management of leiomyomas. Obstet Gynecol. 2008;112(2 Pt 1):387–400.
3. Wise LA, Palmer JR, Harlow BL, Spiegelman D, Stewart EA, Adams-Campbell LL, et al. Reproductive factors, hormonal contraception, and risk of uterine leiomyomata in African-American women: a prospective study. Am J Epidemiol. 2004;159(2):113–23.

4. Marshall LM, Spiegelman D, Goldman MB, Manson JE, Colditz GA, Barbieri RL, et al. A prospective study of reproductive factors and oral contraceptive use in relation to the risk of uterine leiomyomata. Fertil Steril. 1998;70(3):432–9.
5. Tristan M, Orozco LJ, Steed A, Ramirez-Morera A, Stone P. Mifepristone for uterine fibroids. Cochrane Database Syst Rev. 2012;(8):CD007687.
6. Donnez J, Tatarchuk TF, Bouchard P, Puscasiu L, Zakharenko NF, Ivanova T, et al. Ulipristal acetate versus placebo for fibroid treatment before surgery. N Engl J Med. 2012;366(5):409–20.
7. Donnez J, Tomaszewski J, Vazquez F, Bouchard P, Lemieszczuk B, Baro F, et al. Ulipristal acetate versus leuprolide acetate for uterine fibroids. N Engl J Med. 2012;366(5):421–32.
8. Steinauer J, Pritts EA, Jackson R, Jacoby AF. Systematic review of mifepristone for the treatment of uterine leiomyomata. Obstet Gynecol. 2004;103(6):1331–6.
9. Eisinger SH, Bonfiglio T, Fiscella K, Meldrum S, Guzick DS. Twelve-month safety and efficacy of low-dose mifepristone for uterine myomas. J Minim Invasive Gynecol. 2005;12(3):227–33.
10. Fiscella K, Eisinger SH, Meldrum S, Feng C, Fisher SG, Guzick DS. Effect of mifepristone for symptomatic leiomyomata on quality of life and uterine size: a randomized controlled trial. Obstet Gynecol. 2006;108(6):1381–7.
11. Grigorieva V, Chen-Mok M, Tarasova M, Mikhailov A. Use of a levonorgestrel-releasing intrauterine system to treat bleeding related to uterine leiomyomas. Fertil Steril. 2003;79(5):1194–8.
12. Senol T, Kahramanoglu I, Dogan Y, Baktiroglu M, Karateke A, Suer N. Levonorgestrel-releasing intrauterine device use as an alternative to surgical therapy for uterine leiomyoma. Clin Exp Obstet Gynecol. 2015;42(2):224–7.
13. Zapata LB, Whiteman MK, Tepper NK, Jamieson DJ, Marchbanks PA, Curtis KM. Intrauterine device use among women with uterine fibroids: a systematic review. Contraception. 2010;82(1):41–55.
14. Magalhaes J, Aldrighi JM, de Lima GR. Uterine volume and menstrual patterns in users of the levonorgestrel-releasing intrauterine system with idiopathic menorrhagia or menorrhagia due to leiomyomas. Contraception. 2007;75(3):193–8.
15. Carr BR, Marshburn PB, Weatherall PT, Bradshaw KD, Breslau NA, Byrd W, et al. An evaluation of the effect of gonadotropin-releasing hormone analogs and medroxyprogesterone acetate on uterine leiomyomata volume by magnetic resonance imaging: a prospective, randomized, double

blind, placebo-controlled, crossover trial. J Clin Endocrinol Metab. 1993;76(5):1217–23.

16. Marret H, Fritel X, Ouldamer L, Bendifallah S, Brun JL, De Jesus I, et al. Therapeutic management of uterine fibroid tumors: updated French guidelines. Eur J Obstet Gynecol Reprod Biol. 2012;165(2):156–64.

17. Lethaby A, Vollenhoven B, Sowter M. Efficacy of pre-operative gonadotrophin hormone releasing analogues for women with uterine fibroids undergoing hysterectomy or myomectomy: a systematic review. BJOG. 2002;109(10):1097–108.

18. Bozzini N, Rodrigues CJ, Petti DA, Bevilacqua RG, Goncalves SP, Pinotti JA. Effects of treatment with gonadotropin releasing hormone agonist on the uterine leiomyomata structure. Acta Obstet Gynecol Scand. 2003;82(4):330–4.

19. Friedman AJ, Barbieri RL, Doubilet PM, Fine C, Schiff I. A randomized, double-blind trial of a gonadotropin releasing-hormone agonist (leuprolide) with or without medroxyprogesterone acetate in the treatment of leiomyomata uteri. Fertil Steril. 1988;49(3):404–9.

20. Thomas EJ. Add-back therapy for long-term use in dysfunctional uterine bleeding and uterine fibroids. Br J Obstet Gynaecol. 1996;103(Suppl 14):18–21.

21. de Aloysio D, Altieri P, Pretolani G, Romeo A, Paltrinieri F. The combined effect of a GnRH analog in premenopause plus postmenopausal estrogen deficiency for the treatment of uterine leiomyomas in perimenopausal women. Gynecol Obstet Invest. 1995;39(2):115–9.

22. Felberbaum RE, Germer U, Ludwig M, Riethmuller-Winzen H, Heise S, Buttge I, et al. Treatment of uterine fibroids with a slow-release formulation of the gonadotrophin releasing hormone antagonist Cetrorelix. Hum Reprod. 1998;13(6):1660–8.

23. Flierman PA, Oberye JJ, van der Hulst VP, de Blok S. Rapid reduction of leiomyoma volume during treatment with the GnRH antagonist ganirelix. BJOG. 2005;112(5):638–42.

24. Palomba S, Russo T, Orio F, Jr., Tauchmanova L, Zupi E, Panici PL, et al. Effectiveness of combined GnRH analogue plus raloxifene administration in the treatment of uterine leiomyomas: a prospective, randomized, single-blind, placebo-controlled clinical trial. Hum Reprod 2002;17(12):3213–3219.

25. Hilario SG, Bozzini N, Borsari R, Baracat EC. Action of aromatase inhibitor for treatment of uterine leiomyoma in perimenopausal patients. Fertil Steril. 2009;91(1):240–3.

26. Song H, Lu D, Navaratnam K, Shi G. Aromatase inhibitors for uterine fibroids. Cochrane Database Syst Rev. 2013;(10):CD009505.
27. Coutinho EM, Goncalves MT. Long-term treatment of leiomyomas with gestrinone. Fertil Steril. 1989;51(6):939–46.
28. Lethaby A, Duckitt K, Farquhar C. Non-steroidal anti-inflammatory drugs for heavy menstrual bleeding. Cochrane Database Syst Rev. 2013;(1):CD000400.
29. Lethaby A, Farquhar C, Cooke I. Antifibrinolytics for heavy menstrual bleeding. Cochrane Database Syst Rev. 2000;(4):CD000249.
30. Lukes AS, Moore KA, Muse KN, Gersten JK, Hecht BR, Edlund M, et al. Tranexamic acid treatment for heavy menstrual bleeding: a randomized controlled trial. Obstet Gynecol. 2010;116(4):865–75.
31. Gupta JK, Sinha A, Lumsden MA, Hickey M. Uterine artery embolization for symptomatic uterine fibroids. Cochrane Database Syst Rev. 2014;(12):CD005073.
32. Gupta JK, Sinha AS, Lumsden MA, Hickey M. Uterine artery embolization for symptomatic uterine fibroids. Cochrane Database Syst Rev. 2006;(1):CD005073.
33. Kaump GR, Spies JB. The impact of uterine artery embolization on ovarian function. J Vasc Interv Radiol. 2013;24(4):459–67.
34. Hehenkamp WJ, Volkers NA, Broekmans FJ, de Jong FH, Themmen AP, Birnie E, et al. Loss of ovarian reserve after uterine artery embolization: a randomized comparison with hysterectomy. Hum Reprod. 2007;22(7):1996–2005.
35. van der Kooij SM, Bipat S, Hehenkamp WJ, Ankum WM, Reekers JA. Uterine artery embolization versus surgery in the treatment of symptomatic fibroids: a systematic review and metaanalysis. Am J Obstet Gynecol. 2011;205(4):317.e1–18.
36. Spies JB, Bruno J, Czeyda-Pommersheim F, Magee ST, Ascher SA, Jha RC. Long-term outcome of uterine artery embolization of leiomyomata. Obstet Gynecol. 2005;106(5 Pt 1):933–9.
37. Marret H, Cottier JP, Alonso AM, Giraudeau B, Body G, Herbreteau D. Predictive factors for fibroids recurrence after uterine artery embolisation. BJOG. 2005;112(4):461–5.
38. Goodwin SC, Spies JB. Uterine fibroid embolization. N Engl J Med. 2009;361(7):690–7.
39. Edwards RD, Moss JG, Lumsden MA, Wu O, Murray LS, Twaddle S, et al. Uterine-artery embolization versus surgery for symptomatic uterine fibroids. N Engl J Med. 2007;356(4):360–70.
40. SOGC Clinical Practice Guidelines. Uterine fibroid embolization (UFE). Number 150, October 2004. Int J Gynaecol Obstet. 2005;89(3):305–18.

41. McLucas B, Goodwin S, Adler L, Rappaport A, Reed R, Perrella R. Pregnancy following uterine fibroid embolization. Int J Gynaecol Obstet. 2001;74(1):1–7.
42. Goldberg J, Pereira L. Pregnancy outcomes following treatment for fibroids: uterine fibroid embolization versus laparoscopic myomectomy. Curr Opin Obstet Gynecol. 2006;18(4):402–6.
43. Smart OC, Hindley JT, Regan L, Gedroyc WG. Gonadotrophin-releasing hormone and magnetic-resonance-guided ultrasound surgery for uterine leiomyomata. Obstet Gynecol. 2006;108(1):49–54.
44. Gizzo S, Saccardi C, Patrelli TS, Ancona E, Noventa M, Fagherazzi S, et al. Magnetic resonance-guided focused ultrasound myomectomy: safety, efficacy, subsequent fertility and quality-of-life improvements, a systematic review. Reprod Sci. 2014;21(4):465–76.
45. Kim HS, Baik JH, Pham LD, Jacobs MA. MR-guided high-intensity focused ultrasound treatment for symptomatic uterine leiomyomata: long-term outcomes. Acad Radiol. 2011;18(8):970–6.
46. Quinn SD, Vedelago J, Gedroyc W, Regan L. Safety and five-year re-intervention following magnetic resonance-guided focused ultrasound (MRgFUS) for uterine fibroids. Eur J Obstet Gynecol Reprod Biol. 2014;182:247–51.
47. Rabinovici J, David M, Fukunishi H, Morita Y, Gostout BS, Stewart EA. Pregnancy outcome after magnetic resonance-guided focused ultrasound surgery (MRgFUS) for conservative treatment of uterine fibroids. Fertil Steril. 2010;93(1):199–209.
48. Lichtinger M, Hallson L, Calvo P, Adeboyejo G. Laparoscopic uterine artery occlusion for symptomatic leiomyomas. J Am Assoc Gynecol Laparosc. 2002;9(2):191–8.
49. Lichtinger M, Herbert S, Memmolo A. Temporary, transvaginal occlusion of the uterine arteries: a feasibility and safety study. J Minim Invasive Gynecol. 2005;12(1):40–2.
50. Hald K, Langebrekke A, Klow NE, Noreng HJ, Berge AB, Istre O. Laparoscopic occlusion of uterine vessels for the treatment of symptomatic fibroids: initial experience and comparison to uterine artery embolization. Am J Obstet Gynecol. 2004;190(1):37–43.
51. Hald K, Noreng HJ, Istre O, Klow NE. Uterine artery embolization versus laparoscopic occlusion of uterine arteries for leiomyomas: long-term results of a randomized comparative trial. J Vasc Interv Radiol. 2009;20(10):1303–10; quiz 11.

52. Berman JM, Guido RS, Garza Leal JG, Pemueller RR, Whaley FS, Chudnoff SG. Three-year outcome of the halt trial: a prospective analysis of radiofrequency volumetric thermal ablation of myomas. J Minim Invasive Gynecol. 2014;21(5):767–74.

53. Brucker SY, Hahn M, Kraemer D, Taran FA, Isaacson KB, Kramer B. Laparoscopic radiofrequency volumetric thermal ablation of fibroids versus laparoscopic myomectomy. Int J Gynaecol Obstet. 2014;125(3):261–5.

54. Derman SG, Rehnstrom J, Neuwirth RS. The long-term effectiveness of hysteroscopic treatment of menorrhagia and leiomyomas. Obstet Gynecol. 1991;77(4):591–4.

55. Glasser MH, Heinlein PK, Hung YY. Office endometrial ablation with local anesthesia using the HydroThermAblator system: comparison of outcomes in patients with submucous myomas with those with normal cavities in 246 cases performed over 5(1/2) years. J Minim Invasive Gynecol. 2009;16(6):700–7.

56. Hart R, Molnar BG, Magos A. Long term follow up of hysteroscopic myomectomy assessed by survival analysis. Br J Obstet Gynaecol. 1999;106(7):700–5.

57. Pritts EA, Parker WH, Olive DL. Fibroids and infertility: an updated systematic review of the evidence. Fertil Steril. 2009;91(4):1215–23.

58. Sizzi O, Rossetti A, Malzoni M, Minelli L, La Grotta F, Soranna L, et al. Italian multicenter study on complications of laparoscopic myomectomy. J Minim Invasive Gynecol. 2007;14(4):453–62.

59. Jin C, Hu Y, Chen XC, Zheng FY, Lin F, Zhou K, et al. Laparoscopic versus open myomectomy—a meta-analysis of randomized controlled trials. Eur J Obstet Gynecol Reprod Biol. 2009;145(1):14–21.

60. Barakat EE, Bedaiwy MA, Zimberg S, Nutter B, Nosseir M, Falcone T. Robotic-assisted, laparoscopic, and abdominal myomectomy: a comparison of surgical outcomes. Obstet Gynecol. 2011;117(2 Pt 1):256–65.

61. Ascher-Walsh CJ, Capes TL. Robot-assisted laparoscopic myomectomy is an improvement over laparotomy in women with a limited number of myomas. J Minim Invasive Gynecol. 2010;17(3):306–10.

62. Lee JH, Choi JS, Jeon SW, Son CE, Lee SJ, Lee YS. Single-port laparoscopic myomectomy using transumbilical GelPort access. Eur J Obstet Gynecol Reprod Biol. 2010;153(1):81–4.

63. Metwally M, Cheong YC, Horne AW. Surgical treatment of fibroids for subfertility. Cochrane Database Syst Rev. 2012;(11):CD003857.
64. Myomas and reproductive function. Fertil Steril. 2008;90(5 Suppl):S125–30.
65. Sawin SW, Pilevsky ND, Berlin JA, Barnhart KT. Comparability of perioperative morbidity between abdominal myomectomy and hysterectomy for women with uterine leiomyomas. Am J Obstet Gynecol. 2000;183(6):1448–55.

Chapter 4
An 8 cm Subserosal Fibroid in a Patient with Unexplained Infertility and Pain

Maryam Baikpour, Nash S. Moawad, Jennifer S. Eaton, and William W. Hurd

Clinical Case Presentation

A 37-year-old nulligravid woman presents with a chief complaint of a 1-year history of infertility. Prior to this, she used oral contraceptives for 18 years, and she does not currently take any medications. Her menses occur every 28–30 days, are of moderate flow, and last 3–4 days. There have been no recent changes in her menstrual flow volume or duration. She also complains of >6 months of gradually

M. Baikpour, MD
Department of Obstetrics and Gynecology, Duke University School of Medicine, 5704 Fayetteville Rd, Durham, NC 27713, USA
e-mail: bp_maryam@yahoo.com

N.S. Moawad, MD, MS, FACOG
Minimally Invasive Gynecologic Surgery, Department of Obstetrics and Gynecology, University of Florida College of Medicine, Gainesville, FL 32610, USA
e-mail: nmoawad@ufl.edu

J.S. Eaton, MD, MSCI • W.W. Hurd, MD, MPH (✉)
Department of Obstetrics and Gynecology, Duke University School of Medicine, 5704 Fayetteville Rd, Durham, NC 27713, USA
e-mail: jennifer.eaton@dm.duke.edu; william.hurd@duke.edu

N.S. Moawad (ed.), *Uterine Fibroids*,
https://doi.org/10.1007/978-3-319-58780-6_4,
© Springer International Publishing AG 2018

increasing abdominal discomfort that she describes as a feeling of abdominal fullness with weekly episodes of severe cramping pain. Her pain is unrelated to activity or menses. She also complains of urinary frequency, but denies any other urinary symptoms or changes in bowel habits or dyspareunia. Her past medical, surgical, and social histories are unremarkable.

Exam Findings

On physical examination, her vital signs are normal and her BMI is 23 kg/m². Her abdominal examination is remarkable for slight protuberance. Abdominal palpation reveals an 8 cm mobile firm, round, non-tender mass palpated in her right lower abdomen. Her pelvic examination is remarkable for a mobile, irregular uterus of approximately 16 weeks' size that is deviated to the left. She has no tenderness or adnexal masses.

Diagnostic Workup

Her laboratory evaluation included an anti-mullarian hormone (AMH) of 2.2 ng/mL and a hemoglobin of 14 g/dL. Her husband's semen analysis is normal. A transvaginal ultrasound revealed an anteflexed uterus with a thin, symmetrical endometrial stripe and a homogeneous structure originating from the posterior aspect of the uterus that does not impinge upon the uterine cavity. A transabdominal ultrasound reveals an elongated spherical structure arising from the right posterior uterine aspect, measuring 8 cm × 7 cm × 6 cm and consistent with a subserosal fibroid. The ovaries appeared normal. MRI was obtained for preoperative planning and to rule out adenomyoma or other smaller fibroids (Figs. 4.1 and 4.2). A hysterosalpingography (HSG) shows a normal uterine cavity and bilateral tubal patency.

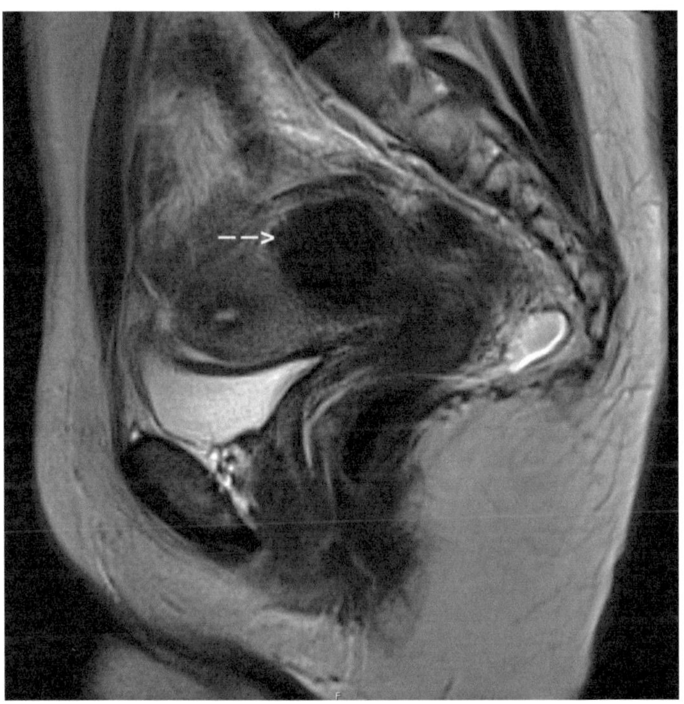

FIGURE 4.1 MRI: Sagittal view showing a posterior subserosal fibroid

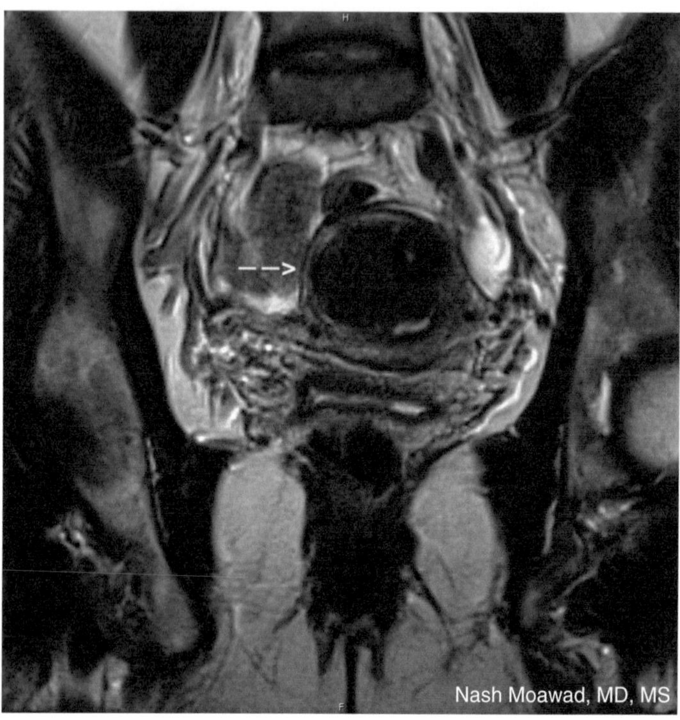

FIGURE 4.2 MRI: Coronal view showing a posterior subserosal fibroid, without distortion of the uterine cavity

Treatment Options

Decisions about when and how to treat uterine fibroids depend on the patient's symptoms, the size and location of the fibroids, and her future fertility plans. For women who want to preserve their fertility, myomectomy is indicated when submucosal fibroids result in distortion of the endometrial cavity or heavy menstrual bleeding, or in the presence of large (>4–5 cm diameter) intramural fibroids [1, 2]. Myomectomy can also be considered with large leiomyoma in any location for treatment of significant abdominal pain or discomfort, or urinary tract symptoms. In the case described above, the patient had both unexplained infertility and abdominal pain. Based on the normal uterine cavity and the subserosal location of the fibroid, her infertility was unlikely to be related to her fibroid. In contrast, her episodic pain and urinary frequency was most likely related to her fibroid.

Uterine fibroids can be treated by both nonsurgical and surgical methods. Nonsurgical treatment options for fibroid treatment are not recommended in women desiring fertility treatment. Medical treatment with GnRH agonists or progesterone receptor antagonist can temporarily reduce fibroid size, but these treatments do not improve fertility [3]. Fibroid size can be more permanently reduced by occluding their blood supply using vascular techniques (e.g., uterine artery embolization or uterine fibroid embolization). Unfortunately, reducing uterine blood supply appears to decrease fertility and dramatically increases the risk of subsequent pregnancy complications [4–8].

Additional minimally invasive techniques have been developed to destroy fibroids without surgically removing them. However, there is not enough data yet available to recommend their use in women desiring future fertility [9–11]. These methods include focused ultrasound guided by either magnetic resonance or ultrasound [12, 13] and laparoscopic ultrasound-guided radiofrequency thermal ablation [14]. Although the effects of these treatments on fertility remain unknown, preliminary data suggests that they dramatically increase the subsequent risk of miscarriage and preterm delivery [9].

Myomectomy remains the standard treatment for women with symptomatic fibroids who wish to retain their fertility. The route and method chosen for myomectomy is based on the location, size, and number of fibroids, as well as the experience and skill of the surgeon. Although many submucosal fibroids can be removed hysteroscopically, an abdominal approach is required for intramural and subserosal fibroids. Abdominal myomectomy can be performed laparoscopically (with or without robotic assistance) or via laparotomy. In addition to the need for different equipment and skill sets, these approaches have other relative advantages and disadvantages.

Laparoscopic myomectomy, using either a standard or robotically assisted technique is the preferred method when feasible. The primary advantages of laparoscopy compared to laparotomy are less postoperative pain and shorter recovery time [15, 16]. The disadvantages are that it requires specialized skill and equipment, closure of subsequent myometrial defect can be difficult using standard laparoscopy without advanced training, and the fibroids must be removed from the abdomen using some type of morcellation.

Standard laparoscopy is used most commonly for removing subserosal or pendunculated fibroids that will not result in large myometrial defects, since such defects can be difficult to close in multiple layers using this technique in the absence of advanced laparoscopic skills. Injection of dilute vasopressin can help minimize blood loss. Dissecting graspers, scissors and both unipolar and bipolar surgical devices or ultrasonic instruments are used to detach fibroids (Fig. 4.3).

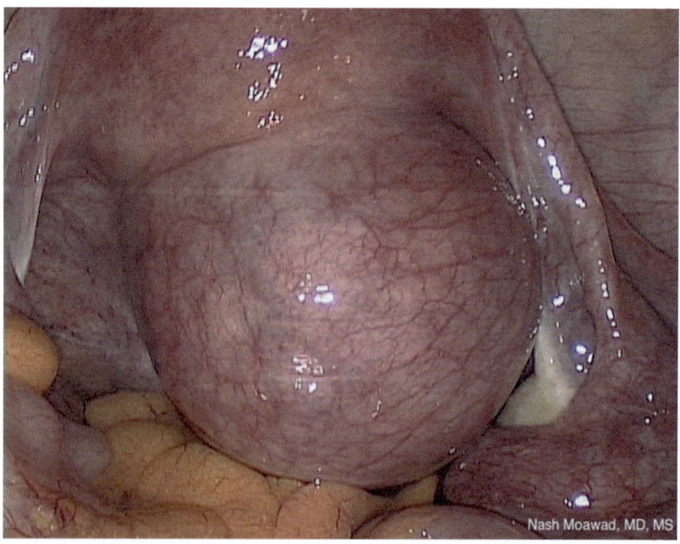

FIGURE 4.3 Laparoscopic view of a posterior subserosal uterine fibroid

Robotically assisted laparoscopy allows more surgeons to perform complex laparoscopic surgeries such as myomectomies [17]. The technical advantages of robotic surgery aid in the careful multilayer closures of myometrial defects after fibroid removal. Special training is required, and this approach is more costly than standard laparoscopy. However, robotically assisted laparoscopic myomectomy is less expensive than a laparotomy approach and is associated with comparatively lower complication rates, less blood loss, and shorter hospitalization periods [18–20] (Fig. 4.4).

Morcellation to remove fibroids from the abdominal cavity has become the most controversial part of laparoscopic myomectomy. In the recent past, "open morcellation" was performed using a power morcellator to cut each fibroid into small pieces within the abdominal cavity as they were withdrawn through a 12 mm port. However, this technique is no longer recommended because of the risk of inadvertent dispersion of small fragments of fibroid tissue within the abdomen during the procedure, which can result in disseminated leiomyomatosis in up to 1% of cases [21, 22]. A much less common, but more serious complication of open morcellation is inadvertent dissemination of an unsuspected leiomyosarcoma. Since these malignant tumors are much less common before menopause, the risk of this occurrence during myomectomy in a reproductive age women is likely to be <0.1% (for detailed discussion of the literature, see Chap. 10). However, since dissemination is likely to worsen the prognosis of this usually fatal disease, open morcellation within the abdominal cavity is no longer recommended.

Several methods have been developed for enclosed morcellation Perhaps, the simplest method is to place the fibroids into a laparoscopic bag, pull the opening of the bag through a 4 cm mini-laparotomy incision, and use scalpel to morcellate the fibroids within the bag [23]. This technique has been termed "laparoscopically assisted myomectomy" by some authors [24, 25]. The disadvantage is that the larger

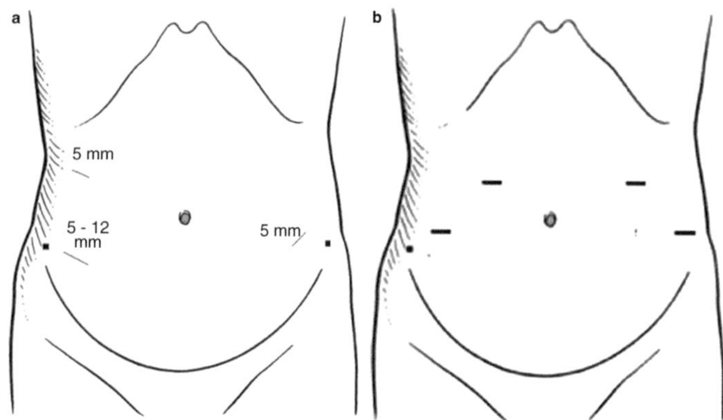

FIGURE 4.4 Trocar placement strategy for (**a**) conventional laparo-scopic myomectomy, and (**b**) robotically assisted laparoscopic myo-mectomy

abdominal incision reduces some of the minimally invasive advantages of the laparoscopic approach.

Other surgeons have recommended power morcellation of fibroids within a bag while still inside the abdomen, termed "enclosed intracorporeal morcellation" [21, 23, 26]. However, since the US Food and Drug Administration strong warnings against intracorporeal morcellation issued in April 2014 [27], some power morcellators have been withdrawn from the market, many surgeons have elected to stop using them, and many hospitals have banned their use. Regardless of whether morcellation is done via mini-lapa-rotomy, using manual morcellation with a scalpel or using a power morcellator, bag-enclosure is recommended to avoid inadvertent dissemination of benign, or in rare cases, malig-nant tissue.

Myomectomy via laparotomy remains an acceptable method, particularly for removing very large or multiple fibroids for women wishing to retain their fertility. This approach is most advantageous for large transmural fibroids and in the presence of a large number of fibroids where an open technique improves the chances of avoiding the uterine cavity and aids in careful closure of the complex myometrial defects compared to a laparoscopic approach, with or without robotic assistance [28, 29].

The advantages of myomectomy via laparotomy are two-fold: morcellation is not required and myometrial defects can be carefully closed in multiple layers. The disadvantages of laparotomy compared to a laparoscopic approach are increased pain, hospital stay, recovery time, and wound infection risk. Blood loss also appears to be increased using the laparotomy approach. However, this is in part related to the differences in types of fibroids relegated to laparotomy compared to laparoscopic treatment is retrospective studies. The use of vasopressin and/or tourniquets with vascular clamps can minimize blood lost during laparotomy myomectomy [30–32].

For the case described above, we utilized laparoscopic myomectomy with enclosed morcellation via a 4 cm mini-laparotomy. The surgery was performed with the patient in a lithotomy position and under general anesthesia. A 5 mm open laparoscopic entry approach was used to place the initial umbilical port [33]. Three additional 5 mm ports were placed under direct visualization, one in the supra-pubic area, a second at McBurney's point on the right, and a third at the corresponding point on the left. Vasopressin (10 U in 100 mL normal saline) was injected into the uterine fundus at the base of the subserous fibroid. The serosa was incised 1 cm above the attachment of the fibroid to the uterus with monopolar electrosurgery. The fibroid was circumferentially detached from the underlying myometrium using a combination of bluntly dissection with grasping forceps and sharp dissection with scissors (Fig. 4.5). The fibroid was temporarily placed in the recto-uterine pouch beneath the uterus.

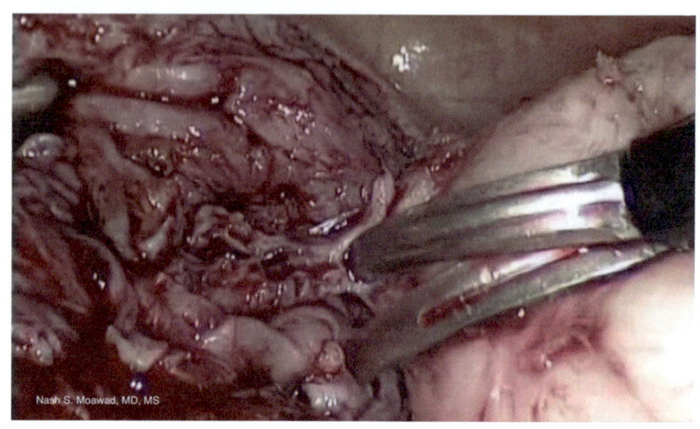

FIGURE 4.5 Laparoscopic myomectomy using cold scissors

After operative site Hemostasis was obtained, the myometrial defect was closed using absorbable barbed suture (v-Loc; Covidien, New Haven, CT) (Fig. 4.6).

To minimize post-myomectomy adhesions and bowel irritation related to barbed suture, the serosal defect was covered with an absorbable adhesions barrier (Interceed; Ethicon, Somerville, NJ) (Fig. 4.7).

The fibroid was subsequently placed in a 50×50-cm isolation bag (3M Steri-Drape Isolation Bag 1003; 3M Corp., St. Paul, MN). The neck of the bag was removed through a 4 cm Pfannenstiel incision made 3 cm cephalad to the symphysis pubis in the midline. The fibroid was carefully morcellated with a scalpel by serially grasping the protruding edge with a towel clip and removing wedge-shaped sections.

The peritoneum beneath the Pfannenstiel incision was closed with 3–0 absorbable monofilament running suture (Biosyn, United States Surgical Corp, Norwalk, CT) to minimized adhesions [34]. The fascia was closed with 0 absorbable braided running suture (Polysorb, United States Surgical Corp).

After hemostasis was verified at the operative and port sites under decreased intra-abdominal pressure, the operative ports and laparoscope were removed from the abdomen.

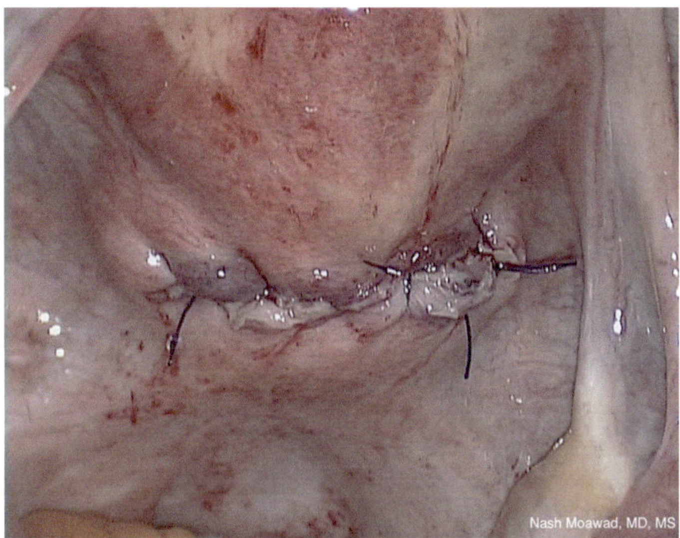

FIGURE 4.6 Laparoscopic view of the closed myomectomy incision after removal of an 8 cm subserosal uterine fibroid

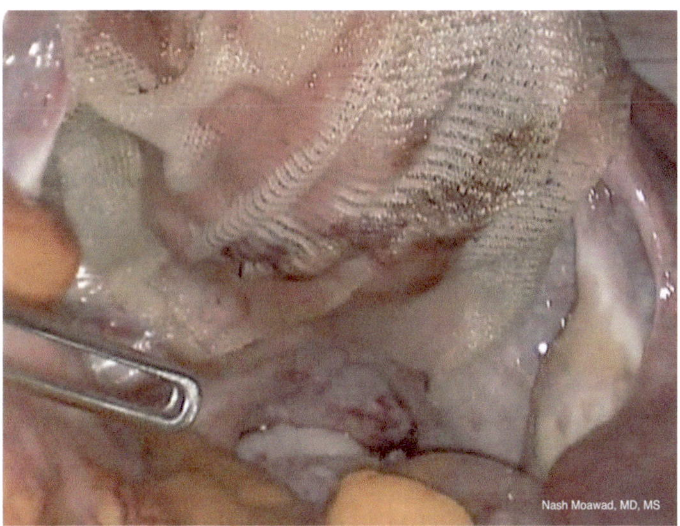

FIGURE 4.7 Laparoscopic view: Interceed was placed after closure of the myomectomy incision to decrease postoperative adhesion formation

Local anesthetic (20 mL of 0.25% bupivacaine) was injected at each port site and into the Pfannenstiel incision beneath the fascia and intradermally. Skin incisions were closed with 4–0 absorbable monofilament running subcuticular suture (Biosyn, United States Surgical Corp) followed by tissue adhesive (Dermabond, Ethicon; Somerville, NJ). The patient was awakened and sent home after a 2 h recovery period.

References

1. Oliveira FG, Abdelmassih VG, Diamond MP, Dozortsev D, Melo NR, Abdelmassih R. Impact of subserosal and intramural uterine fibroids that do not distort the endometrial cavity on the outcome of in vitro fertilization-intracytoplasmic sperm injection. Fertil Steril. 2004;81:582–7.
2. Somigliana E, De Benedictis SD, Vercellini P, Nicolosi AE, Benaglia L, Scarduelli C, et al. Fibroids not encroaching the endometrial cavity and IVF success rate: a prospective study. Hum Reprod. 2011;26:834–9.
3. Hurst BS. Uterine fibroids. Ultrasound imaging in reproductive medicine. New York: Springer; 2014. p. 117–31.
4. Payne JF, Haney AF. Serious complications of uterine artery embolization for conservative treatment of fibroids. Fertil Steril. 2003;79:128–31.
5. Tropeano G, Litwicka K, Di Stasi C, Romano D, Mancuso S. Permanent amenorrhea associated with endometrial atrophy after uterine artery embolization for symptomatic uterine fibroids. Fertil Steril. 2003;79:132–5.
6. Goldberg J, Pereira L, Berghella V, Diamond J, Daraï E, Seinera P, et al. Pregnancy outcomes after treatment for fibromyomata: uterine artery embolization versus laparoscopic myomectomy. Am J Obstet Gynecol. 2004;191:18–21.
7. Walker WJ, McDowell SJ. Pregnancy after uterine artery embolization for leiomyomata: a series of 56 completed pregnancies. Am J Obstet Gynecol. 2006;195:1266–71.
8. Pron G, Mocarski E, Bennett J, Vilos G, Common A, Vanderburgh L, Ontario UFE, Collaborative Group. Pregnancy after uterine artery embolization for leiomyomata: the Ontario multicenter trial. Obstet Gynecol. 2005;105:67–76.

 9. Rabinovici J, David M, Fukunishi H, Morita Y, Gostout BS, Stewart EA, et al. Pregnancy outcome after magnetic resonance-guided focused ultrasound surgery (MRgFUS) for conservative treatment of uterine fibroids. Fertil Steril. 2010;93:199–209.
10. Vilos GA, Daly LJ, Tse BM. Pregnancy outcome after laparoscopic electromyolysis. J Am Assoc Gynecol Laparosc. 1998;5:289–92.
11. Berman JM, Bolnick JM, Pemueller RR, Garza Leal JG. Reproductive outcomes in women following radiofrequency volumetric thermal ablation of symptomatic fibroids. A retrospective case series analysis. J Reprod Med. 2015;60:194–8.
12. Gizzo S, Saccardi C, Patrelli TS, Ancona E, Noventa M, Fagherazzi S, et al. Magnetic resonance-guided focused ultrasound myomectomy safety, efficacy, subsequent fertility and quality-of-life improvements, a systematic review. Reprod Sci. 2013;21(4):465–76.
13. Wang W, Wang Y, Wang T, Wang J, Wang L, Tang J. Safety and efficacy of US-guided high-intensity focused ultrasound for treatment of submucosal fibroids. Eur Radiol. 2012;22(11):2553–8.
14. Brucker SY, Hahn M, Kraemer D, Taran FA, Isaacson KB, Krämer B. Laparoscopic radiofrequency volumetric thermal ablation of fibroids versus laparoscopic myomectomy. Int J Gynecol Obstet. 2014;125(3):261–5.
15. Mettler L, Schollmeyer T, Lehmann-Willenbrock E, Dowaji J, Zavala A. Treatment of myomas by laparoscopic and laparotomic myomectomy and laparoscopic hysterectomy. Minim Invasive Ther Allied Technol. 2004;13(1):58–64.
16. Jin C, Hu Y, X-C C, F-Y Z, Lin F, Zhou K, et al. Laparoscopic versus open myomectomy—a meta-analysis of randomized controlled trials. Eur J Obstet Gynecol Reprod Biol. 2009;145(1):14–21.
17. Holloway R, Patel S, Ahmad S. Robotic surgery in gynecology. Scand J Surg. 2009;98(2):96–109.
18. Advincula AP, Xu X, Goudeau S, Ransom SB. Robot-assisted laparoscopic myomectomy versus abdominal myomectomy: a comparison of short-term surgical outcomes and immediate costs. J Minim Invasive Gynecol. 2007;14(6):698–705.
19. Mansour FW, Kives S, Urbach DR, Lefebvre G. Robotically assisted laparoscopic myomectomy: a Canadian experience. J Obstet Gynaecol Can. 2012;34(4):353–8.
20. Ranisavljevic N, Mercier G, Masia F, Mares P, De Tayrac R, Triopon G. Robot-assisted laparoscopic myomectomy: compari-

son with abdominal myomectomy. J Gynecol Obstet Biol Reprod. 2012;41(5):439–44.

21. Paul PG, Thomas M, Das T, Patil S, Garg R. Contained morcellation for laparoscopic myomectomy within a specially designed bag. J Minim Invasive Gynecol. 2016;23(2):257–60. doi:10.1016/j.jmig.2015.08.004. Epub 2015 Aug 7.

22. Lu B, Xu J, Pan Z. Iatrogenic parasitic leiomyoma and leiomyomatosis peritonealis disseminata following uterine morcellation. J Obstet Gynaecol Res. 2016;42(8):990–9. doi:10.1111/jog.13011.

23. Venturella R, Rocca ML, Lico D, La Ferrera N, Cirillo R, Gizzo S, Morelli M, Zupi E, Zullo F. In-bag manual versus uncontained power morcellation for laparoscopic myomectomy: randomized controlled trial. Fertil Steril. 2016;105(5):1369–76. doi:10.1016/j.fertnstert.2015.12.133. Epub 2016 Jan 19.

24. Nezhat C, Nezhat F, Bess O, Nezhat CH, Mashiach R. Laparoscopically assisted myomectomy: a report of a new technique in 57 cases. Int J Fertil Menopausal Stud. 1993;39(1):39–44.

25. Nezhat C, Nezhat F, Silfen S, Schaffer N, Evans D. Laparoscopic myomectomy. Int J Fertil. 1990;36(5):275–80.

26. Vargas MV, Cohen SL, Fuchs-Weizman N, Wang KC, Manoucheri E, Vitonis AF, Einarsson JI. Open power morcellation versus contained power morcellation within an insufflated isolation bag: comparison of perioperative outcomes. J Minim Invasive Gynecol. 2015;22(3):433–8. doi:10.1016/j.jmig.2014.11.010. Epub 2014 Nov 29.

27. U.S. Food & Drug Administration. Laparoscopic uterine power morcellation in hysterectomy and myomectomy: FDA safety communication. 2014. http://www.fda gov/medicaldevices/safety/alertsandnotices/ucm393576.htm

28. Banas T, Klimek M, Fugiel A, Skotniczny K. Spontaneous uterine rupture at 35 weeks' gestation, 3 years after laparoscopic myomectomy, without signs of fetal distress. J Obstet Gynaecol Res. 2005;31(6):527–30.

29. Parker WH, Iacampo K, Long T. Uterine rupture after laparoscopic removal of a pedunculated myoma. J Minim Invasive Gynecol. 2007;14(3):362–4.

30. Hickman LC, Kotlyar A, Shue S, Falcone T. Hemostatic techniques for myomectomy: an evidence-based approach. J Minim Invasive Gynecol. 2016;23(4):497–504. doi:10.1016/j.jmig.2016.01.026. Review.

31. Conforti A, Mollo A, Alviggi C, Tsimpanakos I, Strina I, Magos A, De Placido G. Techniques to reduce blood loss during open myomectomy: a qualitative review of literature. Eur J Obstet Gynecol Reprod Biol. 2015;192:90–5. doi:10.1016/j.ejogrb.2015.05.027. Review
32. Kongnyuy EJ, Wiysonge CS. Interventions to reduce haemorrhage during myomectomy for fibroids. Cochrane Database Syst Rev. 2014;8:CD005355. doi:10.1002/14651858.CD005355.pub5. Review
33. Pryor KP, Hurd WW. Modified open laparoscopy using a 5-mm laparoscope. Obstet Gynecol. 2016;127(3):535–8.
34. Whitfield R, Huls HR, Crouch JM, Hurd WW. Effects of peritoneal closure and suture material on adhesion formation in a rabbit model. Am J Obstet Gynecol. 2007;197(6):644.e1–5.
35. Wallach EE, Vlahos NF. Uterine myomas: an overview of development, clinical features, and management. Obstet Gynecol. 2004;104(2):393–406.
36. Brady PC, Stanic AK, Styer AK. Uterine fibroids and subfertility: an update on the role of myomectomy. Curr Opin Obstet Gynecol. 2013;25(3):255–9.
37. Casini ML, Rossi F, Agostini R, Unfer V. Effects of the position of fibroids on fertility. Gynecol Endocrinol. 2006;22(2):106–9.
38. Bosteels J, Kasius J, Weyers S, Broekmans FJ, Mol BWJ, D'Hooghe TM. Hysteroscopy for treating subfertility associated with suspected major uterine cavity abnormalities. Cochrane Database Syst Rev. 2015;2
39. Kubinova K, Mara M, Horak P, Kuzel D, Dohnalova A. Reproduction after myomectomy: comparison of patients with and without second-look laparoscopy. Minim Invasive Ther Allied Technol. 2012;21(2):118–24.
40. Soriano D, Dessolle L, Poncelet C, Benifla J, Madelenat P, Darai E. Pregnancy outcome after laparoscopic and laparoconverted myomectomy. Eur J Obstet Gynecol Reprod Biol. 2003;108(2):194–8.
41. Hackethal A, Westermann A, Tchartchian G, Oehmke F, Tinneberg H-R, Muenstedt K, et al. Laparoscopic myomectomy in patients with uterine myomas associated with infertility. Minim Invasive Ther Allied Technol. 2011;20(6):346–53.
42. Paul P, Koshy AK, Thomas T. Pregnancy outcomes following laparoscopic myomectomy and single-layer myometrial closure. Hum Reprod. 2006;21(12):3278–81.

43. Brown JAAGL. Advancing minimally invasive gynecology worldwide: statement to the FDA on power morcellation. The. J Minim Invasive Gynecol. 2014;6(21):970–1.
44. Rimbach S, Holzknecht A, Nemes C, Offner F, Craina M. A new in-bag system to reduce the risk of tissue morcellation: development and experimental evaluation during laparoscopic hysterectomy. Arch Gynecol Obstet. 2015;292(6):1311–20.
45. Takeda A, Watanabe K, Hayashi S, Imoto S, Nakamura H. In-bag manual extraction of excised myomas by surgical scalpel through suprapubic mini-laparotomic incision in laparoscopic-assisted myomectomy. J Minim Invasive Gynecol. 2016;23(5):731–8.
46. Mais V, Ajossa S, Guerriero S, Mascia M, Solla E, Melis GB. Laparoscopic versus abdominal myomectomy: a prospective, randomized trial to evaluate benefits in early outcome. Am J Obstet Gynecol. 1996;174(2):654–8.
47. Doridot V, Dubuisson J-B, Chapron C, Fauconnier A, Babaki-Fard K. Recurrence of leiomyomata after laparoscopic myomectomy. J Am Assoc Gynecol Laparosc. 2001;8(4):495–500.
48. Tropeano G, Amoroso S, Scambia G. Non-surgical management of uterine fibroids. Hum Reprod Update. 2008;14(3):259–74.
49. Wu O, Briggs A, Dutton S, Hirst A, Maresh M, Nicholson A, et al. Uterine artery embolisation or hysterectomy for the treatment of symptomatic uterine fibroids: a cost-utility analysis of the HOPEFUL study. BJOG. 2007;114(11):1352–62.
50. Edwards R, Moss J, Lumsden M, Wu O, Murray L, Twaddle S, et al. Committee of the Randomised Trial of embolisation versus surgical treatment of fibroids. Uterineartery embolization versus surgery for symptomatic uterine fibroids. N Engl J Med. 2007;356(4):360–70.
51. Stewart EA, Rabinovici J, Tempany CM, Inbar Y, Regan L, Gastout B, et al. Clinical outcomes of focused ultrasound surgery for the treatment of uterine fibroids. Fertil Steril. 2006;85(1):22–9.
52. Arcangeli S, Pasquarette MM. Gravid uterine rupture after myolysis. Obstet Gynecol. 1997;89(5):857.
53. Kim Y-W, Park B-J, Ro D-Y, Kim T-E. Single-port laparoscopic myomectomy using a new single-port transumbilical morcellation system: initial clinical study. J Minim Invasive Gynecol. 2010;17(5):587–92.

54. Lee JH, Choi JS, Jeon SW, Son CE, Lee SJ, Lee YS. Single-port laparoscopic myomectomy using transumbilical GelPort access. Eur J Obstet Gynecol Reprod Biol. 2010;153(1):81–4.
55. Einarsson JI, Cohen SL, Fuchs N, Wang KC. In-bag morcellation. J Minim Invasive Gynecol. 2014;21(5):951–3.

Chapter 5
Large Asymptomatic FIGO Type 3–5 Fibroid and Primary Infertility

Paula C. Brady and Antonio R. Gargiulo

Clinical Case

The patient is a 30-year-old healthy nulligravid patient diagnosed with an 8 centimeter (cm) intramural fibroid (FIGO type 3–5) [1].

The patient presents reporting 18 months of primary infertility. She denies pelvic pressure, urinary frequency, dyspareunia, dysmenorrhea, or menorrhagia. She has no significant past medical or surgical history; she has no known family history of gynecologic issues or malignancy. She does not smoke or drink. Her infertility assessment included an anti-Müllerian hormone level of 2.4 ng/mL (indicating normal ovarian reserve), patent fallopian tubes and a normal intrauterine cavity contour by hysterosalpingogram, and a normal semen analysis for her husband, who is also 30 years old, healthy, and without any significant medical or surgical history.

P.C. Brady, MD • A.R. Gargiulo, MD (✉)
Center for Infertility and Reproductive Surgery, Department of Obstetrics, Gynecology and Reproductive Biology, Brigham and Women's Hospital, Harvard Medical School, 75 Francis Street, Boston, MA 02115, USA
e-mail: pbrady2@bwh.harvard.edu; agargiulo@bwh.harvard.edu

N.S. Moawad (ed.), *Uterine Fibroids*,
https://doi.org/10.1007/978-3-319-58780-6_5,
© Springer International Publishing AG 2018

Exam Findings

By physical examination, the patient is well appearing, with normal vital signs and a body mass index of 24 kg/m^2. Bimanual exam reveals an enlarged, 16-week size, mobile uterus, and no adnexal masses.

Diagnostic Workup

Further laboratory testing reveals a negative human chorionic gonadotropin and a normal complete blood count (with hemoglobin of 12.8 g/dL). Based on the patient's physical examination, a pelvic ultrasound is ordered, which reveals an 8 cm intramural fibroid. An MRI is a crucial part of treatment planning in patients with large fibroids, in order to clarify fibroid number and location, to define any encroachment on the endometrium, and to confirm that the suspected fibroid is not an adenomyoma (which would require different management considerations). An MRI reveals an 8 cm intramural fibroid that is adjacent to but does not appear to deform the endometrial cavity.

Images

MRI of 8 cm intramural fibroid. Fibroid is indicated with a star; endometrial cavity is indicated with an arrow (Fig. 5.1).

Treatment Options

The patient is broadly counseled regarding the options for management of uterine fibroids, which include expectant management, medical management with monthly injectable gonadotropin-releasing hormone agonists (GnRHa), uterine artery embolization (UAE), MRI-guided high-intensity

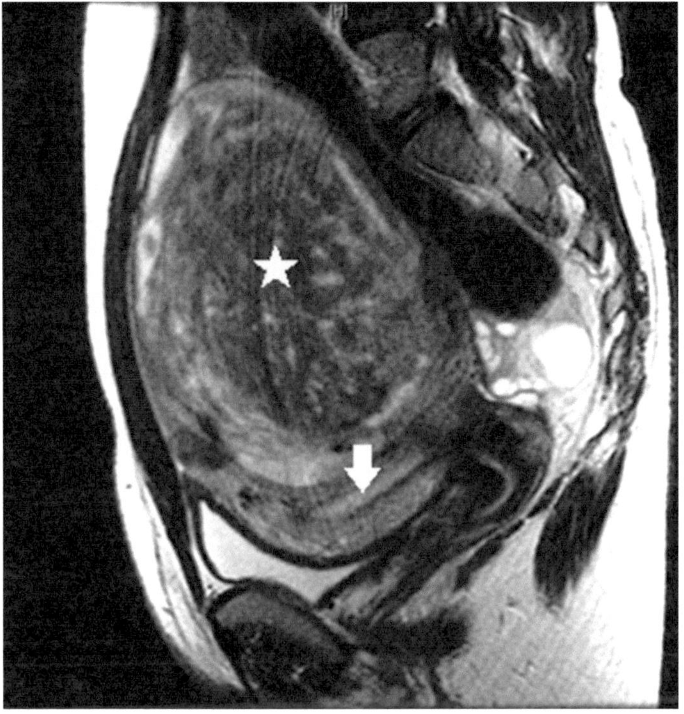

Figure 5.1 MRI of 8 cm intramural fibroid. Fibroid is indicated with a *star*; endometrial cavity indicated with an *arrow*

focused ultrasound, laparoscopic-guided myolysis (using thermal energy, cryoablation, and radiofrequency ablation [RFA]), and laparoscopic, robot-assisted laparoscopic or abdominal myomectomy [2–4].

Hysterectomy is specifically discussed as a method that would provide a definitive cure for this uterine pathology, with the understanding that this is never a first-line management in a patient desiring future fertility. Due to the fact that leiomyosarcomas are a possible finding even in reproductive-aged women (see full discussion below), it is imperative that the decision of not removing the uterus en bloc be made by the patient, not by the surgeon. As a result, a clear discussion about hysterectomy should be had (and should be duly documented) with every reproductive-aged patient.

Expectant management avoids all procedure-related risks and confers the added benefit of not requiring waiting or recovery time before attempting fertility treatments. The presence of an intramural fibroid (over 4–5 cm) may, however, negatively affect implantation rates. Small retrospective studies (approximately 100 patients) have inconsistently shown reduced implantation, ongoing pregnancy, and live birth rates in patients with intramural fibroids [5–8]. A comprehensive meta-analysis confirmed the lower implantation (relative risk [RR] = 0.684; 95% confidence interval [CI], 0.587–0.796), clinical pregnancy (RR = 0.81; 95% CI, 0.696–0.941), and ongoing pregnancy and ongoing pregnancy/live birth rate (RR = 0.703; 95% CI, 0.583–0.848) in women with intramural fibroids not encroaching on the uterine cavity as compared to women without fibroids [9]. A meta-analysis focused on in vitro fertilization (IVF) outcomes in patients with non-cavity-distorting intramural fibroids as compared to patients without fibroids similarly reported a significant decrease in the live birth (RR = 0.79; 95% CI, 0.70–0.88; $P < 0.0001$) and clinical pregnancy rates (RR = 0.85; 95% CI, 0.77–0.94; P = 0.002) [10]. Please refer to the section on myomectomy below for data regarding comparison of expectant management and operative interventions.

Fewer studies have attempted to identify size thresholds for the potentially negative effect of intramural fibroids on pregnancy rates. A retrospective review including 130 women undergoing IVF with intramural fibroids reported that pregnancy rates were lower in women with intramural fibroids over 4 cm in diameter: 29%, as compared to 51% in women with fibroids measuring 2–4 cm and 53% in women with fibroids less than 2 cm ($p < 0.05$) [11]. Conversely, a prospective study of 119 women with intramural fibroids less than 5 cm in diameter and matched controls undergoing IVF demonstrated no significant difference in pregnancy rates and live birth rates [12]. Ultimately, the size of intramural fibroids warranting removal for fertility reasons remains undetermined, and the decision to intervene or proceed expectantly must be individualized and based on patient's age, past reproductive history, associated pathology, and the degree of invasiveness of the tools available to treat the pathology.

The presence of fibroids in pregnancy is also associated with a variety of complications in the antepartum period and at delivery. Expectantly managed intramural fibroids in pregnancy have been associated with a higher rate of pregnancy loss; a meta-analysis of studies of intramural fibroids in early pregnancy (mean diameters of 1.8 cm to over 5 cm) reported a cumulative first trimester spontaneous abortion rate of 20.4% as compared to 12.9% in patients without fibroids (odds ratio [OR], 1.6; 95% CI, 1.30–2.0) [9, 13]. The presence of fibroids in later pregnancy has been associated with preterm premature rupture of membranes, preterm labor, placental abruption, intrauterine growth restriction, malpresentation, and pain due to fibroid degeneration [14]. Large submucosal and retro-placental fibroids confer the greatest risk of pregnancy complications [14]. Fibroids greater than 200 mL in volume, in particular, have been associated with fetal growth below the tenth percentile [15]. In a review of 190 women with singleton gestations, those with fibroids over 5 cm in diameter delivered at a mean gestational age of 36.5 weeks, compared to 38.4 weeks in women with fibroids less than 5 cm ($p = 0.002$) [16]. Finally, intrapartum issues associated with the presence of fibroids include dysfunctional labor, increased risk of cesarean section, hemorrhage, and retained placenta [14].

In patients desiring future fertility, **uterine artery embolization**, **MRI-guided focused ultrasound (MRgFUS)**, and **laparoscopic-guided myolysis** are not currently recommended. The most data have been published regarding pregnancy after UAE, which is performed by interventional radiology specialists and involves the cannulation of the femoral artery followed by catheter-guided delivery of embolic particles to the uterine arteries to induce fibroid necrosis. Risks include pain, infection, and nontarget embolization (including the lower extremities and ovaries) [17]. UAE may also result in endometrial atrophy and scarring or pelvic infection, all of which are potentially devastating complications in a patient desiring fertility [18, 19]. Benefits include avoidance of surgery and resultant fibroid shrinkage of 20–50% [20]. While series of successful pregnancies after UAE have been reported, UAE has also been associated with decreased anti-Müllerian hormone levels (presumed to be due to nontarget embolization of the ovaries), which would be highly detrimental to a patient seeking fertility (particularly in the age range of 35–45 years, which is precisely when most uterine fibroids are found) [21]. In a series of 53 pregnancies conceived after UAE as compared to 139 pregnancies conceived following laparoscopic myomectomy, patients with prior UAE were at increased risk for preterm delivery (odds ratio [OR] 6.2; 95% confidence interval [CI] 1.4–27.7) [22]. Series have also reported that UAE may be associated with an increased risk of miscarriage and abnormal placentation (such as placenta previa or accreta) [23, 24].

MRgFUS entails the targeting of ultrasound waves on fibroids to produce tissue destruction; risks include skin or visceral thermal injury [25, 26]. Small series have reported uncomplicated term deliveries after MRgFUS, but data are currently lacking to support use of this method in women planning pregnancy, while better studied alternatives are available [27]. Data are similarly few regarding pregnancy following laparoscopic myolysis, which involves the introduction of an energy source directly into a fibroid under laparoscopic guidance, to produce thermal damage and involution. While uncomplicated term pregnancies have been reported following myolysis using RFA and bipolar energy, reports of gravid uterine ruptures following myolysis with bipolar energy have also been published [28, 29].

In the age of widespread access to minimally invasive myomectomy (made possible by the many technological improvements in the fields of laparoscopy and robot-assisted laparoscopy), any technique that can only provide partial removal of intramural fibroids, but offer risk and recovery profiles comparable to minimally invasive surgery, lack true value proposition and should only be considered as a possible alternative to invasive surgery (open myomectomy).

Medical management with **GnRHa** alone may result in fibroid shrinkage by 35% or more within 3 months [30]. Patients may also report vasomotor symptoms, and prolonged use (greater than 6 months without progesterone add back) may result in decreased bone mineral density. The further limitation of this treatment modality is that the treatment effect is only sustained as long as the medication is continued [31]. This medication, by disrupting gonadotropin release from the pituitary, is also incompatible with spontaneous conception and may dampen ovarian response to ovulation induction. Furthermore, the myometrium would eventually be exposed to large concentrations of estrogen and progesterone during fertility treatment and even more so in pregnancy, which may counteract pre-pregnancy treatment effect [15]. At the present time, the use of GnRH agonists in reproductive-aged women with fibroids should be limited to preoperative treatment in order to shrink fibroids to a size more amenable to minimally invasive surgery (a decision that depends on the technical skills and preference of the surgeon) and to address preoperative anemia in women with fibroid-related abnormal uterine bleeding [32–35].

The conservative surgical approach to intramural fibroids is determined by fibroid number, size, and surgeon and patient preference. Options include **abdominal (open), laparoscopic**, and **robot-assisted laparoscopic myomectomy.** Any myomectomy is not without risk; perioperative complications include blood loss and infection; adhesions may develop, leading to pain and tubal occlusion [36]. Hospital length of stay, blood loss, and complication rates, however, can be significantly reduced with the adoption of a minimally invasive approach (laparoscopic, with or without robotic assistance) instead of an abdominal approach [37]. Minimally invasive approaches can be achieved even in patients with numerous or large fibroids, at a surgeon's discretion; robot-assisted myomectomy has been reported as safe and feasible for fibroids exceeding 9 cm [38].

In the last decade, robot-assisted laparoscopic myomectomy has gained acceptance as an alternative to conventional laparoscopic myomectomy. Hospital stay, postoperative pain, complication rate, and blood loss are comparable between laparoscopic and robot-assisted myomectomy [37, 39, 40]. Robotic surgery, with its stereoscopic view and articulated instruments, allows for microsurgical uterine dissection and careful suturing of hysterotomies in multiple layers, reducing tissue trauma [34]. This gentle handling of reproductive structures is well suited to an infertility population. Most importantly, recent evidence that surgeons can perfect their robotic surgical technique on a digital simulator presents a significant advantage, particularly for patient safety, in the adoption of this minimally invasive approach to myomectomy [41].

Minimally invasive approaches to myomectomy require fragmentation of the enucleated fibroids, for removal through small incisions. A very small percentage of uterine tumors presenting clinically as fibroids will be malignant, most commonly leiomyosarcoma. Currently, no clinical testing can reliably differentiate between a fibroid and a leiomyosarcoma in a low-risk patient population [42]. Patients undergoing myomectomy should be specifically counseled regarding the possibility of occult malignancy, particularly as the disruption of the fibroid capsule and tumor enucleation within the abdomen is implicit in any myomectomy. It is unknown whether the disease-free survival is affected by the spread of cells and tissue fragments in the abdominal cavity that occurs universally during myomectomy. However, extrapolation from hysterectomy data suggests that en bloc removal of a uterus with leiomyosarcoma (as in open hysterectomy) confers longer disease-free interval, but no overall survival advantage, as compared to patients whose uteri were morcellated [43, 44]. An en bloc myomectomy, however, is a surgical impossibility. As a result, every patient who desires a conservative surgical approach to their fibroids must voluntarily assume a certain degree of risk. The patient's active decision to proceed with conservative surgery for solid uterine masses should be documented in every informed consent that is signed before surgery.

Reproductive-aged patients who do not want a hysterectomy can be helped in their decision-making by offering an estimate of risk of occult malignancy. An FDA advisory in 2014 reported an incidence of occult sarcoma of 1 in 350 hysterectomies (following a methodologically questionable and arguably biased analysis of the literature) [45]. However, the risk of occult leiomyosarcoma was reported as less than 1 in 8000 hysterectomies in the only complete meta-analysis in the current literature [44, 46].

In spite of their exaggerated report of the prevalence of malignant uterine tumors, the FDA advisory specifically allows open morcellation in adequately counseled premenopausal women [45]. However, many surgeons and hospitals fear opportunistic lawsuits and have abandoned open morcellation, resulting in a surge in open pelvic surgery—associated with higher complication rates than minimally invasive approaches—rather than in the adoption of alternative tissue extraction techniques for enucleated fibroids [47, 48]. As an alternative to open morcellation—while novel-contained tissue extraction devices await approval by the FDA—enucleated fibroids can be placed within a containment bag in the abdomen and brought up to a laparoscopic incision that has been extended to 2–3 cm in length to allow for manipulation of the fibroids; the fibroids are then serially incised using a scalpel and removed. The use of intra-abdominal containment bags for tissue extraction may limit fragment spread while allowing patients to enjoy the benefits of a minimally invasive approach [49, 50]. Studies of these containment devices are ongoing.

During both abdominal and minimally invasive myomectomy, intraoperative techniques can be used to minimize myometrial damage and provide an optimal myometrial repair, theoretically limiting later risk of gravid uterine rupture [51]. These intraoperative measures include avoiding electrocautery in favor of less destructive energy tools such as the carbon dioxide (CO_2) laser and the Harmonic® scalpel (Ethicon, Somerville, NJ), thereby limiting thermal damage to the myometrium [51, 52]. Additionally, closing the full depth of myometrial incisions in multiple layers avoids hematoma formation, which results in healing by second intention [53].

The utility of myomectomy in improving delivery rates in women with intramural fibroids continues to be debated because the definitive study—i.e., a randomized study to compare myomectomy with expectant management in IVF cycles—has never been done. Such a study has likely not been undertaken as the evidence for a negative impact of fibroids on IVF outcomes is substantial, and patients (and their clinicians) are likely to resist randomization to a nontreatment group. MRI studies of uterine peristalsis suggest utility of myomectomy for reproductive function. Uterine quiescence, which has been demonstrated to be vital for implantation, has been found to be abnormal in women with intramural fibroids, who have increased luteal phase uterine peristalsis by MRI [54]. In a series of 51 patients with intramural fibroids, those with rare uterine peristalsis had a pregnancy rate of 34% compared to 0% in the high peristalsis group. This abnormal peristalsis may be due to increased estrogen resulting from increased aromatase activity within the fibroids [55]. Altered production of neuropeptides involved in peristalsis in the pseudocapsule, and various growth factors may also play a role [56, 57]. Uterine peristalsis has been shown by MRI to return to normal in a majority of patients after myomectomy for intramural fibroids, associated with increased delivery rates following IVF [58, 59].

Few studies have specifically focused on the utility of myomectomy in improving pregnancy outcomes in patients with intramural fibroids. Of note, studies of intramural fibroids and pregnancy outcomes are variable in their methods of assessing fibroid location and encroachment on the uterine cavity (by ultrasound, MRI, hysteroscopy, or other imaging), which complicates comparison among them. A review of 41 patients with intramural and subserosal fibroids who underwent either laparoscopic or open myomectomies reported significantly improved pregnancy rates after myomectomy (34.1% pre-myomectomy vs. 60.9% post-myomectomy) [60]. Patients who were significantly more likely to conceive after myomectomy were younger and had had intramural fibroids (OR, 12.38) or significantly larger fibroids removed (5.80 cm vs. 4.28 cm; P = 0.0274), via laparoscopic myomectomy. Conversely, in their meta-analysis, Pritts and colleagues reported no differences in clinical pregnancy rate, live birth rate, or spontaneous abortion, when comparing women with intramural fibroids who underwent myomectomy when compared to those who did not [9]. In the only prospective study on the subject, Bulletti and colleagues enrolled 168 women with fibroids greater than 5 cm in diameter that did not deform the intrauterine cavity; patients elected whether or not to have laparoscopic myomectomies before IVF treatment [61]. Delivery rates were significantly different between the two groups, who were similar in age (<35 years): 25% in patients who underwent myomectomy as compared to 12% in women who declined myomectomy.

Preoperative treatment with GnRHa (for 3 months) or misoprostol (immediately preoperatively) may decrease surgical morbidity. Pretreatment with GnRHa may reduce intra-operative blood loss and operative time: A prospective study of 91 women with cumulative fibroid diameter of over 10 cm, treated with 3 months of an injectable GnRHa prior to laparoscopic myomectomy, showed a reduction in blood loss, operative time, and need for blood transfusion [62]. Studies have not consistently reported this finding, particularly as many studies included patients with smaller fibroids [32]. Ultimately, the benefit of GnRHa pretreatment is likely in patients who might otherwise not be eligible for a minimally invasive approach due to fibroid size [34, 35]. Additionally, preoperative treatment with rectal misoprostol has been associated with decreased blood loss and is a prudent, low-risk intervention immediately before myomectomy [63, 64].

Recommended recovery time after myomectomy prior to pursuing pregnancy ranges from 3 to 6 months, depending on several factors including patient age, surgeon preference, and, most importantly, the size of the tumors enucleated and number of myometrial incisions [65]. In patients who have successfully conceived, counseling regarding the recommended mode of delivery after myomectomy also largely depends on the extent of surgical dissection. Cesarean delivery is often recommended due to concern for gravid uterine rupture in patients with extensive dissection, particularly with transmural incisions and entry into the uterine cavity. The risk of uterine rupture after myomectomy is estimated at 0.5–0.7% [66]. Uterine rupture is a potentially highly morbid pregnancy complication for both patient and fetus, requiring emergent delivery.

Recommendation: For this patient, given the size of her fibroid (8 cm) and her otherwise idiopathic infertility, removal of her fibroid is likely prudent prior to embarking on costly and time-consuming fertility treatments. She is not a candidate for UAE, MRgFUS, and myolysis, as these are not currently recommended in women planning pregnancy. Medical management with GnRHa would counteract attempts at inducing ovulation as part of her fertility treatment and is unlikely to confer a lasting benefit for the duration of pregnancy, during which she will be exposed to the increased morbidity associated with a large fibroid in situ. This patient is a good candidate for a minimally invasive myomectomy with contained tissue extraction, particularly given the presence of a single dominant fibroid. Robot-assisted laparoscopic myomectomy, if available, is a favorable choice in this infertility patient, in whom maintaining the integrity of the reproductive organs is paramount and facilitated through the microsurgical precision of myometrial manipulation and suturing in multiple layers [67]. Selection of energy tools with limited thermal spread (ultrasonic scalpel and laser) is also particularly beneficial in these patients.

References

1. Munro MG, Critchley HO, Fraser IS, FIGO Menstrual Disorders Working Group. The FIGO classification of causes of abnormal uterine bleeding in the reproductive years. Fertil Steril. 2011;(95):2204–8, 2208.e1–3.

2. Galen DI, Pemueller RR, Leal JG, Abbott KR, Falls JL, Macer J. Laparoscopic radiofrequency fibroid ablation: phase II and phase III results. JSLS. 2014;18:182–90.
3. Clark NA, Mumford SL, Segars JH. Reproductive impact of MRI-guided focused ultrasound surgery for fibroids: a systematic review of the evidence. Curr Opin Obstet Gynecol. 2014;26:151–61.
4. American College of Obstetricians and Gynecologists. ACOG practice bulletin. Alternatives to hysterectomy in the management of leiomyomas. Obstet Gynecol. 2008;112:387–400.
5. Hart R, Khalaf Y, Yeong CT, Seed P, Taylor A, Braude P. A prospective controlled study of the effect of intramural uterine fibroids on the outcome of assisted conception. Hum Reprod. 2001;16:2411–7.
6. Eldar-Geva T, Meagher S, Healy DL, MacLachlan V, Breheny S, Wood C. Effect of intramural, subserosal, and submucosal uterine fibroids on the outcome of assisted reproductive technology treatment. Fertil Steril. 1998;70:687–91.
7. Surrey ES, Lietz AK, Schoolcraft WB. Impact of intramural leiomyomata in patients with a normal endometrial cavity on in vitro fertilization-embryo transfer cycle outcome. Fertil Steril. 2001;75:405–10.
8. Khalaf Y, Ross C, El-Toukhy T, Hart R, Seed P, Braude P. The effect of small intramural uterine fibroids on the cumulative outcome of assisted conception. Hum Reprod. 2006;21:2640–4.
9. Pritts EA, Parker WH, Olive DL. Fibroids and infertility: an updated systematic review of the evidence. Fertil Steril. 2009;91:1215–23.
10. Sunkara SK, Khairy M, El-Toukhy T, Khalaf Y, Coomarasamy A. The effect of intramural fibroids without uterine cavity involvement on the outcome of IVF treatment: a systematic review and meta-analysis. Hum Reprod. 2010;25:418–29.
11. Oliveira FG, Abdelmassih VG, Diamond MP, Dozortsev D, Melo NR, Abdelmassih R. Impact of subserosal and intramural uterine fibroids that do not distort the endometrial cavity on the outcome of in vitro fertilization-intracytoplasmic sperm injection. Fertil Steril. 2004;81:582–7.
12. Somigliana E, De Benedictis SD, Vercellini P, Nicolosi AE, Benaglia L, Scarduelli C, et al. Fibroids not encroaching the endometrial cavity and IVF success rate: a prospective study. Hum Reprod. 2011;26:834–9.
13. Klatsky PC, Tran ND, Caughey AB, Fujimoto VY. Fibroids and reproductive outcomes: a systematic literature review from conception to delivery. Am J Obstet Gynecol. 2008;198:357–66.

14. Ouyang DW, Economy KE, Norwitz ER. Obstetric complications of fibroids. Obstet Gynecol Clin N Am. 2006;33:153–69.
15. Rosati P, Exacoustòs C, Mancuso S. Longitudinal evaluation of uterine myoma growth during pregnancy. A sonographic study. J Ultrasound Med. 1992;11:511–5.
16. Shavell VI, Thakur M, Sawant A, Kruger ML, Jones TB, Singh M, et al. Adverse obstetric outcomes associated with sonographically identified large uterine fibroids. Fertil Steril. 2012;97:107–10.
17. Bulman JC, Ascher SM, Spies JB. Current concepts in uterine fibroid embolization. Radiographics. 2012;32:1735–50.
18. Payne JF, Haney AF. Serious complications of uterine artery embolization for conservative treatment of fibroids. Fertil Steril. 2003;79:128–31.
19. Tropeano G, Litwicka K, Di Stasi C, Romano D, Mancuso S. Permanent amenorrhea associated with endometrial atrophy after uterine artery embolization for symptomatic uterine fibroids. Fertil Steril. 2003;79:132–5.
20. Pelage JP, Le Dref O, Soyer P, Kardache M, Dahan H, Abitbol M, et al. Fibroid-related menorrhagia: treatment with superselective embolization of the uterine arteries and midterm follow-up. Radiology. 2000;215:428–31.
21. Hehenkamp WJ, Volkers NA, Broekmans FJ, de Jong FH, Themmen AP, Birnie E, et al. Loss of ovarian reserve after uterine artery embolization: a randomized comparison with hysterectomy. Hum Reprod. 2007;22:1996–2005.
22. Goldberg J, Pereira L, Berghella V, Diamond J, Daraï E, Seinera P, et al. Pregnancy outcomes after treatment for fibromyomata: uterine artery embolization versus laparoscopic myomectomy. Am J Obstet Gynecol. 2004;191:18–21.
23. Walker WJ, McDowell SJ. Pregnancy after uterine artery embolization for leiomyomata: a series of 56 completed pregnancies. Am J Obstet Gynecol. 2006;195:1266–71.
24. Pron G, Mocarski E, Bennett J, Vilos G, Common A, Vanderburgh L, Ontario UFE Collaborative Group. Pregnancy after uterine artery embolization for leiomyomata: the Ontario multicenter trial. Obstet Gynecol. 2005;105:67–76.
25. Smart OC, Hindley JT, Regan L, Gedroyc WG. Gonadotrophin-releasing hormone and magnetic-resonance-guided ultrasound surgery for uterine leiomyomata. Obstet Gynecol. 2006;108:49–54.
26. Kim YS, Kim JH, Rhim H, Lim HK, Keserci B, Bae DS, et al. Volumetric MR-guided high-intensity focused ultrasound abla-

tion with a one-layer strategy to treat large uterine fibroids: initial clinical outcomes. Radiology. 2012;263:600–9.

27. Rabinovici J, David M, Fukunishi H, Morita Y, Gostout BS, Stewart EA, et al. Pregnancy outcome after magnetic resonance-guided focused ultrasound surgery (MRgFUS) for conservative treatment of uterine fibroids. Fertil Steril. 2010;93:199–209.

28. Vilos GA, Daly LJ, Tse BM. Pregnancy outcome after laparoscopic electromyolysis. J Am Assoc Gynecol Laparosc. 1998;5:289–92.

29. Berman JM, Bolnick JM, Pemueller RR, Garza Leal JG. Reproductive outcomes in women following radiofrequency volumetric thermal ablation of symptomatic fibroids. A retrospective case series analysis. J Reprod Med. 2015;60:194–8.

30. Jasonni VM, D'Anna R, Mancuso A, Caruso C, Corrado F, Leonardi I. Randomized double-blind study evaluating the efficacy on uterine fibroids shrinkage and on intra-operative blood loss of different length of leuprolide acetate depot treatment before myomectomy. Acta Obstet Gynecol Scand. 2001;80:956–8.

31. Olive DL, Lindheim SR, Pritts EA. Non-surgical management of leiomyoma: impact on fertility. Curr Opin Obstet Gynecol. 2004;16:239–43.

32. United States Food and Drug Administration. http://www.accessdata.fda.gov/drugsatfda_docs/label/2011/019943s032,020011s039lbl.pdf. Revised June 2011. Accessed 7 June 2016.

33. Chen I, Motan T, Kiddoo D. Gonadotropin-releasing hormone agonist in laparoscopic myomectomy: systematic review and meta-analysis of randomized controlled trials. J Minim Invasive Gynecol. 2011;1:303–9.

34. Lewis EI, Gargiulo AR. The role of Hysteroscopic and robot-assisted laparoscopic myomectomy in the setting of infertility. Clin Obstet Gynecol. 2016;59:53–65.

35. Lethaby A, Vollenhoven B, Sowter M. Pre-operative GnRH analogue therapy before hysterectomy or myomectomy for uterine fibroids. Cochrane Database Syst Rev. 2001;(2):CD000547.

36. Bulletti C, Polli V, Negrini V, Giacomucci E, Flamigni C. Adhesion formation after laparoscopic myomectomy. J Am Assoc Gynecol Laparosc. 1996;3:533–6.

37. Pundir J, Pundir V, Walavalkar R, Omanwa K, Lancaster G, Kayani S. Robotic-assisted laparoscopic vs abdominal and laparoscopic myomectomy: systematic review and meta-analysis. J Minim Invasive Gynecol. 2013;20:335–45.

38. Gunnala V, Setton R, Pereira N, Huang JQ. Robot-assisted myomectomy for large uterine myomas: a single center experience. Minim Invasive Surg. 2016;2016:4905292.
39. Advincula AP, Xu X, Goudeau ST, Ransom SB. Robot-assisted laparoscopic myomectomy versus abdominal myomectomy: a comparison of short-term surgical outcomes and immediate costs. J Minim Invasive Gynecol. 2007;14:698–705.
40. Barakat E, Bedaiwy MA, Zimberg S, Nutter B, Nosseir M, Falcone T. Robotic-assisted laparoscopic and abdominal myomectomy: a comparison of surgical outcomes. Obstet Gynecol. 2011;117:256–65.
41. Liu G, Zolis L, Kung R, Melchior M, Singh S, Cook EF. The laparoscopic myomectomy: a survey of Canadian gynaecologists. J Obstet Gynaecol Can. 2010;32:139–48.
42. Oduyebo T, Hinchcliff E, Meserve EE, Seidman MA, Quade BJ, Rauh-Hain JA, George S, Nucci MR, del Carmen MG, Muto MG. Risk factors for occult uterine sarcoma among women undergoing minimally invasive gynecologic surgery. J Minim Invasive Gynecol. 2016;23:34–9.
43. Raine-Bennett T, Tucker LY, Zaritsky E, Littell RD, Palen T, Neugebauer R, et al. Occult uterine sarcoma and Leiomyosarcoma: incidence of and survival associated with Morcellation. Obstet Gynecol. 2016;127:29–39.
44. Pritts EA, Parker WH, Brown J, Olive DL. Outcome of occult uterine leiomyosarcoma after surgery for presumed uterine fibroids: a systematic review. J Minim Invasive Gynecol. 2015;22:26–33.
45. U.S. Food and Drug Administration. UPDATED Laparoscopic Uterine Power Morcellation in Hysterectomy and Myomectomy: FDA Safety Communication. http://www.fda.gov/MedicalDevices/Safety/AlertsandNotices/ucm424443.htm. Updated 24 Nov 2014. Accessed 7 June 2016.
46. Pritts EA, Vanness DJ, Berek JS, Parker W, Feinberg R, Feinberg J, et al. The prevalence of occult leiomyosarcoma at surgery for presumed uterine fibroids: a meta-analysis. Gynecol Surg. 2015;12:165–77.
47. Harris JA, Swenson CW, Uppal S, Kamdar N, Mahnert N, As-Sanie S, et al. Practice patterns and postoperative complications before and after US Food and Drug Administration safety communication on power morcellation. Am J Obstet Gynecol. 2016;214:98.e1–98.e13.

48. Siedhoff MT, Wheeler SB, Rutstein SE, Geller EJ, Doll KM, Wu JM, et al. Laparoscopic hysterectomy with morcellation vs abdominal hysterectomy for presumed fibroid tumors in premenopausal women: a decision analysis. Am J Obstet Gynecol. 2015;212:591.e1–8.
49. Vargas MV, Cohen SL, Fuchs-Weizman N, Wang KC, Manoucheri E, Vitonis AF, et al. Open power morcellation versus contained power morcellation within an insufflated isolation bag: comparison of perioperative outcomes. J Minim Invasive Gynecol. 2015;22:433–8.
50. Cohen SL, Einarsson JI, Wang KC, Brown D, Boruta D, Scheib SA, et al. Contained power morcellation within an insufflated isolation bag. Obstet Gynecol. 2014;124:491–7.
51. Choussein S, Srouji SS, Farland LV, Gargiulo AR. Flexible carbon dioxide laser fiber versus ultrasonic scalpel in robot-assisted laparoscopic myomectomy. J Minim Invasive Gynecol. 2015;22:1183–90.
52. Pitter MC, Gargiulo AR, Bonaventura LM, Lehman JS, Srouji SS. Pregnancy outcomes following robot-assisted myomectomy. Hum Reprod. 2013;28:99–108.
53. Parker WH, Einarsson J, Istre O, Dubuisson JB. Risk factors for uterine rupture after laparoscopic myomectomy. J Minim Invasive Gynecol. 2010;17:551–4.
54. Yoshino O, Hayashi T, Osuga Y, Orisaka M, Asada H, Okuda S, et al. Decreased pregnancy rate is linked to abnormal uterine peristalsis caused by intramural fibroids. Hum Reprod. 2010;25:2475–9.
55. Bulun SE, Imir G, Utsunomiya H, Thung S, Gurates B, Tamura M, et al. Aromatase in endometriosis and uterine leiomyomata. J Steroid Biochem Mol Biol. 2005;95:57–62.
56. Malvasi A, Cavallotti C, Nicolardi G, Pellegrino M, Dell'Edera D, Vergara D, et al. NT, NPY and PGP 9.5 presence in myometrium and in fibroid pseudocapsule and their possible impact on muscular physiology. Gynecol Endocrinol. 2013;29:177–81.
57. Ciarmela P, Islam MS, Reis FM, Gray PC, Bloise E, Petraglia F, et al. Growth factors and myometrium: biological effects in uterine fibroid and possible clinical implications. Hum Reprod Update. 2011;17:772–90.
58. Fanchin R, Righini C, Olivennes F, Taylor S, de Ziegler D, Frydman R. Uterine contractions at the time of embryo transfer alter pregnancy rates after in-vitro fertilization. Hum Reprod. 1998;13:1968–74.

59. Yoshino O, Nishii O, Osuga Y, Asada H, Okuda S, Orisaka M, et al. Myomectomy decreases abnormal uterine peristalsis and increases pregnancy rate. J Minim Invasive Gynecol. 2012;19:63–7.

60. Campo S, Campo V, Gambadauro P. Reproductive outcome before and after laparoscopic or abdominal myomectomy for subserous or intramural myomas. Eur J Obstet Gynecol Reprod Biol. 2003;110:215–9.

61. Bulletti C, DE Ziegler D, Levi Setti P, Cicinelli E, Polli V, Stefanetti M. Myomas, pregnancy outcome, and in vitro fertilization. Ann N Y Acad Sci. 2004;1034:84–92.

62. Chang WC, Chu LH, Huang PS, Huang SC, Sheu BC. Comparison of laparoscopic myomectomy in large myomas with and without leuprolide acetate. J Minim Invasive Gynecol. 2015;22:992–6.

63. Lavazzo C, Mamais I, Gkegkes ID. Use of misoprostol in myomectomy: a systematic review and meta-analysis. Arch Gynecol Obstet. 2015;292:1185–91.

64. Abdel-Hafeez M, Elnaggar A, Ali M, Ismail AM, Yacoub M. Rectal misoprostol for myomectomy: a randomized placebo-controlled study. Aust N Z J Obstet Gynaecol. 2015;55:363–8.

65. Tsuji S, Takahashi K, Imaoka I, Sugimura K, Miyazaki K, Noda Y. MRI evaluation of the uterine structure after myomectomy. Gynecol Obstet Investig. 2006;61:106–10.

66. Landon MB, Lynch CD. Optimal timing and mode of delivery after cesarean with previous classical incision or myomectomy: a review of the data. Semin Perinatol. 2011;35:257–61.

67. Pluchino N, Litta P, Freschi L, Russo M, Simi G, Santoro AN, et al. Comparison of the initial surgical experience with robotic and laparoscopic myomectomy. Int J Med Robot. 2014;10:208–12.

Chapter 6
26-Week Fibroid Uterus, Hydroureter, Hydronephrosis, and Infertility

William Parker

Case Description

A 35-year-old patient with massive 26-week fibroid uterus, mild pressure symptoms, back pain, hydroureter, and hydronephrosis. The patient has been trying to conceive × 8 months. She also describes heavy menstrual bleeding, changing pads every hour for 3 days per month.

Exam Findings

Abdominal exam—a 26-week mass, mobile and non-tender. Pelvic exam—vagina and cervix are normal. Bimanual—a low-lying firm 8 cm mass on right confluent with the uterus, against pelvic sidewall. Left sidewall is clear. Uterus is felt at 5 cm above the umbilicus. No peripheral edema, no calf tenderness or signs of DVT.

W. Parker, MD
Department of Obstetrics and Gynecology, UCLA School of
Medicine, Santa Monica, CA 90401, USA
e-mail: wparker@ucla.edu

N.S. Moawad (ed.), *Uterine Fibroids*,
https://doi.org/10.1007/978-3-319-58780-6_6,
© Springer International Publishing AG 2018

Diagnostic Workup

UTZ—multiple fibroids, largest is 8 cm on right. EEC is not well seen due to three fibroids compressing the endometrial cavity, one of which appears to have an intracavitary component. None of the fibroid has increased vascularity.

Although not usually performed when an abdominal myomectomy is planned, an MRI was ordered by the referring physician to better define the size number and position of the fibroids. The MRI shows an 8 cm anterior type 4 fibroid (FIGO) which deviates and compresses the lower uterine segment. Three type 4 fibroids on the right adjacent to the right pelvic sidewall. A 3 cm type 0.

$$CBC - Hgb = 9.7.$$

$$LDH = 180\left(normal =< 200\right), iso-enzyme\,3 = 20\%\left(normal =< 26\%\right).$$

Treatment Options

The patient wishes future fertility. Due to the type 0 fibroid and multiple type 4 fibroids, some of which about the endometrial cavity, neither observation nor uterine artery embolization (UAE) is recommended. Type 0 fibroids have been shown to decrease fertility by approximately 70% (RR 0.32 CI 0.12–0.85) when compared with infertile controls matched by age. Removal of type 0 fibroids has been shown to return fertility to baseline for infertile age-matched controls (RR 1.13 CI 0.96–1.33) [1]. Although rare, UAE has been associated with spontaneous abortion, placenta accreta, and preterm delivery, and at our institution, it is not recommended for women wishing future fertility [2].

Due to the large size of the uterus and insufficient room for placement of endoscopic ports, neither the laparoscopic nor robotic approach is felt to be technically feasible. In addition, identifying and removing smaller type 4 fibroids without the benefit of palpation at the time of surgery is felt to be difficult.

High-intensity focused ultrasound is felt to be inappropriate due to the overall size of the uterus and presence of the intracavitary fibroid. Fertility data, with likelihood of conception following treatment, is not available, and only minimal pregnancy outcome data are available, and, thus, we have not recommended this modality for women wishing to conceive.

Therefore, abdominal myomectomy is considered the procedure of choice with the best outcome (Figs. 6.1, 6.2, and 6.3).

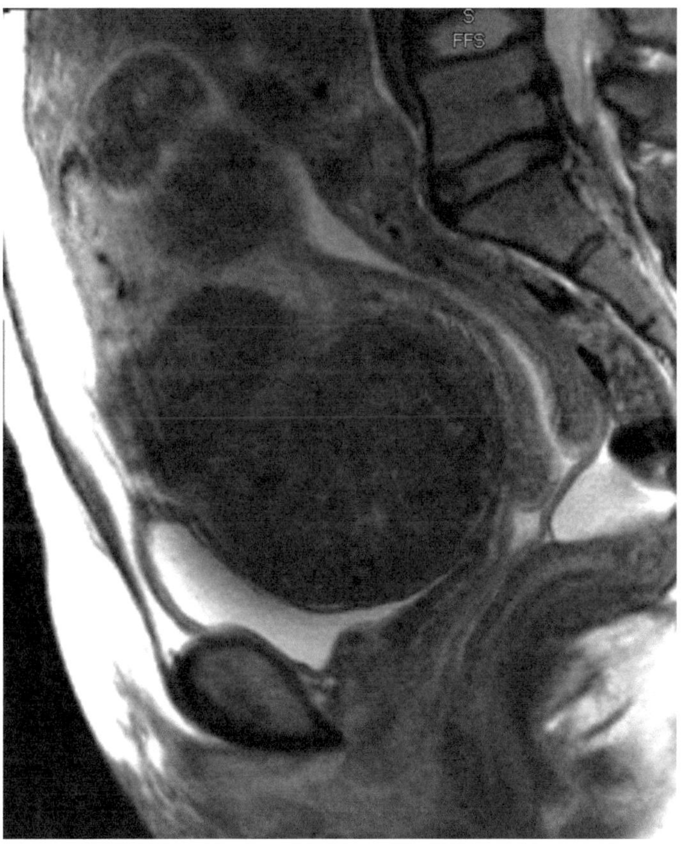

Figure 6.1   MRI, sagittal view, showing multiple large anterior intramural fibroids displacing the uterine cavity posteriorly

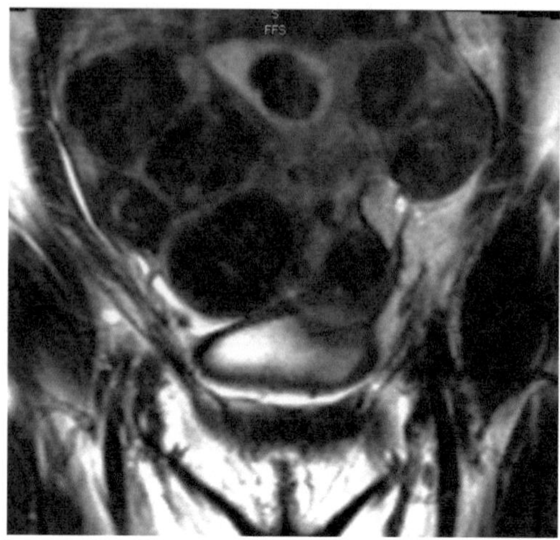

FIGURE 6.2 MRI, coronal view, showing a significantly enlarged uterus with multiple intramural and small submucosal myomas

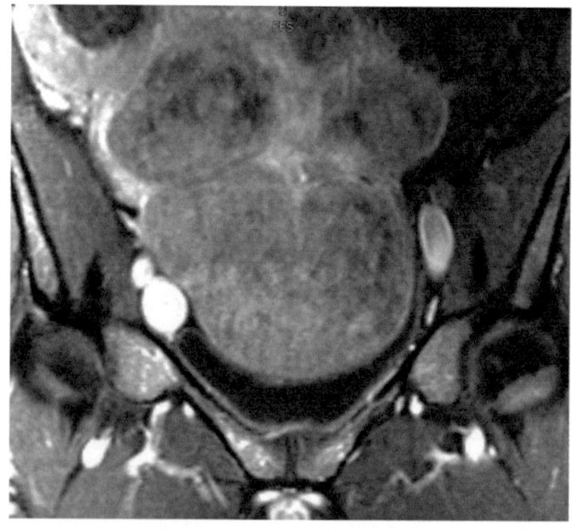

FIGURE 6.3 MRI, coronal view, showing a large lower uterine segment/cervical fibroid compressing the bladder

Preoperative Preparation

Correction of the patient's preoperative anemia was addressed initially. Although we have used either GnRH or erythropoietin in the past, we find that, for women with chronic blood loss anemia, intravenously administered iron infusions are remarkably effective in returning hemoglobin levels to near normal. Intravenous iron avoids the side effects of GnRH agonists (hot flashes, insomnia, vaginal dryness, headaches) and expense of either GnRH agonists or erythropoietin B. Iron sucrose and iron gluconate can be given in a maximal single dose of 200 mg over a minimum infusion time of 30 min.

In order to reduce intraoperative blood loss, we administer preoperative cytotec, 400 μm placed vaginally 3 h before surgery and tranexamic acid 10 mg/kg given IV at the time of the skin incision.

Operative Technique

We perform all of our abdominal myomectomies through low transverse incision. In this case, we would extend the fascial incision cephalad at the lateral borders of the rectus muscles in order to avoid transection of the ilioinguinal nerve. Midline separation of the fascia away from rectus muscles to the level of the umbilicus also allows for more space to exteriorize the uterus.

We place a tourniquet as soon as the uterus is exteriorized and release it approximately every 30 min to allow reperfusion of the uterus and ovaries. Vasopressin 20 U diluted in 100 mL of saline is prepared, and approximately 10 mL (2 U) is injected into the pseudocapsule of each fibroid just prior to each serosal incision. Although not tested together, all four methods of reducing blood loss have independently been shown to reduce blood loss and have different mechanisms of action; we therefore combine the methods.

On rare occasions, for women with low preoperative hemoglobin levels and the possibility of greater than 500 mL operative blood loss due to numerous fibroids, we request a cell saver on standby. This device suctions blood from the operative field, mixes it with heparinized saline, and stores the patient's blood in a canister during surgery. If needed for reinfusion, the cell saver washes the blood with saline, filters and centrifuges it to a hematocrit of approximately 50%, and gives the blood back to the patient intraoperatively via an IV. Consequently, the need for preoperative autologous blood donation or heterologous blood transfusion can often be avoided [3]. The use of cell saver collected blood avoids the risks of infection with HIV or hepatitis or transfusion reaction. The oxygen transport capacity of salvaged red blood cells are equal to, or better than, stored allogeneic red cells, and the survival of red blood cells appears to be at least as good as transfused allogeneic red cells [4]. Also, economic models suggest that the cost of the cell saver should be significantly lower than the cost of blood drawing, testing, processing, storing, and transfusing autologous blood cells.

Uterine incisions can be made either vertically or transversely, since fibroids distort normal vascular architecture, making any attempt to avoid the arcuate vessels impossible [5]. However, careful planning and placement of uterine incisions can avoid inadvertent extension of the incision to the uterine cornua, ascending uterine vessels, or visible large arteries or veins. We extend the uterine incisions through the myometrium and the entire pseudocapsule until the fibroid is clearly seen, which identifies a less vascular surgical plane.

We plan the incisions at the time of surgery in order to facilitate removal of multiple fibroids through each incision, but we avoid tunneling through the myometrium to distant fibroids because hemostasis within these tunnels is difficult. Since excellent hemostasis decreases oozing and adhesion formation, we feel this strategy is important. Multiple uterine incisions may be needed, but we routinely use an adhesion barrier (Seprafilm, Genzyme, Cambridge, MA) to help limit adhesion formation.

One prospective study randomized 127 women undergoing abdominal myomectomy to treatment or no treatment with Seprafilm [6]. During second-look laparoscopy, women treated with Seprafilm had significantly fewer adhesions and lower adhesion severity scores than untreated women.

In order to reduce any rectus diastasis, common with large fibroids distorting the abdominal wall, we reapproximate the rectus abdominis muscles with interrupted sutures. We place an ON-Q catheter (Halyard Health, Alpharetta, Georgia) below the fascial closure and a separate catheter above the fascia in the subcutaneous layer. The catheters are connected to an elastomeric pump filled with 355 mL of bupivacaine which automatically provides 4 mL/h. continuous infusion of local anesthesia to the incision. The ON-Q reservoir provides pain relief for 4 days and has been shown to reduce the need for parenteral or oral narcotics.

Enhanced Recovery

For the past 8 years, we have used the enhanced recovery protocol, initially developed in England, for all of our abdominal myomectomy patients. The protocol has been shown to allow quicker return of bowel and bladder function, shorten length of stay, and decrease postoperative complications, in addition to increasing both nursing and patient autonomy. For the surgeon that translates into fewer days rounding and fewer phone calls, the protocol includes: elimination of bowel preps; preoperative analgesia consisting of celecoxib, 400 mg po and neurontin, 1200 mg po given 1 h before surgery; maintenance of normovolemia during surgery to avoid bowel edema, nausea, and vomiting prophylaxis before the conclusion of surgery which includes dexamethasone 4 mg IV plus ondansetron 4 mg IV; removal of the urinary catheter on the day of surgery; early feeding and ambulation on the day of surgery; and, avoidance of patient-controlled narcotic analgesia [7]. Almost all women are ready for discharge on postoperative day 2. This patient was seen in our office on postoperative day 5 for removal of the ON-Q pain pump. Her 2-week and 6-week postoperative exams were normal, with excellent return of the uterine size to near normal.

References

1. Pritts E, Parker W, Olive D. Fibroids and infertility: an updated systematic review of the evidence. Fertil Steril. 2009;91:1215–23.
2. Mara M, Kubinova K. Embolization of uterine fibroids from the point of view of the gynecologist: pros and cons. Int J Womens Health. 2014;6:623–9.
3. Yamada T, Ikeda A, Okamoto Y, Okamoto Y, Kanda T, Ueki M. Intraoperative blood salvage in abdominal simple total hysterectomy for uterine myoma. Int J Gynaecol Obstet. 1997;59:233–6.
4. Goodnough L, Monk T, Brecher M. Autologous blood procurement in the surgical setting: lessons learned in the last 10 years. Vox Sang. 1996;71:133–41.
5. Discepola F, Valenti DA, Reinhold C, Tulandi T. Analysis of arterial blood vessels surrounding the myoma: relevance to myomectomy. Obstet Gynecol. 2007;110:1301–3.
6. Diamond MP. Reduction of adhesions after uterine myomectomy by Seprafilm membrane (HAL-F): a blinded, prospective, randomized, multicenter clinical study. Seprafilm adhesion study group. Fertil Steril. 1996;66:904–10.
7. Kalogera E, Bakkum-Gamez JN, Jankowski CJ, Trabuco E, Lovely JK, Dhanorker S, Grubbs PL, Weaver AL, Haas LR, Borah BJ, Bursiek AA, Walsh MT, Cliby WA, Dowdy SC. Enhanced recovery in gynecologic surgery. Obstet Gynecol. 2013;122:319–28.

Chapter 7
Submucosal Fibroid, Menorrhagia, Anemia, and Dysmenorrhea

Christina Salazar and Keith Isaacson

Clinical Case: A 32-year-old nulliparous female with a 4 cm submucosal fibroid and with bleeding, anemia, and dysmenorrhea.

Clinical Case Presentation

A 32-year-old nulliparous female presents to the office for gynecologic consultation regarding heavy, painful menstrual periods. Her menstrual periods are regular every 28 days and last 8–10 days, with heavy flow and passage of large clots throughout her menses. These symptoms have been worsening over the past 6 months, whereas her periods were

---

Electronic supplementary material The online version of this chapter (doi:10.1007/978-3-319-58780-6_7) contains supplementary material, which is available to authorized users.

C. Salazar, MD • K. Isaacson, MD (✉)
Minimally Invasive Gynecologic Surgery, Newton Wellesley Hospital, Harvard Medical School, Newton, MA 02462, USA
e-mail: Csalazar3@partners.org; Isaacson.keith@mgh.harvard.edu

N.S. Moawad (ed.), *Uterine Fibroids*,
https://doi.org/10.1007/978-3-319-58780-6_7,
© Springer International Publishing AG 2018

previously normal and lasted 5 days. This patient denies postcoital bleeding, however has recently noticed occasional intermenstrual bleeding. She denies pelvic pressure-type symptoms affecting her bowel or her bladder. Her social, medical, and surgical histories are unremarkable. Her mother and older sister both had hysterectomies for uterine fibroids.

The heavy menstrual bleeding has significantly impacted the quality of her life to the point where she hardly leaves her home while having her period. Three weeks prior to her initial visit, the patient had to leave work early after soaking through several pads and soiling her clothes. The heavy bleeding has also caused her to stop exercising as frequently as she would like. She recently presented to the emergency room after feeling acutely dizzy and lightheaded while on day 9 of her menstrual cycle. At that time, she was found to have iron deficiency anemia. An ultrasound performed in the emergency room revealed an enlarged uterus with a single 4 cm fibroid that appeared to be impacting the cavity. After receiving intravenous fluids for resuscitation of her intravascular volume, her symptoms resolved, and she was given a 5-day "OCP taper" regimen by the ER physician as well as a prescription for iron tablets. It was recommended that she follow up with her gynecologist.

At the time of evaluation of this patient, she was single and had never attempted to conceive, however wished to maintain the option of fertility in the future. For the past 5 years, she has been taking cyclic oral contraceptive pills for purposes of contraception.

Exam Findings

On examination, her abdomen is soft, nontender, and nondistended. A bimanual exam reveals a mobile, nontender uterus enlarged to approximately 10-week size with no palpable adnexal masses. Speculum exam reveals a normal appearing nulliparous cervix without lesions.

Diagnostic Workup

Hematocrit	28.6 (nL range 34.9–44.5)
MCV	71 (nL range 80–96)
Urine pregnancy test	Negative
Pap smear	Normal, high-risk HPV negative

Imaging and Diagnosis

Transvaginal ultrasound performed in the emergency room had revealed an anteverted uterus with a single well-circumscribed 4 cm leiomyoma that appears to be bulging into the uterine cavity, as well as normal adnexa bilaterally (Fig. 7.1).

Vaginoscopic office hysteroscopy is performed with a 3 mm rigid hysteroscope, normal saline, no tenaculum, and no anesthesia (oral or local) for diagnostic workup of abnormal

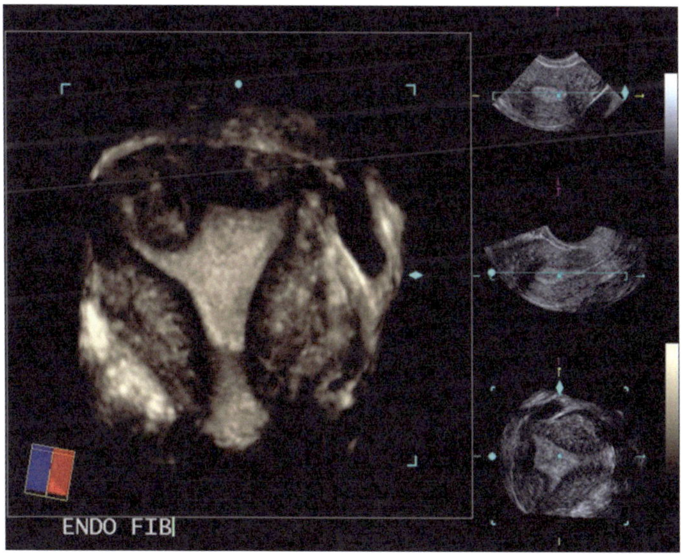

FIGURE 7.1 3-D coronal view of intracavitary fibroid

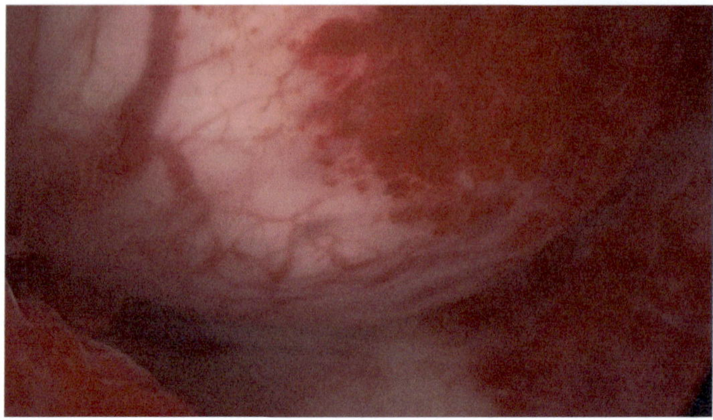

FIGURE 7.2 Type II submucous leiomyoma along the anterior uterine wall visualized hysteroscopically

uterine bleeding [1]. Hysteroscopy reveals normal endometrium and a submucous leiomyoma that appears to be 40% within the cavity; otherwise, no polyps or lesions are noted. Bilateral tubal ostia are visualized, and she has a normal endocervical canal (Fig. 7.2).

Treatment Options

This woman has been diagnosed with a 4 cm Type II submucous leiomyoma which has resulted in abnormal heavy uterine bleeding as well as associated iron deficiency anemia. Strategies for management should be individualized based upon the location, number, and size of leiomyoma while taking into account the severity of symptoms, age, fertility status, and proximity to menopause.

Differential Diagnosis

The differential to consider is leiomyoma, adenomyoma, focal adenomyosis, and leiomyosarcoma. To distinguish between these, we did an evaluation including a bimanual exam, transvaginal ultrasound, and office hysteroscopy. Had the patient been 45 years of age or older, we would have included an endometrial biopsy [2].

Our exam revealed an enlarged, nontender uterus consistent with fibroids and not adenomyosis. We reviewed the ultrasound images from the ED and noted a homogeneous mass with very distinct borders. In the myometrium not affected by the mass, the thickness is similar along the anterior and posterior wall. This would not be expected in patients with adenomyosis. Uteri affected by adenomyosis tend to be globally enlarged and classically have an asymmetric appearance with the posterior uterine wall approximately two times thicker than the anterior uterine wall. Furthermore, uteri affected by adenomyosis tend to be flexed backward in a "hockey stick" position, with the fundus retroflexed toward the posterior cul-de-sac [3].

In comparison, an adenomyoma is a nodular aggregate with an ill-defined border, appears heterogenous in echotexture, and classically contains cystic lakes of endometrial glands and stroma that may retain pockets of old blood. This patient has a mass with a distinct border that suggests a clear pseudocapsule. This pseudocapsule is not seen in adenomyomata.

Uterine leiomyomas are common and malignancy is very rare. For resectoscopic surgery, the incidence of malignancy has been reported as low as 0.13% [4]. This patient's risk may be even lower given her young age.

FIGO Classification System

Classification of the submucous leiomyoma into three subtypes can be useful for guidance and counseling of the patient [5]. The International Federation of Obstetrics and Gynecology (FIGO) put forth one of the most commonly used fibroid classification systems for the extent of myometrial involvement. FIGO describes Type 0 lesions as completely within the endometrial cavity, Type I lesions as those that extend <50% into the myometrium, Type II lesions as those in which ≥50% are within the myometrium, and Type III lesions are 100% intramural and abut the endometrium but do not distort the endometrial cavity. Removal of 100%

of a Type I or II myoma can be safely achieved as long as one stays within the pseudocapsule and does not cut myometrium because a fibroid will displace myometrium and not invade it (as opposed to an adenomyoma). Patients with Type III myomas should only have hysteroscopic resection by very experienced hysteroscopic surgeons.

Surgical Approach

The management of uterine fibroids can generally be approached by a variety of options including medications, surgery, or minimally invasive embolization or ablative techniques [6]. Medical treatment alone is temporary and only effective while on the medication. Fibroid symptoms will recur if medical therapy is discontinued. Likewise, patients with submucous myomas more often experience irregular bleeding on suppressive hormonal therapy. Furthermore, many patients present with heavy bleeding despite already being on combined oral contraceptive pills or levonorgestrel IUD, which should prompt the provider to explore further the etiology of the abnormal uterine bleeding.

Nonsurgical treatment options such as uterine artery embolization (UAE) function by restricting the blood supply of the fibroid and inducing ischemic necrosis within the myoma. Patients should be counseled regarding the risk of reoperation, which is approximately 20% after a successful percutaneous embolization and up to 50% in situations of incomplete infarction [7]. A relative contraindication for UAE is submucous location of the myoma as well as desire for a future pregnancy, as there exists a lack of data ensuring favorable pregnancy outcomes after UAE [8]. One randomized control trial suggests myomectomy is favorable over UAE in regard to rates of successful pregnancy resulting in delivery [9].

A nonsurgical and minimally invasive option that utilizes high-frequency ultrasound is also available for therapeutic treatment of uterine fibroids. The high-intensity focused ultrasound beams is magnetic resonance-guided focused ultrasound (known as MRgFUS) and utilizes thermal ablation to induce myoma shrinkage via tissue necrosis. However, concerns about detrimental impact on future fertility remain with this approach [10], as well as risk of needing a subsequent fibroid surgery within 2 years of having the procedure performed [11]. Of note, these methods also do not allow for histological evaluation of the pathology.

Another minimally invasive treatment option exists that utilizes laparoscopic ultrasound-guided radiofrequency volumetric thermal ablation (RFTVA) and has received FDA approval in the United States (Acessa; Halt Medical, Inc., Brentwood, CA, USA) as well as in Europe. The role of RFTVA is still being evaluated, as patient outcomes including quality of life as well as pregnancy outcomes are currently being followed longitudinally. A recently published 24-month interim analysis data suggest safety as well as efficacy when compared to laparoscopic myomectomy [12].

In this clinical case presentation, the submucosal location of the Type II fibroid lends itself to be an excellent candidate for transcervical resection as it is a definitive and minimally invasive surgical treatment approach.

There are three main techniques for performing hysteroscopic myomectomy: monopolar and bipolar electrosurgical loops, mechanical shavers, and vaporization which is performed with a large surface area electrode (actually, it is a very small surface area in contact with the tissue which produces the high power density that vaporizes the intracellular water of the cells causing bursting of the tissue and vaporization). Due to their side opening cutting design, the hysteroscopic morcellators have limited utility in cases with myomas that have deep involvement into the myometrium. For this case presentation at hand, a 24 French bipolar resectoscope (7.5 mm diameter) with a 12° viewing angle would be recommended for complete resection of the leiomyoma.

Should focal adenomyosis or an adenomyoma be encountered during hysteroscopic resection, there may be no clear pseudocapsule to dissect as there would be with a pure fibroid. Instead, continue resection of the hypertrophied smooth muscle associated with the focal nodule of adenomyosis until normal myometrium is visualized.

Fluid Management Considerations

When performing hysteroscopic myomectomy, one should recognize the risk of excess fluid absorption and be mindful of the fluid management guidelines published in 2013 by the American Association of Gynecologic Laparoscopists (AAGL). AAGL guidelines for operative hysteroscopy using isotonic distention media such as normal saline recommend limiting the fluid deficit to 2500 mL in order to restrict intravasation of significant volumes of fluid and thereby prevent the onset of dangerous sequelae associated with fluid overload such as right-sided heart failure, hypoxia, difficulty with ventilation, and pulmonary edema [13]. Electrolyte-rich fluids can be used with bipolar radiofrequency surgical instruments and mechanical shavers but are not an appropriate fluid choice for monopolar radiofrequency surgical instruments due to the dispersion of current. The key to minimizing fluid overload is to keep the intrauterine pressure at the lowest level that allows for adequate flow and distention. If it is feasible to keep the intracavitary pressure lower than the patient's mean arterial pressure, then the risk of significant fluid intravasation is drastically reduced. Additional methods of decreasing fluid absorption include pretreatment with gonadotropin-releasing hormone agonists (GnRHa) as well as administration of vasopressin.

Pretreatment with GnRH Agonists

Premenopausal women are more susceptible than postmenopausal women to hyponatremic hypotonic encephalopathy secondary to estrogen's inhibition of the Na^+/K^+-ATPase pump and so are more likely to die or have permanent brain damage [14]. When planning to perform resectoscopic surgery, some clinicians will pretreat with GnRHa in order to decrease the circulating levels of estrogen [15] and thereby decrease the estrogen-related suppression of the Na^+/K^+-ATPase pump. However, there is conflicting evidence regarding the effect of GnRHa on fluid intravasation, and its use should be at the discretion of the provider.

Intracervical Vasopressin Administration

Intracervical injection of 8 mL of a dilute solution of vasopressin (0.05 U/mL of normal saline) has been shown to decrease fluid absorption during resectoscopic surgery via its primary mechanism of inducing vasoconstriction [16]. The dilute injection can be repeated at 20-min intervals. Care should be taken to avoid intravascular injection, as systemic absorption can result in vagal-mediated bradycardia as well as coronary artery vasospasm provoking cardiac arrest.

Surgical Technique

After successful entry into the uterine cavity, the surgical technique for hysteroscopic myomectomy begins with unroofing the myoma. You should visualize the fibroid as dense, white fibers that are distinct from the appearance of the surrounding pink myometrium. Shave the fibroid evenly down to the level of the endometrium. Identification of the pseudocapsule is the next critical step, as this provides an excellent guide to the boundaries of the myoma for the remainder of the resection. Complete resection of 100% of the myoma is the goal for hysteroscopic myomectomy. Long-term studies indicate that transcervical resection of myomas has a high rate of success >94% [17]. Rates of requiring a second completion surgery is related to the overall size of the fibroid, depth of myometrial invasion, as well as the location and number of fibroids.

References

1. van Dongen H, de Kroon CD, Jacobi CE, Trimbos JB, Jansen FW. Diagnostic hysteroscopy in abnormal uterine bleeding: a systematic review and meta-analysis. BJOG. 2007;114(6):664–75.
2. Committee on Practice B-G. Practice bulletin no. 128: diagnosis of abnormal uterine bleeding in reproductive-aged women. Obstet Gynecol. 2012;120(1):197–206.
3. Alabiso G, Alio L, Arena S, Barbasetti di Prun A, Bergamini V, Berlanda N, et al. Adenomyosis: what the patient needs. J Minim Invasive Gynecol. 2016;23(4):476–88.
4. Vilos GA, Edris F, Abu-Rafea B, Hollett-Caines J, Ettler HC, Al-Mubarak A. Miscellaneous uterine malignant neoplasms detected during hysteroscopic surgery. J Minim Invasive Gynecol. 2009;16(3):318–25.
5. American Association of Gynecologic Laparoscopists: Advancing Minimally Invasive Gynecology W. AAGL practice report: practice guidelines for the diagnosis and management of submucous leiomyomas. J Minim Invasive Gynecol. 2012;19(2):152–71.
6. Zupi E, Centini G, Sabbioni L, Lazzeri L, Argay IM, Petraglia F. Nonsurgical alternatives for uterine fibroids. Best Pract Res Clin Obstet Gynaecol. 2016;34:122–31.
7. Kroencke TJ, Scheurig C, Poellinger A, Gronewold M, Hamm B. Uterine artery embolization for leiomyomas: percentage of infarction predicts clinical outcome. Radiology. 2010;255(3):834–41.
8. Donnez J, Dolmans MM. Uterine fibroid management: from the present to the future. Hum Reprod Update. 2016;22(6):665–86.
9. Mara M, Maskova J, Fucikova Z, Kuzel D, Belsan T, Sosna O. Midterm clinical and first reproductive results of a randomized controlled trial comparing uterine fibroid embolization and myomectomy. Cardiovasc Intervent Radiol. 2008;31(1):73–85.
10. Clark NA, Mumford SL, Segars JH. Reproductive impact of MRI-guided focused ultrasound surgery for fibroids: a systematic review of the evidence. Curr Opin Obstet Gynecol. 2014;26(3):151–61.
11. Jacoby VL, Kohi MP, Poder L, Jacoby A, Lager J, Schembri M, et al. PROMISe trial: a pilot, randomized, placebo-controlled trial of magnetic resonance guided focused ultrasound for uterine fibroids. Fertil Steril. 2016;105(3):773–80.
12. Kramer B, Hahn M, Taran FA, Kraemer D, Isaacson KB, Brucker SY. Interim analysis of a randomized controlled trial comparing

laparoscopic radiofrequency volumetric thermal ablation of uterine fibroids with laparoscopic myomectomy. Int J Gynaecol Obstet. 2016;133(2):206–11.
13. Worldwide AAMIG, Munro MG, Storz K, Abbott JA, Falcone T, Jacobs VR, et al. AAGL practice report: practice guidelines for the Management of Hysteroscopic Distending Media: (Replaces Hysteroscopic fluid monitoring guidelines. J Am Assoc Gynecol Laparosc. 2000;7:167–168). J Minim Invasive Gynecol. 2013;20(2):137–48.
14. Ayus JC, Wheeler JM, Arieff AI. Postoperative hyponatremic encephalopathy in menstruant women. Ann Intern Med. 1992;117(11):891–7.
15. Muzii L, Boni T, Bellati F, Marana R, Ruggiero A, Zullo MA, et al. GnRH analogue treatment before hysteroscopic resection of submucous myomas: a prospective, randomized, multicenter study. Fertil Steril. 2010;94(4):1496–9.
16. Corson SL, Brooks PG, Serden SP, Batzer FR, Gocial B. Effects of vasopressin administration during hysteroscopic surgery. J Reprod Med. 1994;39(6):419–23.
17. Polena V, Mergui JL, Perrot N, Poncelet C, Barranger E, Uzan S. Long-term results of hysteroscopic myomectomy in 235 patients. Eur J Obstet Gynecol Reprod Biol. 2007;130(2):232–7.

Chapter 8
Intramural Fibroid Impinging on the Uterine Cavity

Andrew Deutsch, Aarathi Cholkeri-Singh, and Charles E. Miller

Abbreviations

ACOG	American College of Obstetrics Gynecology
BMI	Body mass index
BP	Blood pressure
CBC	Complete blood count
FDA	Food and drug administration
GnRH	Gonadotropin-releasing hormone
Hct	Hematocrit
Hgb	Hemoglobin
HPV	Human papillomavirus
LUAO	Laparoscopic uterine artery occlusion
MRgFUS	Magnetic resonance-guided focused ultrasound

A. Deutsch, MD, MS
Department of Gynecology, Advocate Lutheran General Hospital, 1775 Dempster Street, Park Ridge, IL 60540, USA
e-mail: andrew.deutsch@advocatehealth.com

A. Cholkeri-Singh, MD, FACOG
C.E. Miller, MD, FACOG (✉)
The Advanced Gynecologic Surgery Institute, 120 Osler Drive, Suite 100, Naperville, IL 60540, USA
e-mail: acholkeri@gmail.com; chuckmillermd@gmail.com

N.S. Moawad (ed.), *Uterine Fibroids*,
https://doi.org/10.1007/978-3-319-58780-6_8,
© Springer International Publishing AG 2018

MRI	Magnetic resonance imaging
OCPs	Oral contraceptive pills
PDS	Polydioxanone
RFVTA	Radiofrequency volumetric thermal ablation
T	Temperature
TSH	Thyroid-stimulating hormone
UAE	Uterine artery embolization

Clinical Case Presentation

A 37-year-old G0 African-American female with progressive, worsening heavy menstrual bleeding leading to anemia over the past few years. Her past medical, gynecologic, and surgical histories are otherwise unremarkable. She desires future fertility. Office ultrasound and hysteroscopy revealed an anterior fundal fibroid impinging on the endometrial cavity. She was referred by her Reproductive Endocrinologist to see Dr. Miller.

Exam Findings

General: well-developed, well-nourished
Vital signs: BMI 30, BP 110s/80s, T 37.6, RR 12, P 90s
Abdominal exam: soft, non-tender, enlarged irregular mass palpated suprapubically
Pelvic exam: normal appearing labia, vagina, and cervix; uterus enlarged (about 12–14 weeks sized) and irregular; unable to palpate the ovaries

Diagnostic Workup

B-hCG: negative
TSH: 1.2 mIU/L
CBC: Hgb 9.5 and Hct 29
Iron studies: microcytic hypochromic red blood cells, RBC 3.9, transferrin 400 µg/dL, ferritin 20 ng/mL

Pap smear: negative for intraepithelial malignancy, adequate for evaluation, HPV negative
Endometrial biopsy: proliferative endometrium
Transvaginal ultrasound: anterior fundal fibroid impinging on the endometrial cavity
Saline infusion sonohysterogram: anterior and fundal transmural myoma

Management Options

There are several management options to consider when one approaches a fibroid uterus: expectant, medical, radiologic, and surgical. Multiple factors are important to consider when determining which option is best for each patient. Each decision should be based upon the size, number, location, and symptoms of the fibroids. Furthermore, the patient's age and desire for fertility should be taken into account. Thus, the management options can be further subdivided into fertility sparing versus conception contraindicated. The plan for the case above was a dragnostic hysteroscopy and laparoscopic myomectomy. The different management options are discussed in detail below.

Expectant Management

The prevalence of fibroids in the general female population is difficult to determine. Pathologists report finding fibroids in 77% of women status post hysterectomy, but severity depends upon race [1]. Only 25% of the Caucasian population develops clinically significant disease with a higher incidence, approaching the prevalence, in the African-American population [1]. Thus, there is an unknown percentage of fibroids that are asymptomatic. If watchful waiting was considered in the case above, then preconception counseling is important. Fibroids may enlarge during pregnancy or potentially degenerate and subsequently cause pain. A CBC to assess for anemia should be performed and subsequent hematologic workup undertaken. Microcytic hypochromic red blood cells, increased transferrin, and decreased ferritin confirm iron deficiency anemia due to blood loss. Hemoglobin should be optimized with iron replacement as necessary. Ultrasound evaluation, ideally transvaginal, is important to confirm the location of the fibroids. If necessary, further workup may require sono-hysterogram or MRI with or without contrast.

Counseling regarding submucosal fibroids' impingement on the uterine cavity and the potential for infertility, spontaneous abortion, or preterm birth should be discussed. Pritts et al. performed a metamanalysis of randomized trials and concluded that submucosal and intramural fibroid cause problems with fertility, and their removal has been shown to confer a benefit. However, no significant difference in pre-term delivery was observed [2]. Anatomic changes due to fibroids can result in malpresentation, dysfunctional labor, or placental abruption. Thus, Cesarean delivery has been reported to increase by over 30% in those affected by fibroids [3]. The same anatomic abnormalities can in theory predispose to an increased risk of postpartum hemorrhage, although reports are conflicting [3]. Thus, several experts recommend that in a patient desiring pregnancy, hysteroscopically resectable fibroids should be removed [3, 4].

Further counseling about infertility is especially important in patients of advanced maternal age. Someone contemplating a future pregnancy with a preexisting potential infertility factor, such as fibroids, should be counseled about oocyte cryopreservation.

Adjunctive Medical Therapy

Currently, in the United States, there is no long-term medical treatment for fibroids. Symptoms caused by fibroids do not begin to resolve naturally until menopause alters the hormonal state. Thus, relatively young patients remote from menopause should be counseled that greater than 50% of women using medical treatment undergo surgery within 2 years [5].

Gonadotropin-Releasing Hormone Agonists (GnRH)

GnRH agonists are the most effective medical therapy currently available in the United States. The use of GnRH agonists can shrink a fibroid by 30–40%, stop bleeding, and improve anemia [6]. However, the mechanism of action, feedback inhibition, ultimately results in a hypogonadotropic hypogonadal state. This causes a pseudo-menopausal hypoestrogenic state with side effects such as amenorrhea, hot flashes, bone loss, and sleep and mood disruptions. If used for an extended period of time (greater than 6 months), one must provide add back therapy with progesterone alone or in combo with estrogen to prevent bone loss and vasomotor problems. Ultimately, once GnRH agonist therapy concludes there is a rapid return of the fibroid to pretreatment size. These drugs are not approved by the FDA to decrease fibroid size; the only FDA approved use of GnRH agonists in the treatment of fibroids is to treat anemia. A typical regimen is 3.75 mg leuprolide acetate® every month for 3 months with iron supplementation. A statistically significant elevation in post-op hemoglobin has been seen in GnRH agonist-treated groups; however, there was no difference in transfusion requirements [7]. Further, preoperative treatment with GnRH agonists causes degenerative changes of the fibroids capsule. These changes result in a more difficult surgical resection, which translates to increased operative times [8, 9]. One use of GnRH agonists at this time is to shrink a large fibroid while optimizing hemoglobin in an attempt to convert an open procedure to a minimally invasive approach.

Aromatase Inhibitors

Aromatase inhibitors work to suppress estrogen but, unlike GnRH agonists, avoid the initial flare. Due to a paucity of research on aromatase inhibitors, the treatment of fibroids with these medications is currently an off-label use [10]. However, there are case reports that show efficacy in the treatment of fibroids [11]. Further data is needed before the routine use of aromatase inhibitors to treat symptomatic fibroids is recommended.

Other Medications

There is a plethora of other medications that have been used to treat fibroids and its symptoms. In a patient attempting pregnancy, several of these are contraindicated. Progesterone receptor modulators, such as ulipristal acetate and mifepristone, have shown efficacy in shrinking fibroids and reducing symptoms [12, 13]. However, unwanted side effects are seen such as amenorrhea, endometrial hyperplasia, and transient elevations of transaminases. These side effects severely limit its usefulness. Levonorgestrel intrauterine device can also decrease vaginal bleeding, but intracavitary fibroids are a relative contraindication due to a higher rate of expulsion [5]. Oral estrogen-progesterone contraceptive pills (OCPs) have several known non-contraceptive benefits: a decrease in the risk of ovarian and endometrial cancer and treatment of acne, menorrhagia, and dysmenorrhea. Long-term longitudinal studies show that women who used OCPs for 10 years had a 31% reduction in fibroid risk [14]. Clinically, they have been used to successfully improve anemia in patients with menorrhagia. However, evidence of efficacy in treating women with symptomatic fibroids is scarce and of low quality [15]. A trial of OCPs can be attempted in women who do not currently desire pregnancy.

Radiologic Treatment

Several radiologic treatment modalities that combine radiologic imaging with a minimally invasive approach are in various stages of development.

Uterine Artery Embolization (UAE)

UAE is the nonsurgical systematic occlusion of blood flow to the uterus performed by interventional radiologists. This procedure has been shown to cause a 30–40% decrease in fibroid size [16]. The upper limit of fibroid or uterine size safely treated with UAE has not been established. Pedunculated fibroids or a large fibroid burden (dominant fibroid >10 cm and/or uterine volume of >700 cm^3) is a relative contraindication due to early case reports of ischemic uterine artery injury which manifests as severe pain and infection [17]. Thirty percent of fibroids recur, and between 15 and 32% require surgery within 2 years of UAE [16, 18].

A retrospective cohort by Goldberg et al. compared pregnancy following UAE to pregnancies following laparoscopic myomectomy. They concluded that surgical treatment is superior since most patients end up needing surgery after treatment. They also found that pregnancies post UAE were at increased risk of preterm delivery and malpresentation [18]. Due to a lack of research in women desiring fertility after UAE, pregnancy post UAE is relatively contraindicated per ACOG [19]. However, there are case reports of patients becoming pregnant after UAE and carrying to term without complications [20]. At this time, UAE should be reserved for patients who no longer desire fertility and wish to avoid surgery.

Magnetic Resonance-Guided Focused Ultrasound (MRgFUS)

One of the newer modalities used by interventional radiology is the use of thermoablative ultrasound energy to destroy fibroids. MRgFUS was FDA approved in 2004 and uses MRI mapping to deliver a focused ultrasound beam to fibroid tissue. The advantages of same day outpatient therapy with no incisions are appealing. However, several aspects of this time-consuming and costly procedure are yet to be elucidated. Preliminary case reports show that post-procedure pregnancy is possible, but the risk of rupture during pregnancy is unknown [21]. Another question that remains to be answered is the upper limit of fibroid size that can be ablated by this procedure. Contraindications to an MRI or Gadolinium use exclude patients from MRgFUS treatment. Side effects such as skin burns and bowel injury are possible. This is another example of a treatment modality in its infancy. Further data is needed before recommendations can be made.

Myolysis

Myolysis refers to the use of thermal, radiofrequency, or cryoablative energy to destroy fibroids. Laparoscopic radiofrequency volumetric thermal ablation (RFVTA) is now FDA approved for such use. The current technique involves 5–10 mm laparoscopic incisions; one to insert a laparoscopic ultrasound probe and another to introduce a handpiece that will deliver the energy. The fibroids are mapped with the ultrasound, and then the energy source is applied to the fibroid under ultrasound guidance. The technique has improved with the recent FDA approval of a guidance system. One prospective, single-center study concluded that RFVTA decreased intraoperative blood loss, decreased length of stay, and treated more fibroids, when compared to laparoscopic myomectomy [22]. The landmark 3-year prospective, multicenter, international trial of 135 premenopausal women demonstrated a repeat intervention rate of 11% [23]. There is also a concern for increased risk of adhesion formation. Case reports of viable term pregnancies after myolysis do exist [24]. However, some studies suggest an increased risk of uterine rupture during pregnancy [25]. Further data is needed before universally recommending myolysis as a first-line treatment.

Surgical Therapy

Surgery is the mainstay of treatment for fibroids in the gynecologic armamentarium. The benefit of surgery versus other modalities is the opportunity for pathologic evaluation of tissue to confirm a benign, atypical, or malignant pathology. Indications for surgery include heavy and/or abnormal uterine bleeding, bulk-related issues (heaviness, bloating, pain, urinary frequency), infertility, and recurrent pregnancy loss. Minimally invasive surgery is ideal due to the known benefits of decreased pain, blood loss, adhesion formation, infection, hospital stay, and superior patient satisfaction when compared to an open approach [4, 26].

Myomectomy

Myomectomy is the standard of care for women with symptomatic fibroids who desire fertility. The goal of a myomectomy is to remove fibroids while preserving the uterus. In patients desiring fertility, it is important to distinguish which fibroids to remove. Studies have shown that removal of fibroids confer a significantly higher pregnancy rate and decreased spontaneous abortion rate [2]. Post myomectomy pregnancy rates are highest in women without other identifiable infertility factors [27, 28]. The data on the removal of subserosal fibroids is mixed. Theoretically, subserosal fibroids can impinge on the fallopian tubes, cause distortion of the uterine cavity, or interfere with uterine contractility. The removal of subserosal fibroids have been shown to increase pregnancy rates however not significantly [2, 29]. Thus, consideration should be given to the removal of subserosal fibroids that present with bulk symptoms, or its position and site impact the ability to achieve pregnancy. One large case series retrospectively looked at pain and bleeding post laparoscopic myomectomy. The mean preoperative pain score decreased from 6.9 to 1.7, NSAID use dropped in 67% and hormone use in 87% in those that underwent myomectomy for pain. While 86% with preop abnormal bleeding reported no bleeding post-procedure [30]. Myomectomy is not a definitive treatment. A 33% recurrence rate at 27 months has been reported in the literature [19]. However, one can counsel patients that only about 6.7% at 5 years and 16% at 8 years require a repeat procedure [19]. The greater the number of fibroids present, the greater the risk of recurrence [31].

Hysteroscopic Myomectomy

The ideal procedure for a submucosal fibroid is a hysteroscopic myomectomy. Patients that become pregnant following hysteroscopic removal of fibroids can attempt a trial of labor as long as a transmural incision did not occur [19]. Hysteroscopic myomectomy does have risks of perforation, excessive fluid absorption, bleeding, and adhesions. However, complication rates are less than 3% [32]. In one study, 20% of hysteroscopically removed fibroids recurred, 21% required a repeat surgery at 4 years, and 0% thereafter [33]. Submucosal fibroids can be classified based upon their depth of invasion into the myometrium: Type 0 with no myometrial extension, Type I < 50%, and Type II > 50% within the myometrium [34]. The rate of complete resection depends upon fibroid type, with a greater chance of failure when attempting to remove fibroids with more myometrial involvement [35]. This explains the wide variation in success. Reports estimate that 65–100% of fibroids are completely removed at initial hysteroscopy [19].

Several hysteroscopic techniques exist for submucosal fibroid removal: resectoscopic dissection, morcellation. and vaporization. One review of the literature concludes that the monopolar wire loop resectoscope continues to be the gold standard for the removal of Type 0 fibroids [36]. However, morcellation or loop resection can be used for Type 0 or I fibroids, and loop resection is ideal for Type II. A nonionic nonconductive distension media is a necessity when using the monopolar energy absorption of which puts the patient at risk of hyponatremia. Physicians and companies are moving toward bipolar and less monopolar to reduce that fluid absorption risk. The resectoscope and vaporization carry a risk of thermal injury while the morcellator utilizes a rotary blade, thus no risk of thermal injury. Studies have shown that morcellation takes less operating time when compared to the resectoscope [37]. Vaporization of a fibroid leaves no tissue for pathologic assessment.

Laparoscopic Myomectomy

Laparoscopic myomectomy can be combined with hysteroscopic myomectomy to remove as many fibroids as possible or as a lone procedure to reduce bulk symptoms. This procedure is associated with postoperative pregnancy rates greater than 57% [38]. In patients with no other infertility factors, more than 60% of women successfully conceive after laparoscopic myomectomy [39,40]. Further, data supports a decrease in pelvic pain and a decrease in abnormal uterine bleeding following laparoscopic myomectomy [30].

As mentioned above, a minimally invasive approach is far superior to an open surgery with benefits of decreased blood loss, decreased adhesion formation, and a faster recovery with a shorter hospital stay [4, 26]. The decision to perform a laparoscopic versus open myomectomy is based upon several factors. Factors, such as the number, size, and location of fibroids, prior abdominal surgery, medical comorbidities, concern of malignancy, inability to perform morcellation secondary to hospital policy, and a surgeon's comfort level with the procedure, should be taken into account when deciding between an open versus minimally invasive approach. The most important factor is a surgeon's experience and comfort with the case. Varying operative expertise between attending physicians is the reason guidelines differ across institutions. Consideration should be given to an open case if the primary surgeon feels that operative time would be excessive, exposing a patient to prolonged anesthesia, or increased blood loss. A rule of thumb is to consider every patient a suitable candidate for laparoscopy if there is access to an experienced minimally invasive surgical team. One exception would be a rapidly enlarging uterus which is suspicious for malignancy, and intact removal of the uterus would be warranted.

Patients with a prior laparoscopic myomectomy are at risk of uterine rupture during a subsequent pregnancy, but the incidence is low (less than 1%) [29, 39, 40]. Nevertheless, ACOG recommends patients with a prior myomectomy undergo elective Cesarean delivery between 37 and 38 6/7 weeks' gestational age [41].

The use of ultrasonic energy is preferred over monopolar and especially bipolar energy due to less thermal injury to healthy tissue, but regardless of energy use, the time of energy on tissue needs to be minimal to reduce thermal tissue damage. Vertical incisions on the uterus avoid the adnexa and periuterine vessels, while horizontal incisions reduce the number of uterine vessels transected (these are pearls that apply to open procedures as well). During laparoscopic multiple myomectomy, one concern is the loss of specimen within the abdominal cavity. By introducing a Keith needle transabdominally, one can string fibroids along a suture and hold them in place until all the fibroids are removed.

Meticulous wound approximation without hematoma formation results in better wound healing and a stronger scar [39, 40]. This is why closure of multiple layers is important. In our practice, uterine defects are closed with interrupted sutures of 3–0 PDS to reapproximate the endometrium, with care taken to avoid stitches in the endometrium. A delayed absorbable 3–0 V-Loc running stitch is used for the myometrial layers to minimize dead space. A baseball stitch of 4–0 or 3–0 V-Loc is used for the serosa to minimize suture exposure in an attempt to decrease adhesion formation.

Adhesions post abdominal surgery are known to cause complications such as pain, bowel obstruction, and infertility. The purpose of adhesion barriers, like sodium hyaluronate-carboxymethylcellulose and oxidized regenerated cellulose, is to prevent adhesion formation. A retrospective cohort study of 62,563 individuals undergoing myomectomy revealed that surgeons used an adhesion barrier 5.4% of the time [42]. The same study identified a slightly increased risk of fever and ileus associated with the use of an adhesion barrier. Currently, the use of adhesion barriers for laparoscopic surgery is off-label.

Minimizing blood loss is another concern during myomectomy. Intramyometrial vasopressin injected into the incision site for each fibroid is not FDA approved to decrease blood loss during myomectomy but has been used with great success. A systematic review of the data concluded with moderate-quality evidence that vasopressin can reduce bleeding during myomectomy [43]. To minimize the risk of cardiovascular side effects, the use of a dilute solution and avoidance of intravascular injection are paramount. Intravascular injection has been known to cause vasoconstriction resulting in peripheral or myocardial ischemia, bronchial constriction, and even anaphylaxis. A cumulative total dose of 4–6 units has been suggested as an upper limit [44]. If one dilutes 20 units vasopressin in 100 mL of saline, then 20–30 mL of this dilute solution will deliver 4–6 units of vasopressin. However, the relatively short half-life of vasopressin, 10–20 min, allows repetitive doses if not all given at once. In the author's practice, the use of 30 units of vasopressin in 100 mL of saline and injections 40–80 cm^3 at a time (12–24 units) has no anatomic effect.

Laparoscopic Uterine Artery Occlusion (LUAO)

Laparoscopic uterine artery occlusion is another technique that can be performed at the time of laparoscopic myomectomy and is useful in a patient with several small fibroids. Case reports of successful pregnancy after LUAO are available, with outcomes similar to uterine artery embolization [45]. Like UAE, which is discussed below, LUAO is not recommended at this time for patients that desire fertility.

Robotic Myomectomy

Recent literature comparing robotic versus laparoscopic myomectomy has shown no significant difference in operative time, blood loss, complication rate, overnight admission, or fibroid number on postoperative ultrasound [46]. Robotic myomectomy pregnancy rates are similar to those after laparoscopy [47]. The decision to proceed with robotic versus laparoscopic myomectomy must take into account operator comfort with each modality and cost-effectiveness at that institution.

Case Conclusion

In the United States, ACOG has issued guidelines for alternatives to hysterectomy in the management of leiomyomas [19]. However, no comprehensive guidelines exist in the

United States to guide clinicians in the treatment of fibroids. At this time, due to the lack of effective medications, and the paucity of data on pregnancy following other procedures, myomectomy is the recommended treatment for women who desire to maintain their fertility. The patient presented above underwent a hysteroscopy, operative laparoscopy with myomectomy, uterine reconstruction, lysis of adnexal adhesions, excision of deep infiltrating endometriosis, morcellation in a bag, and a uterine uplift. Hysteroscopy revealed two fibroids: a Type 2 submucosal fibroid that entered the uterine cavity and a 3 cm Type 1 submucosal fibroid entering the cavity. She was advised to wait 3 months prior to getting pregnant, and then when she goes into labor, she would need a Cesarean section. She subsequently became pregnant and is currently 11 weeks gestational age.

References

1. Walker CL, Parker EA. Uterine fibroids: the elephant in the room. Science. 2005;308:1589–92.
2. Pritts EA, Parker WH, Olive DL. Fibroids and infertility: an updated systematic review of the evidence. Fertil Steril. 2009;91:1215–23.
3. Klatsky PC, Tran ND, Caughey AB, Fujimoto VY. Fibroids and reproductive outcomes: a systematic literature review from conception to delivery. Am J Obstet Gynecol. 2008;198:357–66. doi:10.1016/j.ajog.2007.12.039.
4. Miller CE. Myomectomy: comparison of open and laparoscopic techniques. Obstet Gynecol Clin N Am. 2000;27:407–20.
5. Marjoribanks J, Lethaby A, Farquhar C. Surgery versus medical therapy for heavy menstrual bleeding. Cochrane Database Syst Rev. 2006:CD003855.
6. Olive DL, Lindheim SR, Pritts EA. Non-surgical management of leiomyoma: impact on fertility. Curr Opin Obstet Gynecol. 2004;16:239–43.
7. Lethaby A, Vollenhoven B, Sowter M. Efficacy of pre-operative gonadotropin hormone releasing analogues for women with uterine fibroids undergoing hysterectomy or myomectomy: a systematic review. BJOG. 2002;109:1097–108.

8. Hickman LC, Kotlyar A, Shue S, Falcone T. Hemostatic techniques for myomectomy: an evidence-based approach. J Minim Invasive Gynecol. 2016;23(4):497–504. doi:10.1016/j.jmig.2016.01.026.

9. Zullo F, Pellicano M, De Stefano R, Zupi E, Mastrantonio P. A prospective randomized study to evaluate leuprolide acetate treatment before laparoscopic myomectomy: efficacy and ultrasonographic predictors. Am J Obstet Gynecol. 1998;178:108–12.

10. Song H, Lu D, Navaratnam K, Shi G. Aromatase inhibitors for uterine fibroids. Cochrane Database Syst Rev. 2013:CD009505. doi:10.1002/14651858.

11. Varelas FK, Papanicolaou AN, Vavatsi-Christaki N, Makedos GA, Vlassis GD. The effect of anastrazole on symptomatic uterine leiomyomata. Obstet Gynecol. 2007;110:643–9.

12. Donnez J, Tatarchuk TF, Bouchard P, Puscasiu L, Zakharenko N, Ivanova T, et al. Ulipristal acetate versus placebo for fibroid treatment before surgery. N Engl J Med. 2012;366:409–20.

13. Steinauer J, Pritts EA, Jackson R, Jacoby AF. Systematic review of mifepristone for the treatment of uterine leiomyomata. Obstet Gynecol. 2004;103:1331–6.

14. Ross RK, Pike MC, Vessey MP, et al. Risk factors for uterine fibroids: reduced risk associated with oral contraceptives. Br Med J (Clin Res Ed). 1986;293:359.

15. Moroni RM, Martins WP, Dias SV, Vieira CS, Ferriani RA, Nastri CO, et al. Combined oral contraceptive for treatment of women with uterine fibroids and abnormal uterine bleeding: a systematic review. Gynecol Obstet Investig. 2015;79:145–52.

16. Gupta JK, Sinha AS, Lumsden MA, Hickey M. Uterine artery embolization for symptomatic uterine fibroids. Cochrane Database Syst Rev. 2014:CD005073. doi:10.1002/14651858.

17. Smeets AJ, Nijenhuis RJ, Jan van Rooij W, Weimar E, Boekkooi PF, Lampmann LE, et al. Uterine artery embolization in patients with a large fibroid burden: long-term clinical and MR follow-up. Cardiovasc Intervent Radiol. 2010;33:943–8.

18. Goldberg J, Pereira L, Berghella V, Diamond J, Darai E, Seinera P, et al. Pregnancy outcomes after treatment for fibromyomata: uterine artery embolization versus laparoscopic myomectomy. Am J Obstet Gynecol. 2004;191:18–21.

19. American College of Obstetricians and Gynecologists. ACOG practice bulletin no. 96: alternatives to hysterectomy in the Management of Leiomyomas. Obstet Gynecol. 2008;112:387–400.

20. Ravina JH, Vigneron NC, Aymard A, Le Dref O, Merland JJ. Pregnancy after embolization of uterine myoma: report of 12 cases. Fertil Steril. 2000;73:1241–3.
21. Rabinovici J, David M, Fukunishi H, Marita Y, Gostout B, Stewart E. Pregnancy outcome after magnetic resonance-guided focused ultrasound surgery (MRgFUS) for conservative treatment of uterine fibroids. Fertil Steril. 2010;93:199–209.
22. Brucker S, Hahn M, Kraemer D, Taran F, Isaacson K, Kramer B. Laparoscopic radiofrequency volumetric thermal ablation of fibroids versus laparoscopic myomectomy. Int J Gynecol Obstet. 2014;125:261–5.
23. Berman J, Guido R, Garza Leal J, Pemueller R, Whaley F, Chudnoff S. Three-year outcome of the halt trial: a prospective analysis of radiofrequency volumetric thermal ablation of myomas. J Minim Invasive Gynecol. 2014;21:767–74.
24. Berman J, Bolnick JM, Pemueller RR, Garza Leal JG. Reproductive outcomes in women following radiofrequency volumetric thermal ablation of symptomatic fibroids. A retrospective case series analysis. J Reprod Med. 2015;60:194–8.
25. Arcangeli S, Pasquarette MM. Gravid uterine rupture after myolysis. Obstet Gynecol. 1997;89:857.
26. Falcone T, Parker WH. Surgical management of leiomyomas for fertility or uterine preservation. Obstet Gynecol. 2013;121:856–68.
27. Miller CE, Johnston M, Rundell M. Laparoscopic myomectomy in the infertile woman. J Am Assoc Gynecol Laparosc. 1996;3(4):525–32.
28. Samejima T, Koga K, Nakae H, Wada-Hiraike O, Fujimoto A, Fujii T, et al. Identifying patients who can improve fertility with myomectomy. Eur J Obstet Gynecol Reprod Biol. 2015;185:28–32.
29. Casini ML, Rossi F, Agostini R, Unfer V. Effect of the position of fibroids on fertility. Gynecol Endocrinol. 2006;22:106–9.
30. Hoffman MR, Johnston M, Terplan M, Smith EJ, Cholkeri-Singh A, Miller CE. Laparoscopic myomectomy for abnormal uterine bleeding and pain - preliminary results from a large case series. J Minim Invasive Gynecol. 2009; doi:10.1016/j.jmig.2009.08.182.
31. Emanuel MH, Wamsteker K, Hart AA, Metz G, Lammes FB. Long-term results of hysteroscopic myomectomy for abnormal uterine bleeding. Obstet Gynecol. 1999;93:743–8.
32. Polena V, Mergui JL, Perrot N, et al. Long-term results of hysteroscopic myomectomy in 235 patients. Eur J Obstet Gynecol Reprod Biol. 2007;130:232.

33. Hart R, Molnar BG, Magos A. Long term follow up of hysteroscopic myomectomy assessed by survival analysis. Br J Obstet Gynecol. 1999;106(7):700–5.
34. American Association of Gynecologic Laparoscopists (AAGL): Advancing Minimally Invasive Gynecology Worldwide. AAGL practice report: practice guidelines for the diagnosis and management of submucous leiomyomas. J Minim Invasive Gynecol. 2012;19:152–71. doi:10.1016/j.jmig.2011.09.005.
35. Wamsteker K, Emanuel MH, de Kruif JH. Transcervical hysteroscopic resection of submucous fibroids for abnormal uterine bleeding: results regarding the degree of intramural extension. Obstet Gynecol. 1993;82:736–40.
36. Di Spiezio Sardo A, Mazzon I, Bramante S, Bettocchi S, Bifulco G, Guida M, et al. Hysteroscopic myomectomy: a comprehensive review of surgical techniques. Hum Reprod Update. 2008;14:101–19.
37. Rubino RJ, Lukes AS. Twelve-month outcomes for patients undergoing hysteroscopic morcellation of uterine polyps and myomas in an office or ambulatory surgical center. J Minim Invasive Gynecol. 2015;22:285–90. doi:10.1016/j.jmig.2014.10.015.
38. Altgassen C, Kuss S, Berger U, Loning M, Diedrich K, Schneider A. Complications in laparoscopic myomectomy. Surg Endosc. 2006;20:614–8.
39. Dubuisson JB, Fauconnier A, Babaki-Fard K, Chapron C. Laparoscopic myomectomy: a current view. Hum Reprod Update. 2000;6:588–94.
40. Dubuisson JB, Fauconnier A, Chapron C, Kreiker G, Norgaard C. Reproductive outcome after laparoscopic myomectomy in infertile women. J Reprod Med. 2000;45:23–30.
41. American College of Obstetricians and Gynecologists. ACOG Committee opinion no. 560: medically indicated late-preterm and early-term deliveries. Obstet Gynecol. 2013;121:908–10.
42. Tulandi T, Closon F, Czuzoj-Shulman N, Abenhaim H. Adhesion barrier use after myomectomy and hysterectomy: rates and immediate postoperative complications. Obstet Gynecol. 2016;127:23–8.
43. Kongnyuy EJ, Wiysonge CS. Interventions to reduce haemorrhage during myomectomy for fibroids. Cochrane Database Syst Rev. 2011:CD005355. doi:10.1002/14651858.
44. Frishman G. Vasopressin: if some is good, is more better? Obstet Gynecol. 2009;113:476–7.

45. Holub Z, Mara M, Kuzel D, Jabor A, Maskova J, Eim J. Pregnancy outcomes after uterine artery occlusion: prospective multicentric study. Fertil Steril. 2008;90:1886–91.
46. Sasaki KJ, Cholkeri-Singh A, Sulo S, Miller CE. Comparison of laparoscopic and robotic-assisted myomectomy: operative and peri-operative results. J Minim Invasive Gynecol. 2014;21:S209.
47. Pitter MC, Gargiulo AR, Bonaventura LM, Lehman JS, Srouji SS. Pregnancy outcomes following robot-assisted myomectomy. Hum Reprod. 2012;28:99–108.

Chapter 9
The Prolapsed Myoma

Richard Guido, Mallory Stuparich, and Nash S. Moawad

Case Description

A 37-year-old patient presented to the emergency department with heavy bleeding, cramping, lightheadedness, and dizziness. She appeared pale and fatigued, with tachycardia to a heart rate of 119 bpm and normal blood pressure and temperature. Upon speculum examination, she was noted to be actively bleeding with moderate amount of blood in the vagina. She was noted to have a large fungating mass protruding from the cervical os, which was

---

The original version of this chapter was revised. An erratum to this chapter can be found at https://doi.org/10.1007/978-3-319-58780-6_20

R. Guido, MD, CIP (✉) • M. Stuparich, MD
Department of Obstetrics, Gynecology and Reproductive Sciences, University of Pittsburgh, Magee-Womens Hospital of the UPMC Health System, 300 Halket St, Pittsburgh, PA 15213, USA
e-mail: rguido@mail.magee.edu

N.S. Moawad, MD, MS, FACOG
Minimally Invasive Gynecologic Surgery, Department of Obstetrics and Gynecology, University of Florida College of Medicine, Gainesville, FL, USA
e-mail: nmoawad@ufl.edu

N.S. Moawad (ed.), *Uterine Fibroids*,
https://doi.org/10.1007/978-3-319-58780-6_9,
© Springer International Publishing AG 2018

quite dilated to about 4–5 cm. The cervical rim itself appeared normal without focal lesions. On bimanual examination, the uterus was enlarged to approximately10 weeks in size, and was difficult to assess due to the likely prolapsed mass. No Pap or endometrial biopsy was obtainable in the presence of the mass.

The patient was noted to be very anemic with hemoglobin of six and required admission to the hospital and transfusion of 3 units of packed red blood cells. The patient reported she has been suffering with heavy bleeding for 6 weeks, along with severe pelvic cramping pain and dyspareunia.

The patient has had a hysteroscopic myomectomy of a large submucosal fibroid 4 years prior. She was to have a staged procedure but felt better after 75% of the fibroid was resected during the initial myomectomy and elected not to have the second procedure. She tried hormonal management of the irregular heavy periods, using oral progesterone that did not adequately control her symptoms and caused emotional side effects. She subsequently had a levonorgestrel IUD placed, and her symptoms were much better for 1 year, when she had a heavy period and the IUD was expelled. Her bleeding has gotten progressively worse since then.

Her pelvic ultrasound showed an enlarged uterus that measured $10.4 \times 6.5 \times 6.4$ cm. Multiple uterine fibroids were noted, including a 2.5 cm submucosal fibroid in the posterior uterine fundus and a subserosal posterior uterine fibroid measuring up to 2.5 cm. A posterior lower uterine segment fibroid measured up to 4.3 cm (Fig. 9.1). Endometrial thickness was 10 mm. The ovaries appeared normal on ultrasound.

Due to the patient's significant anemia, the decision was made to defer surgical intervention until her anemia has been corrected. The patient received Lupron 3.75 mg IM and was discharged home on daily Provera 40 mg.

The patient's bleeding slightly improved but persisted. She was seen in the office for follow-up, where the decision was made to perform a vaginal myomectomy in an attempt to improve the bleeding.

After a comprehensive discussion of the risks and benefits of the procedure, and the acceptable alternatives, an informed consent was obtained. The vagina and cervix were prepped

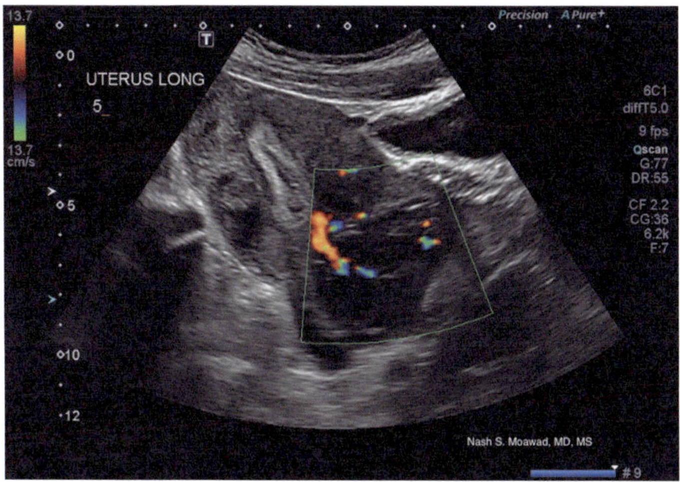

FIGURE 9.1 Transabdominal ultrasound showed a 10-week size uterus with multiple fibroids, the largest of which was a 4.3 cm pedunculated submucosal fibroid arising from the lower uterine segment

with betadine. Three successive Polysorb Endoloops® (Ethicon Inc., Somerville, NJ) were placed as high up into the uterine cavity as possible, around the mass. Bleeding was well controlled and the mass appeared pale. The mass was truncated with scissors. A large, 6 × 5 × 4 cm mass was removed (Fig. 9.2). Excellent hemostasis was noted. Silver nitrate was applied to the stalk for added security.

The patient tolerated the procedure well and blood loss was minimal. The specimen was submitted to pathology and was confirmed to be a degenerating leiomyoma partially coated with benign endometrium. Focal areas of cystic degeneration, myxoid degeneration, hemorrhage, and infarct-type necrosis were noted. No coagulative tumor cell necrosis was noted.

The patient did well on follow-up, and she subsequently underwent cervical cytology screening and an endometrial biopsy after the cervix has restituted and appeared fairly normal. The Pap test showed no evidence of intraepithelial

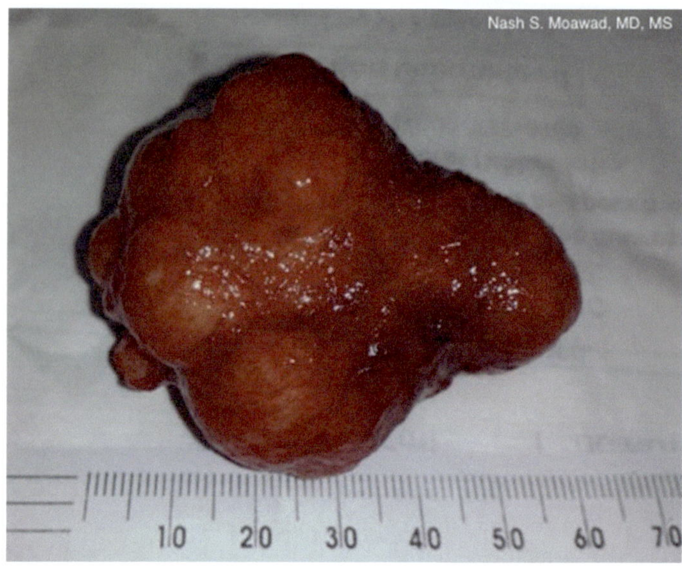

FIGURE 9.2 A large pedunculated prolapsed submucosal myoma was resected

lesions or malignancy and was negative for high-risk HPV. The endometrial biopsy showed benign endometrium with chronic endometritis. The patient was treated with antibiotics and reported her bleeding has significantly improved.

Discussion

Uterine fibroids are one of the most common benign tumors of women. It is estimated between 50 and 70% of women in the reproductive age will experience fibroids. Most patients are asymptomatic. The symptoms a patient experiences depend upon the location of her fibroids. Submucosal fibroids can produce significant bleeding symptoms and constitute 15–20% of all fibroids [1]. Submucosal fibroids can be classi- fied by the amount of the fibroid that protrudes into the uterine cavity. Type 0 fibroids are entirely in the uterine cavity, type 1 have more than 50% in the uterine cavity, and type 2 fibroids have less than or equal to 50% in the uterine cavity. Uterine contractions over time can elongate the attachment of fibroids resulting in the eventual prolapse of a fibroid through the cervical canal. Prolapsed uterine fibroids have been found in up to 3.8% of women undergoing surgery for fibroids [2].

Most women (90%) with a prolapsed uterine fibroid have symptoms, while a few women may be identified on physical examinations that are asymptomatic. Vaginal bleeding is seen in 70–84% of women [2, 3]. Symptomatic women can experience menometrorrhagia, menorrhagia, or postmenopausal bleeding. Women may also experience abdominal cramping or weakness and up to 42.8% may be anemic [2]. The presence of the fibroid in the vagina can produce a pressure sensation, vaginal discharge, or in rare circumstances voiding dysfunction.

Women who have symptomatic fibroids frequently have multiple fibroids resulting in enlargement of the uterus. In one of the larger series describing women treated for prolapsed fibroid, 59% of the women had a uterus greater than 10-week size, and 65% of the women had a prolapsed fibroid greater than 3 cm [3]. Rarely, a prolapsed fibroid has been reported as large as 3.5 kg [4].

The differential diagnosis of a mass protruding from the cervix includes a fibroid emanating from the uterine cavity or the cervix, uterine polyp, cervical polyp, cervical cancer, endometrial adenocarcinoma, endometrial stromal sarcoma, adenosarcoma, and leiomyosarcoma. It is often difficult to assess the nature of a prolapsed mass as the process of prolapsing through the cervix with the resulting restriction of blood flow due to elongation of the stalk results in ischemic necrosis. Clinical management should await final pathology as intraoperative frozen section diagnosis is challenging in the setting of necrosis.

The physical examination of the patient with a prolapsed uterine fibroid typically results in the correct diagnosis.

Speculum placement may be very difficult in such patients, as the fibroid may obstruct the vaginal canal and the cervix is often not visible. Depending on the size and location of the fibroid, it may not be possible to identify or palpate the entire cervix. If the fibroid is small and does not completely obscure the cervix, it may be possible to reduce the fibroid and thereby identify if it originates from the cervix or the uterine cavity. It is not uncommon, however, for the fibroid to be greater than 3 cm and prevent adequate assessment of the cervical anatomy.

Prolapsed uterine fibroids may originate from the uterine cavity, cervix, or lower uterine segment. Depending on the length of time, the fibroid has been prolapsed the elongated stalk to the uterus may be very long, with the longest reported case being 76 cm [5]. This unusual case was notable for the fact that the prolapsed section of the fibroid originated not directly from the endometrial cavity or cervix but from a 6 cm submucosal fibroid. Fibroids often have multiple small fibroids contained within an outer capsule. In this case the prolapsing portion was only one part of the fibroid.

Management

Patients that have prolapsing fibroids will require surgical intervention; therefore, it is important to image the uterus to completely investigate the uterine anatomy for surgical planning. Clinically it is very helpful to assess the entire uterus so as to provide accurate counseling to the patient regarding the ability of the planned procedure to alleviate the patient's symptoms. The objective of imaging is to identify the origin of the fibroid for surgical planning as well as evaluate the entire uterus for the overall fibroid burden. A pelvic ultrasound is the most cost-effective first step in the evaluation. If the ultrasound does not provide adequate information, a pelvic MRI can provide greater detail of the uterine anatomy. A soft tissue stalk connecting a cervical mass to the uterine cavity identified on MRI has been termed the "broccoli sign." This finding is not specific to a prolapsed fibroid and has been associated with endometrioid adenocarcinoma, carcinosarcoma, and adenosarcoma [6].

Management of a prolapsed uterine fibroid is generally successful with minimal complications. The success rate for vaginal myomectomy ranges from 70 to 96.6% in two large series [2, 3]. Generally, the success rate approaches 100% in women when the fibroid is <5 cm. Caglar's series included 40 women with prolapsed fibroids ≥5 cm, where 30% underwent a hysterectomy. It is not clear if this was due to patient and clinician choice or technical difficulties with the procedure. The majority of women treated by excision will require no further intervention; however, up to 13.7% of women undergo a hysterectomy following a vaginal myomectomy at some future time [3]. In a retrospective series of 46 women treated for prolapsed uterine fibroid, 43 of 46 were successfully treated at initial presentation, with the three failures requiring abdominal procedures, two for very large fibroids. Long-term follow-up with a median of 5.5 years demonstrated that 8.9% of the patients required a repeat vaginal myomectomy and 5.9% underwent a hysterectomy [7].

Surgical excision can be conducted either in the operating room or the office. The decision to treat in the office or the operating room is dependent on several factors: the comfort level of the surgeon, the size of the fibroid, the position of the fibroid, the width of the stalk, the support in the office, and the ability of the patient to tolerate the procedure. In general, an office procedure should be conducted when the size of the fibroid is <4 cm, the stalk is palpable, the physician feels comfortable with the approach and has appropriate support in the office, and the patient has adequate pelvic exposure. If the clinical situation is not ideal for an office procedure, the patient should be taken to the operating room. The majority of these procedures can be done with IV sedation and local anesthetic. General anesthesia may be required depending on the medical history of the patient and the nature of the prolapsed fibroid.

The majority of vaginal myomectomies can be accomplished by exposure and ligation of the stalk. Exposure of the stalk is dependent on the length and width of the stalk, along with the degree of dilation of the cervix and the origin of the fibroid. Those fibroids where the stalk can be accessed easily can be ligated by placing a clamp across the stalk followed by suture ligation. Access to the stalk is improved by placing a single tooth clamp in the fibroid and applying gentle traction. Care must be taken to avoid excessive traction that may result in evulsion of the fibroid. It is unlikely that evulsion will result in significant bleeding, as only 10% of women required suturing of the stalk to treat excessive bleeding when rotation and evulsion was used as the primary technique [7]. It is not uncommon for access to the stalk to be difficult. In these settings, a pre-tied suture such as an Endoloop® (Ethicon Inc., Somerville, NJ) can be placed over the fibroid to access the stalk that is not accessible by direct visualization. The loop can be used to try to strangulate the stalk, followed by sharp dissection to release the fibroid. The use of vasoconstrictive agents can also be injected into the fibroid before the ligation process to further reduce the chance of blood loss during the procedure. If the stalk is not readily accessible, it is possible to perform a vaginal myomectomy by making an incision in the capsule of the fibroid and using traditional surgical techniques typically used during abdominal myomectomy to debulk the fibroid. This should be conducted with a vasoactive agent and will lead to access to the stalk of the fibroid that can then be ligated. This technique can also be used to address a fibroid with a wide base or those emanating from the cervix. Enlarging the cervix to allow access to the stalk can be achieved by making incisions in the cervix at 2, 6, and 10:00 o'clock (Dührssen's incisions) [1]. Rarely, in situations where there is excessive bleeding or sepsis, the fibroid has been pushed back into the uterine cavity with closure of the cervix followed by an abdominal hysterectomy [8].

Following the removal of the fibroid, the surgeon may use hysteroscopy to evaluate the origin of the stalk and the inside of the uterine cavity. This step may not be necessary depending on the specific clinical situation. There are also a number of challenges to doing hysteroscopy following a vaginal myomectomy. The cervix is dilated, and therefore expanding the uterine cavity may be difficult and require clamping the cervix to allow for distention. If there is a substantial portion of the stalk remaining and it is physically possible to remove it, then resection can be conducted using electrical loop or mechanical morcellating devices.

There has been a variety of case reports describing unusual clinical situations associated with prolapsed uterine fibroids. Prolapsed uterine fibroids associated with pregnancy have had mixed result with regard to the ability to successfully remove the fibroid and successfully maintain the pregnancy. Care must be undertaken when assessing the treatment of a prolapsed fibroid in pregnancy. MRI is recommended to fully assess the origin and nature of the fibroid, as determining the location of the fibroid by clinical exam may be challenging as the cervix is very soft during pregnancy. Close observation is recommended unless the fibroid represents an immediate health risk for bleeding, infection, or urinary retention. If the fibroid is asymptomatic and it appears that the fibroid will obstruct delivery, a C-section is advised. Case reports of vaginal myomectomy for prolapsed fibroid emanating from either the cervix or the endometrial canal have described either successful treatment with subsequent uneventful delivery or PROM and miscarriage [9, 10]. Consultation with an experienced gynecologist and a maternal fetal medicine specialist is recommended in any prolapsed fibroid in pregnancy.

Rare cases of prolapsed fibroids resulting in a uterine inversion that required removal of the fibroid and potentially a hysterectomy have been described. These clinical situations require expertise in dealing with complicated surgical cases as well as extensive individualized counseling with the patient [11].

In summary, prolapsed uterine fibroids represent a small percentage of fibroids; however, given the high frequency of fibroids in the general population, most obstetrician/gynecologists will encounter this clinical situation in their career. It is important to perform a full history and careful physical examination before embarking on therapy. It is important to image the uterus to assess the location of the fibroid and its attachment to the uterus as well as the fibroid burden when planning treatment. The majority of patients can undergo a vaginal myomectomy with good results. The patient should be counselled about the procedure, the rate of success, and the possibility of a hysterectomy. Each clinical situation should be individualized to best serve the patient.

References

1. Parker WH, Barbieri RL, Sharp HT. Prolapsed uterine fibroid. In J.A. Melin (ed.), Up to date. Retrieved June 1 2017, From http://www.uptodate.com/Contents/Prolapsed-Uterine-lecomyoma-fibroid
2. Caglar GS, Tasci Y, Kayikcioglu F. Management of prolapsed pedunculated myomas. Int J Gynaecol Obstet. 2005;89(2):146–7.
3. Golan A, Zachalka N, Lurie S, Sagiv R, Glezerman M. Vaginal removal of prolapsed pedunculated submucous myoma: a short, simple, and definitive procedure with minimal morbidity. Arch Gynecol Obstet. 2005;271(1):11–3.
4. Ikechebelu JI, Eleje GU, Okpala BC, Onyiaorah IV, Umeobika JC, Onyegbule OA, Ejikeme BT. Vaginal myomectomy of a prolapsed gangrenous cervical leiomyoma. Niger J Clin Pract. 2012;15(3):358–60.
5. Usta IM, Hobeika EM, Nassar AH. A tale of 2 pedunculated myomas. Am J Obstet Gynecol. 2005;193(5):1753–5.
6. Jha P, Chang ST, Rabban JT, Chen LM, Yeh BM, Coakley FV. Utility of the broccoli sign in the distinction of prolapsed uterine tumor from cervical tumor. Eur J Radiol. 2012;81(8):1931–6.
7. Ben-Baruch G, Schiff E, Menashe Y, Menczer J. Immediate and late outcome of vaginal myomectomy for prolapsed pedunculated submucous myoma. Obstet Gynecol. 1988;72(6):858–61.
8. Brooks GG, Stage AH. The surgical management of prolapsed pedunculated submucous leiomyomas. Surg Gynecol Obstet. 1975;141(3):397–8.

9. Kilpatrick CC, Adler MT, Chohan L. Vaginal myomectomy in pregnancy: a report of two cases. South Med J. 2010;103(10):1058–60.
10. Obara M, Hatakeyama Y, Shimizu Y. Vaginal myomectomy for semipedunculated cervical Myoma during pregnancy. AJP Rep. 2014;4(1):37–40.
11. Pieh-Holder KL, Bell H, Hall T, DeVente JE. Postpartum prolapsed leiomyoma with uterine inversion managed by vaginal hysterectomy. Case Rep Obstet Gynecol. 2014;2014:435101. doi:10.1155/2014/435101.

Chapter 10
The Fibroid with Red Flags!

Kristine Zanotti and Randi Shae Connor

A 33-year-old nulliparous patient who desires fertility presents with a 6-month history of deep dyspareunia. She reports a history of renal cell carcinoma and heavy periods but is otherwise healthy. Her exam is significant for multiple cutaneous nodules and a mildly enlarged uterus. Pelvic ultrasound shows a 7 cm lower uterine segment subserosal fibroid.

K. Zanotti, MD (✉)
Division of Gynecologic Oncology, Department of Obstetrics and Gynecology, University Hospitals Cleveland Medical Center, 11100 Euclid Ave, Cleveland, OH 44106, USA
e-mail: Kristin.Zanotti@uhhospitals.org

R.S. Connor, MD
Department of Gynecologic Oncology, University Hospitals Seidman Cancer Center, 11100 Euclid Ave,
Cleveland, OH 44106, USA
e-mail: randi.connor@uhhospitals.org

N.S. Moawad (ed.), *Uterine Fibroids*,
https://doi.org/10.1007/978-3-319-58780-6_10,
© Springer International Publishing AG 2018

Epidemiology

As the debate over power morcellation in gynecologic surgery has swelled in recent years, the risk of occult malignancy in women with presumed leiomyomata has become the subject of intense scrutiny and clinical research. Still, the available scientific data is incomplete, and many experts disagree about the optimal evaluation and management of this common benign condition, given the relatively small risk of a rare cancer. It is clear, however, that the possibility of an occult sarcoma should be considered when weighing medical and surgical treatment options for patients with fibroids. Clinicians should understand the risk of malignancy in meaningful terms, be able to identify possible risk factors, appreciate the utility and limitations of diagnostic testing, and individualize treatment based on a comprehensive interpretation of the clinical scenario.

Uterine sarcomas are rare, accounting for fewer than 8% of all uterine cancers [1, 2]. Furthermore, histologic criteria have evolved in recent decades, making it difficult to determine the true prevalence and histologic distribution of these uncommon malignancies. Although carcinosarcoma was previously classified as a mesenchymal tumor, it is now widely considered a high-grade carcinoma, which is reflected in the revised 2009 FIGO staging system [3]. When carcinosarcomas are excluded, leiomyosarcomas account for more than two-thirds of uterine sarcomas [2]. Although they can be difficult to distinguish from leiomyomas preoperatively, leiomyosarcomas do not usually result from malignant transformation of benign fibroids but rather arise de novo. Despite the fact that most leiomyosarcomas are confined to the uterus at the time of diagnosis, these cancers have a remarkably poor prognosis. Five-year overall survival for stage I disease is only 57%, and that number drops precipitously with advancing stage [4].

Women with leiomyosarcomas tend to be slightly younger than patients with endometrial cancers, with the median reported ages ranging from 48 to 57 years [2, 4–7]. The incidence of leiomyosarcoma is higher in African Americans than in white women, although the racial disparity is not as great as that seen in uterine carcinosarcoma; the reported age-adjusted incidence of leiomyosarcoma is 1.5 per 100,000 for black women, compared to 0.9 per 100,000 for white women [8]. More than half of patients present with abnormal vaginal bleeding (53%), followed closely by an abdominopelvic mass (48%) and pain (23%) [2]. Rapid uterine enlargement, arbitrarily defined by various criteria, has historically been considered a possible sign of underlying malignancy; however, numerous retrospective reviews have suggested that this conjecture is likely inaccurate [9, 10]. The rate of sarcoma in women identified as having rapid uterine enlargement is actually quite low, ranging from 0.27 to 2.6% across studies [9, 11].

Grossly, leiomyosarcoma is usually a solitary, poorly circumscribed, fleshy intramural mass with its epicenter located within the myometrium [2]. Areas of necrosis and hemorrhage are common. Microscopically, leiomyosarcomas are characterized by tumor cell necrosis, cytologic atypia, and abundant mitoses [2, 9].

Risk Factors

In addition to age and race, several other risk factors for uterine sarcomas have been identified, including postmenopausal status, hormonal exposure, and hereditary predisposition [2]. Although prior pelvic radiation increases the risk of developing carcinosarcoma, it is not considered a risk factor for leiomyosarcoma [2, 12]. A recent analysis of data from the Finnish Cancer Registry found a significant association between combination hormone replacement therapy and elevated risk of leiomyosarcoma; in the study of 243,857 women, use of estradiol-progestin combination therapy for 5 years or more was associated with an 80% increase in the risk for leiomyosarcoma (standardized incidence ratio (SIR), 1.8; 95% CI, 1.3–2.4) [13]. Despite an elevated relative risk, however, the absolute risk of uterine sarcomas is still exceedingly low. The authors of the Finnish study concluded that there is an absolute risk of two to three additional uterine sarcoma cases per 10,000 long-term estradiol-progestin users [13]. A possible association between tamoxifen therapy for breast cancer and subsequent carcinosarcoma has also been suggested [14, 15], but tamoxifen has not been implicated as a risk factor for leiomyosarcoma.

Genetic predisposition to uterine sarcomas has been suggested, but the risk of leiomyosarcoma attributed to certain hereditary syndromes is still unclear. Although Lynch syndrome is typically associated with endometrial carcinomas, a recent analysis of 164 families in the Danish HNPCC-register suggests a possible association with leiomyosarcoma as well [16]. It has also been postulated that women with hereditary retinoblastoma have an elevated risk of uterine leiomyosarcoma, which increases dramatically with age [17]. The patient depicted at the beginning of this chapter has findings consistent with hereditary leiomyomatosis and renal cell carcinoma (HLRCC), which should raise concern for the possibility of an underlying sarcoma. HLRCC is a recently described tumor predisposition syndrome caused by heterozygous germline mutations in the fumarate hydratase (*FH*) gene on chromosome 1q [18, 19]. The syndrome is characterized by benign cutaneous and uterine leiomyomas, renal cell carcinoma, and uterine leiomyosarcomas. One recent study reported a 71-fold increased risk of uterine leiomyosarcoma compared to the general population [19]. The predilection primarily affected younger patients, with the excess risk being concentrated in the 15–29 and 30–44 years age groups [19].

Preoperative Diagnosis

The true incidence of leiomyosarcoma in women with presumed fibroids has been the subject of much debate in recent years, largely due to concern about the potential dissemination of malignant tissue when power morcellation is used in minimally invasive gynecologic surgery. In November 2014, the US Food and Drug Administration (FDA) released recommendations to curtail the use of power morcellators in women undergoing hysterectomy or myomectomy for presumed fibroids, citing an incidence of occult sarcoma of 1 in 350 in this population [20]. Many authors have raised concerns about the quality of data used by the FDA to reach these conclusions and suggested that the incidence of occult malignancy is actually much lower [10, 21–26]. The best available data from a recent meta-analysis suggests the rate of occult sarcoma in women undergoing surgery for fibroids is closer to 1 in 2000 [22], although that data is imperfect as well. Both the American Congress of Obstetricians and Gynecologists (ACOG) and the Society of Gynecologic Oncology (SGO) have issued statements questioning the FDA's research methodology, disputing the Administration's conclusions regarding incidence and risk and advocating for the continued responsible use of morcellation in gynecologic surgery [10, 26].

This professional and public debate is fueled by the unfortunate reality that diagnosing leiomyosarcoma preoperatively is inherently difficult. There are no reliable serum tumor markers for uterine sarcoma [2] nor are there any imaging modalities that can definitively distinguish leiomyosarcoma from benign uterine tumors [10]. The pretest probability of any diagnostic test is directly related to the prevalence of disease in the population; because uterine leiomyosarcoma is rare, even in women with presumed leiomyomas, the pretest probability of detecting it with conventional means is necessarily limited. There are, however, several tools the clinician can use to estimate the risk of occult sarcoma preoperatively and proceed with management in the safest manner possible.

First, a thorough assessment of the patient's history and risk factors should be completed, with particular attention given to increasing age, postmenopausal status, prior hormone use or radiation exposure, and evidence of hereditary cancer syndromes. ACOG has issued guidance to clinicians recommending that women at risk for Lynch syndrome or HLRCC not undergo surgery involving morcellation due to their increased risk of malignancy [10]. Secondly, the preoperative evaluation for a woman with abnormal uterine bleeding should include current cervical cytology and endometrial sampling, and consideration should be given to pelvic imaging. Cervical cytology is important to exclude cervical pathology, and it may occasionally detect endometrial carcinoma or preinvasive disease. In one small series, the presence of atypical endometrial cells on cytology had a modest positive predictive value of 50% for endometrial cancer [27]. Leiomyosarcoma and other uterine sarcomas, however, are highly unlikely to be detected by Pap smear alone. Similarly, endometrial sampling by office pipelle or dilation and curettage has excellent sensitivity for detecting endometrial carcinomas (95–97.5% in symptomatic women), but rather low sensitivity in the diagnosis of leiomyosarcoma [11]. The reported sensitivity for detecting leiomyosarcoma on endometrial biopsy is approximately 35% [28, 29], and it depends greatly on tumor location. In one study, all of the leiomyosarcomas identified by preoperative biopsy were submucosal in location [29].

Pelvic ultrasound is often the first step in the assessment of gynecologic symptoms, but its usefulness in identifying uterine sarcomas is limited. Color Doppler has been evaluated as a potential adjunct to gray-scale ultrasonography in the preoperative diagnosis of leiomyosarcoma, but the available studies are small and results are inconsistent. An early report by Kurjak et al. compared color Doppler findings prior to planned hysterectomy in 2010 women, ten of whom were later diagnosed with uterine sarcoma on final pathology. All of the leiomyosarcoma cases were associated with abnormal blood vessels, demonstrating a significantly lower resistance index (RI) than those of normal or myomatous uteri. Using a cutoff point of 0.40 for RI, the researchers were able to distinguish leiomyosarcoma from benign myometrial tumors with a sensitivity of 90.91%, specificity of 99.82%, positive predictive value of 71.43%, and negative predictive value of 99.96% [30]. Unfortunately, these findings have not proven reproducible. In a study of 111 women, 98 with confirmed leiomyomas, six with leiomyosarcoma, and seven with carcinosarcoma, Aviram et al. observed a significant difference between the mean RI of leiomyoma (0.59 ± 0.01) and carcinosarcoma (0.41 ± 0.06) ($p < 0.001$), but no difference between leiomyoma and leiomyosarcoma (0.49 ± 0.18) [31]. Hata et al. were also unable to detect a significant difference in RI between benign and malignant processes but noted that the peak systolic velocity (PSV) was significantly higher in uterine sarcomas than in leiomyomas. Using a cutoff value for PSV that was two standard deviations greater than the mean PSV observed in benign fibroids, the detection rate for uterine sarcomas was 80.0%, with a false-positive rate of 2.4% [32]. In contrast, Szabó et al. found that mean RI and pulsatility index (PI) were significantly lower, and intratumoral PSV was significantly higher in uterine sarcomas than leiomyomas, but noted that these findings were also present in benign leiomyomas that demonstrated large size and/or necrotic, degenerative, or inflammatory changes. Using a cutoff value of 0.5 for RI, the detection rate for uterine sarcoma in that study was only 67%, and the false-positive rate was 11.8% [33]. Furthermore, given the small sample sizes in each of these studies, even positive results are difficult to extrapolate to the general population. While ultrasound findings may increase one's suspicion of a malignant process, they cannot be relied on to diagnosis leiomyosarcoma definitively.

Pelvic MRI offers superior anatomic detail compared to ultrasound and has therefore been the focus of much research. Findings suggestive of leiomyosarcoma on magnetic resonance imaging include areas of low attenuation suggestive of hemorrhage or necrosis, irregular or poorly defined margins, lack of calcifications, and tissue heterogeneity [11]. An early study by Schwartz et al. demonstrated 100% sensitivity, specificity, positive predictive value, and negative predictive value for differentiating uterine sarcoma from benign tumors using conventional MRI [34]. That study, however, included only four cases of leiomyosarcoma and has not been reproduced. Other studies have reported sensitivities and specificities ranging from 56% to 100% and 88% to 100%, respectively [35–37]. Of note, most studies have evaluated the ability of MRI to differentiate clearly benign lesions from either leiomyosarcomas or smooth muscle tumors of uncertain malignant potential (STUMPs), even though the natural history and prognosis of STUMPs are far different from those of leiomyosarcoma. A recent study from the University of Michigan determined that leiomyosarcoma could not be accurately diagnosed by either ultrasound or conventional MRI [38].

Contrast-enhanced (CE) and diffusion-weighted (DWI) MRI, however, have emerged as superior diagnostic tools. Tanka et al. described well-demarcated unenhanced pocket-like areas on CE-MRI suggestive of leiomyosarcoma or STUMP. Although the study included only nine leiomyosarcomas and three STUMPs, the results are particularly important because these tumors were compared to 12 clinically suspicious cases, in which gynecologists expressed high preoperative suspicion for leiomyosarcomas. Overall, the authors reported an accuracy of 87%, sensitivity of 73%, and a specificity of 100% for CE-MRI [35]. Several studies have investigated the use of DWI to differentiate benign from malignant uterine tumors [36, 39, 40], suggesting that intravenous administration of gadolinium contrast medium may be unnecessary. A recent study in Taiwan compared CE-MRI and DWI in a consecutive cohort of eight LMS/STUMP cases and 25 benign leiomyomas and found that CE-MRI yielded a significantly higher specificity (0.96 vs. 0.35) and greater diagnostic accuracy (0.94 vs. 0.52) than DWI ($p < 0.05$) while maintaining similar sensitivity [41]. The authors noted, however, that combining DWI and apparent diffusion coefficient (ADC) values achieved a comparable diagnostic accuracy to that of CE-MRI.

DWI is based on differences in the motion of water molecules between tissues. The degree of restriction to water diffusion is inversely related to tissue cellularity and the integrity of cell membranes; therefore, water molecule diffusion is more restricted in tumor tissue, which has a high cellular density associated with numerous intact cell membranes [37]. This type of imaging can be performed quickly within a few minutes, does not require administration of intravenous contrast, and provides both qualitative and quantitative information that can be used to evaluate tumor characteristics. Qualitatively, malignant tumors appear as areas of heterogeneous hyperintensity on DWI (Fig. 10.1) [41].

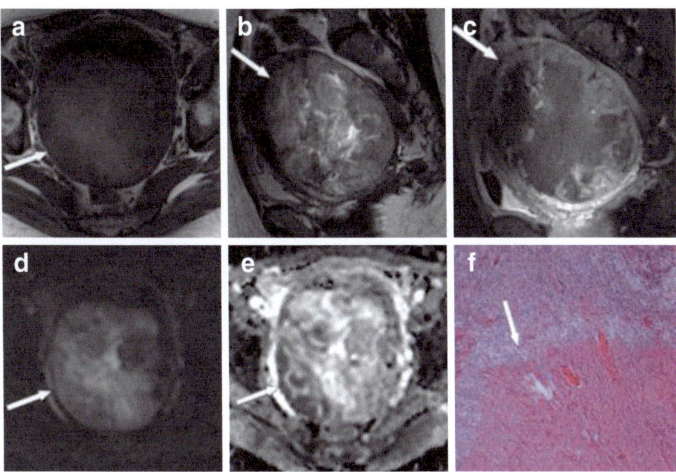

FIGURE 10.1 Lin G, Yang L, Huang Y, et al. Comparison of the diagnostic accuracy of contrast-enhanced MRI and diffusion-weighted MRI in the differentiation between uterine leiomyosarcoma/smooth muscle tumor with uncertain malignant potential and benign leiomyoma. *J Magn Reson Imaging*. 2016;43:333–342

Varying the gradient amplitude, or "b value," can further characterize a mass; often the necrotic center of a malignant tumor will demonstrate attenuation of signal intensity with increasing b values due to less cellularity and less restricted water diffusion, while the outer rim of the mass, which is more cellular, shows little attenuation [37]. Calculating the ADC value allows for quantitative assessment of tumor properties. In general, ADCs are lower for leiomyosarcomas than for leiomyomas, but there is not yet consensus regarding an optimal cutoff value to distinguish benign from malignant uterine tumors [36, 37, 39–41]. The available literature supports the use of ADC values for discriminating benign from malignant uterine tumors with a sensitivity of 1.00, specificity of 0.94–1.00, positive predictive value of 0.67, negative predictive value of 1.00, and diagnostic accuracy of 0.92–0.95 [37, 40, 42]. It should be noted, however, that due to the rarity of uterine sarcomas, all of the available studies include small sample sizes and heterogeneous histopathologies. It is difficult to define an optimal cutoff value for ADC because the various studies reported considerable overlap between ADC values for leiomyosarcomas and those for benign leiomyomas with atypical features, such as increased cellularity or degeneration. Furthermore, it is unclear if the reported diagnostic accuracy would translate into the general population due to the variable experience and expertise of radiologists in the community setting.

Some have advocated for the use of serum lactate dehydrogenase (LDH) as a potential serum biomarker for distinguishing uterine sarcomas from benign tumors, particularly as an adjunct to MR imaging [2, 11, 43]. LDH is often elevated in leiomyosarcoma due to coagulative necrosis of tumor cells. Goto et al. compared CE-MRI alone to CE-MRI combined with serum LDH assessment in a prospective trial of 140 patients, ten with confirmed leiomyosarcoma and 130 with benign leiomyomas. The investigators found that combining CE-MRI and serum LDH offered superior diagnostic accuracy. The reported sensitivity for each modality was 100%, but the specificity, positive predictive value, negative predictive value, and diagnostic accuracy increased from 93.8%, 83.3%, 100%, and 95.2%, respectively, with CE-MRI alone to 100% across the board with the combination of CE-MRI and LDH [43].

Treatment Options

The goals of treating any human disease are to prolong life and alleviate symptoms while minimizing treatment-related morbidity and mortality. When a woman presents with a symptomatic uterine mass, this necessarily involves the reasonable exclusion of life-threatening malignancy. Although most patients are eager for expeditious symptom relief, all management options must be weighed in terms of potential risks and likelihood of benefit.

Expectant management is always an option for women with minimally symptomatic uterine fibroids, but there is no data to inform the expectant management of uterine sarcoma. The presence of metastatic disease at the time of diagnosis is an important prognostic indicator for patients with leiomyosarcoma. Although still poor, patients with disease confined to the uterus have the best overall survival [4]; therefore, expectant management of presumed fibroids carries the inherent risk of delaying diagnosis of malignancy. Furthermore, hysterectomy with surgical cytoreduction is the only intervention that has ever been proven to improve survival in uterine leiomyosarcoma [44]. Although previously advocated by some experts, serial imaging to exclude a rapidly enlarging uterine mass is not helpful since the incidence of sarcoma in these patients is actually not increased [45]. The absolute risk of delayed diagnosis is unclear since there is no data on the risk of progression based on tumor characteristics such as lesion size or growth rate.

Over the last two decades, conservative management of symptomatic fibroids with selective uterine artery embolization (UAE) has become increasingly popular, and there are several published case reports of women who have been subsequently diagnosed with leiomyosarcoma after undergoing UAE for presumed leiomyomas [46–48]. The true incidence of uterine sarcoma in women undergoing UAE is impossible to determine, but it is reasonable to assume that it is similar to women undergoing myomectomy or hysterectomy for presumed fibroids. It is unclear how embolization of an occult sarcoma affects the tumor's potential for growth and dissemination, but UAE certainly delays diagnosis. One review of the available case reports suggested a mean diagnostic delay of 8 months (range 1 day to 15 months) and noted that younger patients were more likely to experience longer delays [46]. All of the women in that review presented with continued abnormal uterine bleeding in the months following their procedures; therefore, it is reasonable to consider early failure of UAE an indication for further evaluation as it may be suggestive of occult malignancy.

Similarly, there are multiple case reports of leiomyosarcomas inadvertently treated with leuprolide acetate [49–51]. Over 40% of leiomyosarcomas express estrogen and progesterone receptors [52]; therefore they may initially respond to the hypoestrogenic effects of gonadotropin-releasing hormone analogues in a fashion similar to leiomyomas. One case report identified similar microscopic degenerative and vascular changes such as hyalinization, fibrosis, and narrowing of blood vessel lumens as those seen in leuprolide-treated benign leiomyomas [51]. In each of the reported cases, surgical management was eventually indicated due to treatment failure [49–51]. Again, the greatest risk associated with medical management is likely diagnostic delay. Continued or increased vaginal bleeding, worsening pelvic pain, or increasing uterine size while receiving treatment with leuprolide acetate should prompt concern for a possible undiagnosed malignancy.

Myomectomy is often considered the definitive treatment option for women with symptomatic leiomyoma who wish to retain their fertility. The dissemination of uterine tissue, both benign and malignant, has long been recognized as a potential complication of myomectomy. Leiomyomatosis, or the dissemination of benign tissue fragments, has been observed in open and laparoscopic myomectomies both with and without morcellation, and there is no data to describe a difference in incidence between the two modalities [53]. One can reasonably infer that malignant tissue is disseminated in a similar fashion following myomectomy. The impact of tumor morcellation at the time of either myomectomy or hysterectomy has been the subject of much debate in recent years. Unfortunately, the data is difficult to interpret due to the rarity of occult malignancy and the heterogeneous nature of surgical interventions performed in various studies. For example, one of the largest studies available reviewed 56 cases of early stage leiomyosarcoma, 25 of which underwent some form of tumor morcellation and 31 of which had intact specimen removal. Park et al. concluded that tumor morcellation of occult sarcoma increased the rate of abdominopelvic dissemination and negatively affected disease-free (40% vs. 65%) and overall (46% vs. 73%) survival at 5 years [5]. In that analysis, however, no distinctions were made among the variety of surgical procedures, including transvaginal coring with a scalpel and myomectomy with minilaparotomy. Although much interest has focused on the dangers of power morcellation, it is likely that only one case of power morcellation was included in Park's 2011 study [53]. Similarly, Perri et al. reported a significantly higher recurrence rate and lower overall survival in women treated with anything other than total hysterectomy. The hazard ratios for recurrence and survival for total hysterectomy compared to any other surgical intervention, including myomectomy, morcellation, and supracervical hysterectomy, were 0.39 and 0.36, respectively [54]. From this limited data, it is possible that any tumor disruption, including myomectomy without morcellation, can disseminate disease and worsen prognosis in cases of occult leiomyosarcoma. In addition, the accuracy of intraoperative frozen section for leiomyosarcoma is particularly poor with estimates ranging from 11 to 38% [11]. Therefore, myomectomy should be reserved for well-selected patients determined to be at low risk for occult malignancy who have a strong desire to retain fertility. In one review of 41 cases of iatrogenic parasitic myoma, investigators noted that lesions were localized to the dependent portions of the abdomen; therefore, copious irrigation with position changes has been proposed as a theoretical mechanism to reduce tissue dissemination [55]. Given the minimal increase in operative time required for irrigation, this seems to be a reasonable technique if myomectomy is performed, with or without morcellation.

Hysterectomy is the gold standard for both diagnosis and treatment of leiomyosarcoma, and it is the only intervention that has been shown to improve survival. It is reasonable to offer hysterectomy as one of several options to any medically operable woman with symptoms related to presumed leiomyomata, and hysterectomy should be preferred and strongly recommended in women with clinical risk factors or imaging characteristics concerning for malignancy. Although most experts perform bilateral salpingoophorectomy as part of the definitive surgery, there is no data to suggest that this practice decreases mortality. In a review of SEER data including 341 women under 50 years old with early stage leiomyosarcoma, removing the tubes and ovaries had no impact on 5-year disease-specific survival [44]. Despite a lack of supportive data, one reasonable strategy is to consider salpingoophorectomy in women whose tumors are estrogen or progesterone receptor positive. Although beyond the scope of this review, it should be noted that there is no clear benefit to routine lymphadenectomy in patients with leiomyosarcoma limited to the uterus and clinically normal lymph nodes as the risk of occult nodal metastasis is less than 3% [2].

For women diagnosed with an occult leiomyosarcoma after total hysterectomy for presumed fibroids, there does not appear to be any benefit to a secondary surgery, either to remove the ovaries or complete staging. For women who underwent myomectomy or subtotal hysterectomy, however, completion surgery is recommended. Additionally, in women who underwent tumor morcellation, there appears to be a role for reexploration and secondary cytoreduction. In a small study investigating the utility of secondary surgical intervention in women with no evidence of extrauterine spread at the time of initial surgery who underwent morcellation and were subsequently diagnosed with leiomyosarcoma, three of eight women had disseminated intraperitoneal disease at immediate reexploration [56]. Reexploration therefore offers prognostic information and may improve survival if complete cytoreduction can be accomplished [57].

The optimal surgical approach to hysterectomy in women with fibroids is a matter of intense debate. Minimally invasive pelvic surgery offers superior patient outcomes in terms of reduced morbidity and mortality, but often large fibroid uteri cannot be removed through the vagina or laparoscopic port sites without tissue morcellation, which confers the risk of disseminating benign or occult malignant tissue, as described previously. Certainly, in cases that are highly suspicious for uterine sarcoma, the entire uterus should be removed intact. The majority of leiomyosarcomas, however, are not diagnosed preoperatively. Although it appears that patient outcomes are worse when uterine sarcomas are inadvertently morcellated, it should be remembered that current understanding of this phenomenon is extrapolated from two small studies that did not define the method of tumor disruption [54, 58]. Subjecting every woman with a large uterus to conventional laparotomy will result in increased morbidity for patients and overall increases in healthcare costs. Both the American Congress of Obstetricians and Gynecologists and the Society of Gynecologic Oncology continue to support minimally invasive surgery, including the use of power morcellation, in appropriately selected patients undergoing myomectomy or hysterectomy for presumed fibroids [10, 26]. Recently, there has been much interest in contained morcellation as a means of reducing risk related to iatrogenic dissemination of tissue. Contained morcellation refers to the use of a surgical bag or containment system, into which an intact specimen is placed prior to morcellation. Theoretically, morcellation within a bag would decrease tissue dissemination, but there is little data to support improved outcomes in patients undergoing contained morcellation compared to conventional techniques [53]. Contained power morcellation is not well studied and may pose increased risks due to limited visibility of the tissue being morcellated and surrounding organs [10]. One review of 152 patients undergoing total laparoscopic hysterectomy found a statistically significant increase in operative time of 20 min with contained versus non-contained electromechanical morcellation, but the study was underpowered to detect differences in other complications [59]. Recently, a single case report suggested improved outcomes at 2 years of follow-up for a patient who underwent contained morcellation of an occult leiomyosarcoma compared with historical data [60], but no retrospective or prospective trials have specifically investigated patient outcomes or survival.

Conclusion

Although uterine leiomyosarcoma is rare, its incidence among women undergoing surgery for presumed leiomyoma is likely higher than historically thought, and the consequences of delayed diagnosis or surgical mismanagement can be devastating for patients. Clinicians should maintain a high index of suspicion for occult malignancy in women with symptomatic uterine masses. They should be aware of the risk factors associated with uterine sarcomas and understand the utility and limitations of available imaging modalities. It would be cost-prohibitive to perform an exhaustive preoperative evaluation for every patient with suspected fibroids, but gynecologists should be cognizant of the tools available to them. For a patient deemed to be high risk for occult malignancy based on clinical risk factors, a history of failed medical management or UAE, or concerning ultrasound findings, further evaluation is indicated. CE-MRI and DWI, possibly with determination of serum LDH, are reasonable investigations. In cases of suspected sarcoma, hysterectomy with intact specimen removal is the preferred management option.

References

1. Kosary CL. Cancer of the corpus uteri. In: Ries LAG, Young JL, Keel GE, Eisner MP, et al., editors. SEER survival monograph: cancer survival among adults: U.S. SEER program, 1988–2001, patient and tumor characteristics. Bethesda, MD: National Cancer Institute, SEER Program, NIH pub. No. 07–6215; 2007. p. 123–32.
2. Leitao MM Jr, Tornos C, Wolfson AH, O'Cearbhaill R. Corpus: mesenchymal tumors. In: Barakat RR, et al., editors. Principles and practice of gynecologic oncology. 6th ed. Philadelphia: Lippincott Williams & Wilkins; 2013. p. 715–56.
3. FIGO Committee On Gynecologic Oncology. FIGO staging for uterine sarcomas. Int J Gynecol Cancer. 2009;104:179.

4. Zivanovic O, Leitao MM, Iasonos A, et al. Stage-specific outcomes of patients with uterine leiomyosarcoma: a comparison of the International Federation of Gynecology and Obstetrics and American joint committee on cancer staging systems. J Clin Oncol. 2009;27:2066–72.

5. Park J, Kim D, Suh D, et al. Prognostic factors and treatment outcomes of patients with uterine sarcoma: analysis of 127 patients at a single institution, 1989-2007. J Cancer Res Clin Oncol. 2008;134:1277–87.

6. Garg G, Shah JP, Liu R, et al. Validation of tumor size as staging variable in the revised International Federation of Gynecology and Obstetrics stage I leiomyosarcoma: a population-based study. Int J Gynecol Cancer. 2010;20:1201–6.

7. Pautier P, Genestie C, Rey A, et al. Analysis of clinicopathologic prognostic factors for 157 uterine sarcomas and evaluation of grading score validated for soft tissue sarcoma. Cancer. 2000;88:1425–31.

8. Brooks SE, Zhan M, Cote T, et al. Survival epidemiology and end results analysis of 267 cases of uterine sarcomas, 1989–1999. Gynecol Oncol. 2004;93:204–8.

9. Tzu-I W, Tzu-Chen Y, Chyong-Huey L. Clinical presentation and diagnosis of uterine sarcoma, including imaging. Best Pract Res Clin Obstet Gynaecol. 2011;25:681–9.

10. American College of Obstetricians and Gynecologists. Power morcellation and occult malignancy in gynecologic surgery: a special report. 2014. http://www.acog.org/Resources-And-Publications/Task-Force-and-Work-Group-Reports/Power-Morcellation-and-Occult-Malignancy-in-Gynecologic-Surgery. Accessed 30 June 2016.

11. Lynam S, Young L, Morozov V, et al. Risk, risk reduction and management of occult malignancy diagnosed after uterine morcellation: a commentary. Womens Health. 2015;11:929–44.

12. Giuntoli RL, Metzinger DS, DiMarco CS, et al. Retrospective review of 208 patients with leiomyosarcoma of the uterus: prognostic indicators, surgical management, and adjuvant therapy. Gynecol Oncol. 2003;89:460–9.

13. Jaakkola S, Lyytinen HK, Pukkala E, et al. Use of estradiol-progestin therapy associates with increased risk for uterine sarcomas. Gynecol Oncol. 2011;122:260–3.

14. Lavie O, Barnett-Griness O, Narod SA, et al. The risk of developing uterine sarcoma after tamoxifen use. Int J Gynecol Cancer. 2008;18:352–6.

15. Hoogendoorn WE, Hollema H, van Boven HH, et al. Prognosis of uterine corpus cancer after tamoxifen treatment for breast cancer. Breast Cancer Res Treat. 2008;112:99–108.
16. Nilbert M, Therkildsen C, Nissen A, et al. Sarcomas associated with hereditary nonpolyposis colorectal cancer: broad anatomical and morphological spectrum. Familial Cancer. 2009;8:209–13.
17. Francis JH, Kleinerman RA, Seddon J, et al. Increased risk of secondary uterine leiomyosarcoma in hereditary retinoblastoma. Gynecol Oncol. 2012;124:254–9.
18. Launonen V, Vierimaa O, Kiuru M, et al. Inherited susceptibility to uterine leiomyomas and renal cell cancer. Proc Natl Acad Sci U S A. 2001;98:3387–92.
19. Lehtonen HJ, Kiuru M, Ylisaukko-oja SK, et al. Increased risk of cancer in patients with fumarate hydratase germline mutation. J Med Genet. 2006;43:523–6.
20. U.S. Food and Drug Administration. Updated laparoscopic uterine power morcellation in hysterectomy and myomectomy: FDA safety communication. http://www.fda.gov/MedicalDevices/Safety/AlertsandNotices/ucm424443.htm. Accessed 30 June 2016.
21. Parker WH, Kaunitz AM, Pritts EA, et al. U.S. Food and Drug Administration's guidance regarding morcellation of leiomyomas: well-intentioned, but is it harmful for women? Obstet Gynecol. 2016;127:18–22.
22. Pritts EA, Vanness DJ, Berek JS, et al. The prevalence of occult leiomyosarcoma at surgery for presumed uterine fibroids: a meta-analysis. Gynecol Surg. 2015;12:165–77.
23. Wright JD. Electric power morcellation in gynecology: the path forward. Obstet Gynecol. 2016;127:7–9.
24. Paul PG, Rengaraj V, Das T, et al. Uterine sarcomas in patients undergoing surgery for presumed leiomyomas: 10 years' experience. J Minim Invasive Gynecol. 2016;23:384–9.
25. Rodriguez AM, Asoglu MR, Sak ME, et al. Incidence of occult leiomyosarcoma in presumed morcellation cases: a database study. Eur J Obstet Gynecol Reprod Biol. 2016;197:31–5.
26. Society of Gynecologic Oncology. Statement of the Society of Gynecologic Oncology to the Food and Drug Administration's Obstetrics and Gynecology Medical Devices Advisory Committee concerning safety of laparoscopic power morcellation; 2014. https://www.sgo.org/wp-content/uploads/2014/04/SGO-Testimony-to-FDA-on-Power-Morcellation-FINAL.pdf. Accessed 1 July 2016.

27. Van den Bosch T, Vandendael A, Wranz PA, et al. Cervical cytology in menopausal women at high risk for endometrial disease. Eur J Cancer Prev. 1998;7:149–52.
28. Schwartz L, Diamond M, Schwartz P. Leiomyosarcomas: clinical presentation. Am J Obstet Gynecol. 1993;168:180–3.
29. Hinchcliff EM, Esselen KM, Watkins JC, et al. The role of endometrial biopsy in preoperative detection of uterine leiomyosarcoma. J Minim Invasive Gynecol. 2016;23:567–72.
30. Kurjak A, Kupesic S, Shalan H, et al. Uterine sarcoma: a report of 10 cases studied by transvaginal color and pulsed Doppler sonography. Gynecol Oncol. 1995;59(3):342–6.
31. Aviram R, Oscshom Y, Markovitch O, et al. Uterine sarcoma versus leiomyomas: gray-scale and Doppler sonographic findings. J Clin Ultrasound. 2005;33(1):10–3.
32. Hata K, Hata T, Maruyama R, Hirai M. Uterine sarcoma: can it be differentiated from uterine leiomyoma with Doppler ultrasonography? A preliminary report. Ultrasound Obstet Gynecol. 1997;9(2):101–4.
33. Szabó I, Szánthó A, Csabay L, et al. Color Doppler ultrasonography in the differentiation of uterine sarcomas from uterine leiomyosarcomas. Eur J Gynaecol Oncol. 2002;23(1):29–34.
34. Schwartz LB, Zawin M, Carcangiu ML, et al. Does pelvic magnetic resonance imaging differentiate among the histologic subtypes of uterine leiomyomata? Fertil Steril. 1998;70(3):580–7.
35. Tanaka YO, Nishida M, Tsunoda H, et al. Smooth muscle tumors of uncertain malignant potential and leiomyosarcomas of the uterus: MR findings. J Magn Reson Imaging. 2004;20(6):998–1007.
36. Namimoto T, Yamashita Y, Awai K, et al. Combined use of T2-weighted and diffusion-weighted 3-T MR imaging for differentiating uterine sarcomas from benign leiomyomas. Eur Radiol. 2009;19(11):2756–64.
37. Koh D, Collins DJ. Diffusion-weighted MRI in the body: application and challenges in oncology. AJR Am J Roentgenol. 2007;188:1622–35.
38. Gaetke-Udager K, McLean K, Sciallis AP, et al. Diagnostic accuracy of ultrasound, contrast-enhanced CT, and conventional MRI for differentiating leiomyoma from leiomyosarcoma. Acad Radiol. 2016;23(10):1290–7. doi:10.1016/j.acra.2016.06.004.
39. Tamai K, Koyama T, Saga T, et al. The utility of diffusion-weighted MR imaging for differentiating uterine sarcomas from benign leiomyomas. Eur Radiol. 2008;18:723–30.

40. Sato K, Yuasa N, Fujita M, Fukushima Y. Clinical application of diffusion-weighted imaging for preoperative differentiation between uterine leiomyoma and leiomyosarcoma. Am J Obstet Gynecol. 2014;210(4):368.
41. Lin G, Yang L, Huang Y, et al. Comparison of the diagnostic accuracy of contrast-enhanced MRI and diffusion-weighted MRI in the differentiation between uterine leiomyosarcoma/smooth muscle tumor with uncertain malignant potential and benign leiomyoma. J Magn Reson Imaging. 2016;43:333–42.
42. Thomassin-Naggara I, Dechoux S, Bonneau C, et al. How to differentiate benign from malignant myometrial tumours using MR imaging. Eur Radiol. 2013;23:2306–14.
43. Goto A, Takeuchi S, Sugimura K, Maruo T. Usefulness of Gd-DTPA contrast-enhanced dynamic MRI and serum determination of LDH and its isozymes in the differential diagnosis of leiomyosarcoma from degenerated leiomyoma of the uterus. Int J Gynecol Cancer. 2002;12(4):354–61.
44. Kapp DS, Shin JY, Chan JK. Prognostic factors and survival in 1396 patients with uterine leiomyosarcomas: emphasis on impact of lymphadenectomy and oophorectomy. Cancer. 2008;112(4):820–30.
45. Parker WH, YS F, Berek JS. Uterine sarcoma in patients operated on for presumed leiomyoma and rapidly growing leiomyoma. Obstet Gynecol. 1994;83:414–8.
46. Papadia A, Salom EM, Fulcheri E, Ragni N. Uterine sarcoma occurring in a premenopausal patient after uterine artery embolization: a case report and review of the literature. Gynecol Oncol. 2007;104(1):260–3.
47. Goldberg J, Burd I, Frederic VP, et al. Leiomyosarcoma in a premenopausal patient after uterine artery embolization. Am J Obstet Gynecol. 2004;191:1733–5.
48. Al-Badr A, Fraught W. Uterine artery embolization in an undiagnosed uterine sarcoma. Obstet Gynecol. 2001;97:836–7.
49. Hitti IF, Glasberg SS, McKenzie C, Meltzer BA. Uterine leiomyosarcoma with massive necrosis diagnosed during gonadotropin-releasing hormone analog therapy for presumed uterine fibroid. Fertil Steril. 1991;56:778–80.
50. Meyer WR, Mayer AR, Diamond MP, et al. Unsuspected leiomyosarcoma: treatment with a gonadotropin-releasing hormone analogue. Obstet Gynecol. 1990;75:529–31.
51. Mesia AF, Williams FS, Yan Z, Mittal K. Aborted leiomyosarcoma after treatment with leuprolide acetate. Obstet Gynecol. 1998;92:664–6.

52. Leitao MM Jr, Hensley ML, Barakat RR, et al. Immunohistochemical expression of estrogen and progesterone receptors and outcomes in patients with newly diagnosed uterine leiomyosarcoma. Gynecol Oncol. 2012;124(3):558–62.
53. Noel NL, Isaacson KB. Morcellation complications: from direct trauma to inoculation. Best Pract Res Clin Obstet Gynaecol. 2016;35:37–43. doi:10.1016/j.bpobgyn.2015.12.002.
54. Perri T, Korach J, Sadetzki S, et al. Uterine leiomyosarcoma: does the primary surgical procedure matter? Int J Gynecol Cancer. 2009;19:257–60.
55. Huang PS, Chang WC, Huang SC. Iatrogenic parasitic myoma: a case report and review of the literature. Taiwan J Obstet Gynecol. 2014;53(3):392–6.
56. Oduyebo T, Rauh-Hain AJ, Meserve EE, et al. The value of re-exploration in patients with inadvertently morcellated uterine sarcoma. Gynecol Oncol. 2014;132(2):360–5.
57. Leitao MM Jr, Zivanovic O, Chi DS, et al. Surgical cytoreduction in patients with metastatic uterine leiomyosarcoma at the time of initial diagnosis. Gynecol Oncol. 2012;125:409–13.
58. Park JY, Park SK, Kim DY, et al. The impact of tumor morcellation during surgery on the prognosis of patients with apparently early leiomyosarcoma. Gynecol Oncol. 2011;122(2):255–9.
59. Winner B, Porter A, Velloze S, Biest S. Uncontained compared with contained power morcellation in total laparoscopic hysterectomy. Obstet Gynecol. 2015;126(4):834–8.
60. Boruta DM, Shibley T. Power morcellation of unsuspected high grade leiomyosarcoma within an inflated containment bag: 2-year follow-up. J Minim Invasive Gynecol. 2016;23(6):1009–11.

Chapter 11
The Broad Ligament Fibroid

Jonathan Y. Song, Carlos Rotman, and Edgardo L. Yordan

Clinical Case Presentation

A 31-year-old woman (gravida 2, para 1) with secondary infertility was seen in consultation for a laparoscopic approach to remove a 36-cm right broad ligament leiomyoma. She was experiencing dyspareunia, numbness, and weakness of the right thigh and was found to have a right tubal occlusion from previous records. The patient wished to avoid a laparotomy and presented for a second opinion.

Electronic supplementary material The online version of this chapter (doi:10.1007/978-3-319-58780-6_11) contains supplementary material, which is available to authorized users.

J.Y. Song, MD, FACOG, FACS (✉)
Robotics and Minimally Invasive Surgery,
Northwestern Medicine Delnor Hospital, TLC Medical Group,
S.C. 2455 Dean St. (Suite A), St. Charles, IL 60175, USA
e-mail: Jsong3972@gmail.com

C. Rotman, MD, FACOG, FACS
E.L. Yordan, MD, FACOG, FACS
Department of Gynecology, Weiss Memorial Hospital,
4646 N. Marine Dr. (Suite A-3300), Chicago, IL 60640, USA
e-mail: Ombu29@hotmail.com; Edgardoyordan668@gmail.com

N.S. Moawad (ed.), *Uterine Fibroids*,
https://doi.org/10.1007/978-3-319-58780-6_11,
© Springer International Publishing AG 2018

Exam Findings

The patient had a visibly large abdomen with what appeared to be a 34–36 week size uterus on pelvic exam. Even with gentle palpation, she experienced pelvic pressure and had decreased motor strength of the right lower extremity and complained of significant lower back pain.

Diagnostic Work-Up

Pelvic ultrasound with a pelvic MRI with contrast confirmed the presence of a massive right broad ligament fibroid, with a mild right hydroureter and hydronephrosis. No suspicious features suggestive of a possible sarcoma were present. LDH isoenzyme studies revealed normal levels, and Doppler studies were negative for blood clots. A hysterosalpingogram performed by the patient's gynecologist revealed a right isthmic tubal occlusion.

Discussion

Leiomyomas (fibroids) are the most common benign neoplasms of the female reproductive system [1]. Although the etiology of fibroids remains uncertain, there is convincing evidence that estrogens and progestogens play a role in the proliferation of tumor growth [2, 3]. Fibroids are rarely found in young patients prior to menarche, and they regress in size after menopause; therefore, leiomyomas essentially affect women of the reproductive age [4, 5].

Although the majority of women with fibroids do not experience any symptoms, women who do may encounter significant discomfort such as pain, heavy bleeding, and even infertility [6, 7], leading to the need for surgical treatments in some cases. Leiomyomas serve as the most common indication for hysterectomy in the United States [8–10]. This does not sound surprising since fibroids are found to occur commonly in

women with a prevalence of 5–77% [11]. A significant variation in the prevalence rate occurs since available data are difficult to compare due to differences in the study population
and screening methods used [12–15].

There are numerous studies that show a higher incidence
of leiomyomas in Black women compared to White women.
The literature also implies that Black women are more likely
to have larger and more symptomatic fibroids than White
women at the time of treatment [16–21]. In the authors' personal experience, the largest fibroids removed laparoscopically were from patients of Asian, Hispanic, and Caucasian
decent. This only adds to the fact that we still do not know the
details and intricacies of the pathophysiology of this common
tumor.

Given the high prevalence of fibroids in women, and the
fact that most exhibit no particular symptoms, ascribing
symptomatology specifically to fibroids can become challenging. If we take into consideration the rare but obvious exis-
tence of extrauterine fibroids, accurate diagnosis becomes
more difficult to establish. Extrauterine fibroids can occur on
the cervix, fallopian tube, ovary, urethra, and vaginal and vul-
var regions [22]. Although broad ligament fibroids are the
most common of the extrauterine fibroids, they are rare with
an incidence of approximately 1% [23, 24]. Their location can
cause unusual presentations and potentially compromise the
accuracy of a preoperative diagnosis [25].

Given its proximity, broad ligament fibroids can sometimes be difficult to discern and can be confused with an
adnexal mass. Since the tumor is located outside of the uterus,
patients may not experience significant bleeding (Fig. 11.1).
Depending on the size, patients may encounter urinary symptoms such as increased frequency or urinary retention, dyspareunia, pelvic pain and pressure, and lower back pain. In rare
circumstances, if significantly large enough, a massive broad
ligament leiomyoma can cause numbness and weakness of
the lower extremity of the affected side if the obturator nerve
is compressed (Fig. 11.2), as well as causing ipsilateral hydroureter and/or hydronephrosis [26].

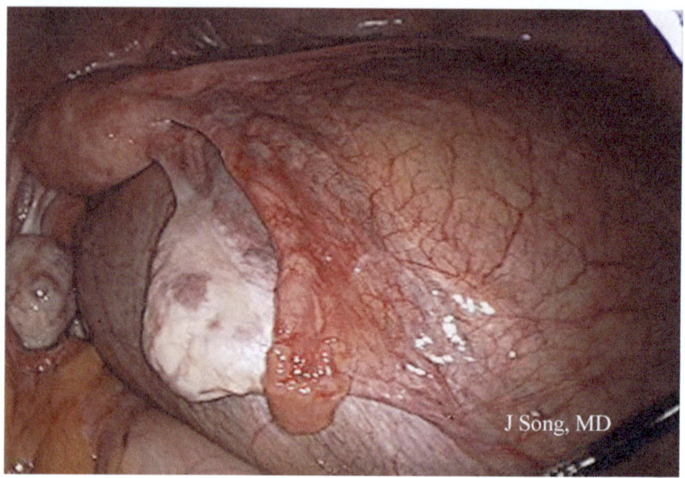

FIGURE 11.1 Large broad ligament leiomyoma

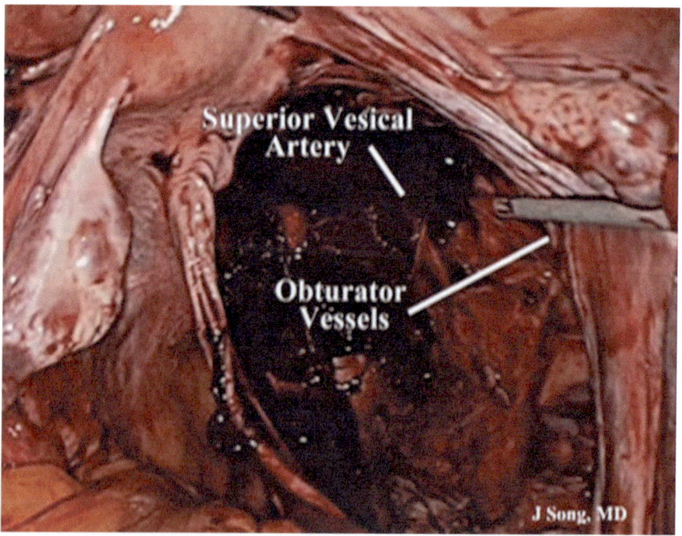

FIGURE 11.2 Retroperitoneal space with identified structures

Establishing an accurate diagnosis can be challenging given the factors mentioned, and because of this reason, it is crucial to proceed with a thorough work-up. When the patient presents for a consultation, a meticulous history must first be obtained. As stated, due to the location of the fibroid, these patients may not necessarily present with menorrhagia or be anemic; it is not uncommon for these patients to present with what may sound like orthopedic complaints. Patients may experience lower back pain or "tail bone" pain, as well as encounter dull achy discomfort when getting into and out of a car, or getting in or out of bed, affecting potentially what appear to be weight-bearing joints such as the hip.

For all patients with uterine fibroids presenting for a potentially minimally invasive surgical approach for removal, a systematic method is utilized. Since the authors perform almost exclusively laparoscopic and robot-assisted procedures, some type of morcellation will be required to extract these large specimens. Therefore, we have established an algorithm that we follow to screen for appropriate cases where morcellation (whether manual or using power morcellators) can safely be performed. The authors' institutions and hospitals also refer to this algorithm to assist and guide their OB/GYN departments in determining which cases would be applicable for power morcellators to be used. Our patients are also informed that, unfortunately, there are no preoperative assessments that are available that would allow us to *confidently* rule out an unidentified malignant process, and a consent form stating this understanding is signed by all patients prior to proceeding with surgery.

Given that the authors see a vast number of patients for second and third opinions, as part of our work-up for very large or what appears to be a rapidly growing fibroid (primarily in postmenopausal women), in addition to performing our own pelvic ultrasounds, we obtain a pelvic MRI with contrast to rule out any suspicious features for a possible sarcoma [27, 28]. We also order a lactate dehydrogenase isoenzyme panel (LDH isoenzymes) to complete our work-up [29, 30].

Any abnormalities involving the MRI or LDH isoenzyme levels may potentially heighten our suspicion for a possible sarcoma, and a gynecologic oncology consultation may be requested.

Following the pelvic ultrasound, pelvic MRI with contrast, and LDH isoenzyme assessment, all patients undergo endometrial sampling (endometrial biopsy or dilatation and curettage if biopsy is inconclusive) prior to the myomectomy. Depending on the presence of potential risk factors for a possible sarcoma such as Black women over the age of 40 years [31, 32], history of previous pelvic radiation [33, 34], Tamoxifen usage exceeding 5 years [35–37], childhood retinoblastoma, renal cell carcinoma, certain hereditary cancer syndromes (e.g., Lynch Syndrome) [38–40], and tumor growth after menopause regardless of hormone replacement therapy [41–44], the algorithm the authors developed is used to help delineate which patients would be applicable to undergo morcellation in a safe manner (Table 11.1).

When working with massive broad ligament fibroids laparoscopically, one must keep in mind several key factors. The retroperitoneal space can serve as a reservoir, which can house a very large specimen. The surgeon should therefore be aware that the specimen can be much larger than its initial appearance. This space can also hold significant amount of blood, and hence, meticulous hemostasis early in the case is vital [45]. Since the location is peculiar due to the complex anatomy in this region (i.e., ureters, internal iliac and obturator vessels and nerves), the surgeon must pay close attention during dissection. Mass effect due to size can compress the vessels and nerves in this region and can cause weakness and numbness of the affected side as was the case in this patient.

After the mentioned work-up has been completed and all appropriate consents have been obtained, the patient is scheduled for surgery under general anesthesia. The patient is examined and is prepped and draped in the normal sterile fashion. A Foley catheter is then inserted. All patients undergo our modified open laparoscopy technique [46], and the abdominal and pelvic anatomy is carefully assessed.

TABLE 11.1   Algorithm for work-up and determining proper candidates to undergo morcellation

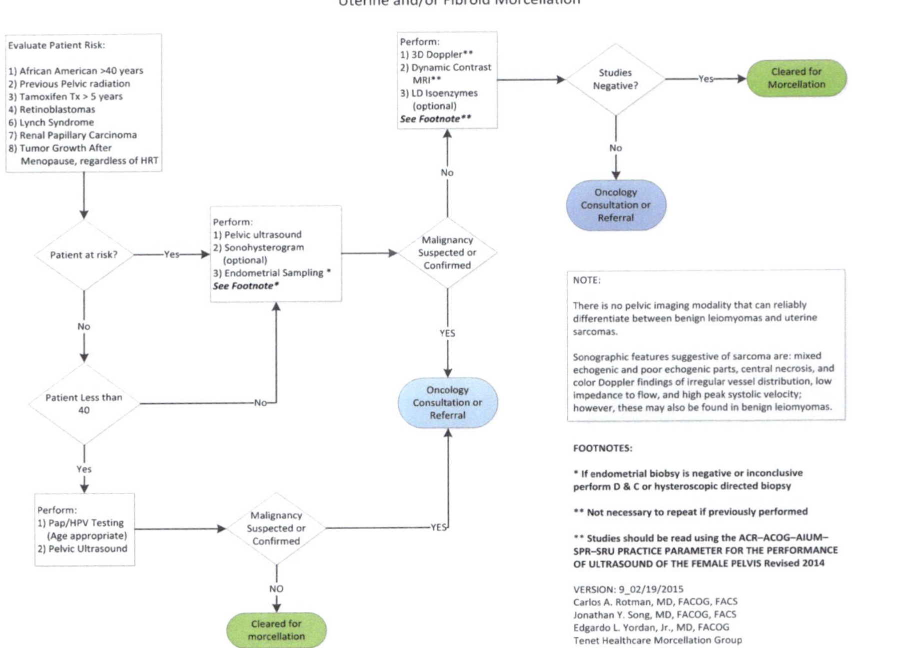

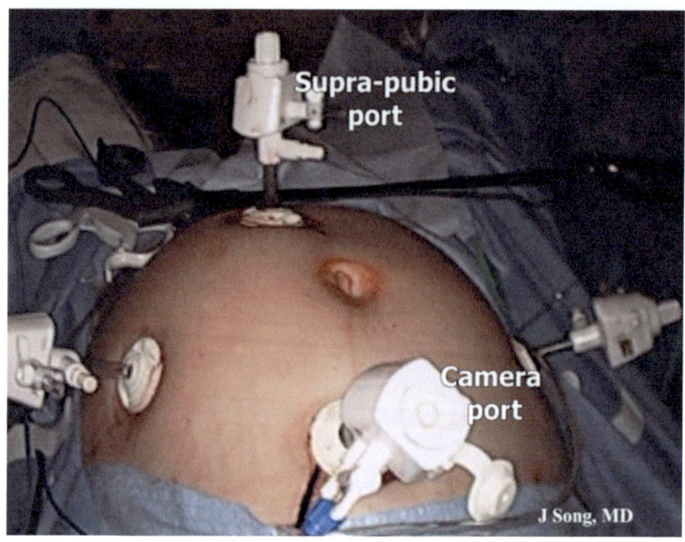

Figure 11.3 Appropriate trocar placements for large pelvic pathology

The presence of potential adhesions and/or the size of the pathology will determine where our ancillary trocars will be placed. For large specimens as in this case, the trocars should be placed cephalad to the large fibroid to facilitate surgical maneuvers. This may mean placing the camera port several centimeters above the umbilicus if need be (Fig. 11.3). After this step has been completed, three ancillary 5 mm trocars are placed. If adhesiolysis is required, this step is executed next.

Based on the authors' experience, careful dissection and location of the ureter of the affected side would be helpful for small tumors. However, in cases such as this where the broad ligament fibroid is extremely large, the surgeon will not know exactly how the ureter has been displaced (laterally, superiorly, inferiorly, etc.), and therefore, attempts for locating and dissecting out the ureter may be futile and dangerous since the anatomy can be significantly distorted. We therefore recommend that the surgeon should "hug" the fibroid and stay

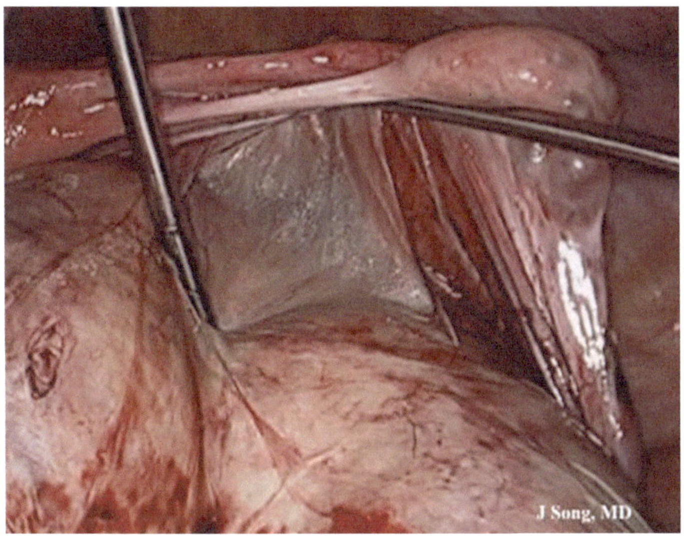

FIGURE 11.4 Dissection of the large broad ligament fibroid

close while dissecting and enucleating the tumor (Fig. 11.4). This way, as the peripheral structures are falling away from the specimen, visualization of the surrounding anatomy may become more familiar.

As the fibroid is being dissected and pulled out of the broad ligament, one can try to "walk the specimen" as the surgeon can cross over with laparoscopic grasper with teeth or tenaculum, to enhance grip providing traction, which will enhance visualization beyond the edge and horizon of the tumor (Fig. 11.5). It can become challenging at times to see clearly when dealing with large tumors, and the authors find this tip to be helpful.

After the fibroid is resected, careful dissection would lead to minimal bleeding. If moderate oozing is observed, hemostatic agents can be used to facilitate hemostasis. Bipolar cautery can also be used as long as the surgeon is mindful of the anatomy in this region. Zero absorbable polyglactin suture on a straight needle is used to close the peritoneum (Fig. 11.6).

In order to remove the specimen, we utilize our simplified laparoscopic abdominal morcellation ("SLAM") technique. It is

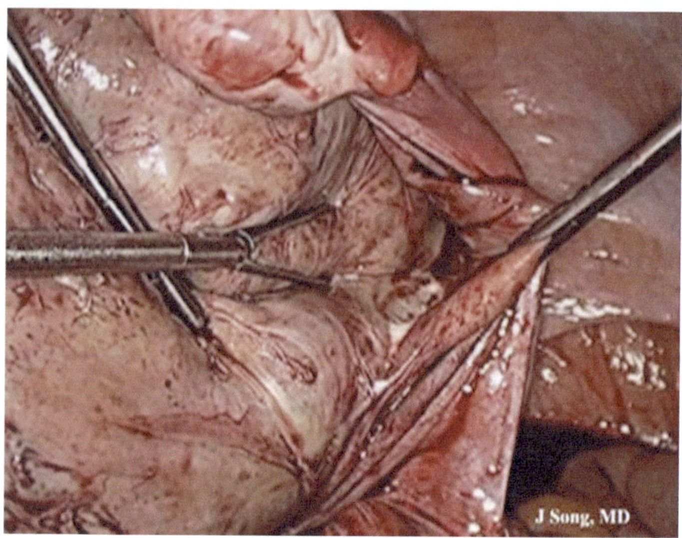

FIGURE 11.5 Walking the specimen and "hugging" the fibroid given its large size

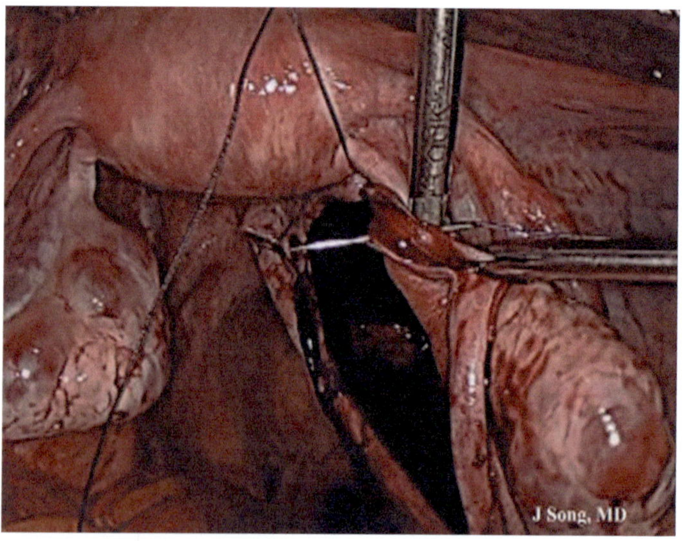

FIGURE 11.6 Closure of the peritoneum after the fibroid has been removed

a technique that Carlos Rotman has developed in the early 1990s to remove large specimen in a safe and efficient manner [47]. The large fibroid is held under tension by using either two laparoscopic tenaculums or graspers with teeth, inserted from the left and right side. Grasping the large specimen initially with tenaculums may facilitate the handling of the large pathology especially when beginning the SLAM. The suprapubic trocar is removed and an 11-blade is inserted (Fig. 11.7). With forward motion, and with the blade always facing away from pelvic organs, the large fibroid is cut into longitudinal strips, which are carefully counted as they are being cut and stored for later extraction. This would prevent creating crumbs or debris of tissue unlike the automated morcellators, which can lead to unwanted seeding, and large specimens can be expeditiously removed. Abdominal wall tissues are generally forgiving, and thus, the small skin incision can be extended just slightly and the specimen can be removed as it is pulled out using a Kocher clamp (Figs. 11.8 and 11.9), making sure that all pieces are accounted for. Long strips of tissue can be removed quite rapidly in this fashion.

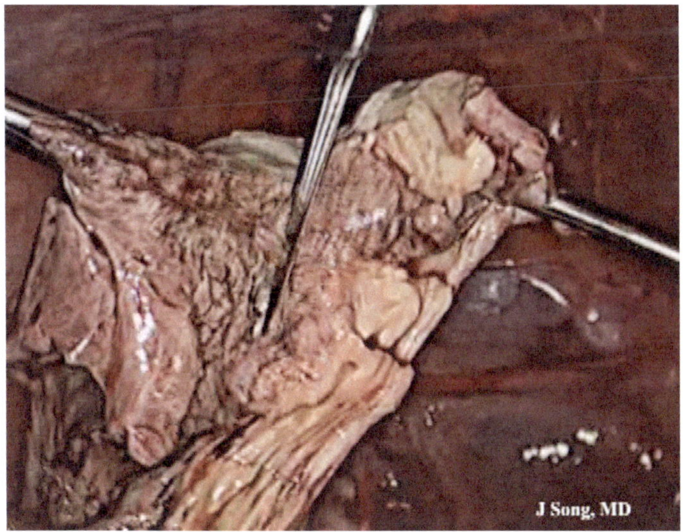

FIGURE 11.7 Demonstrating the SLAM technique

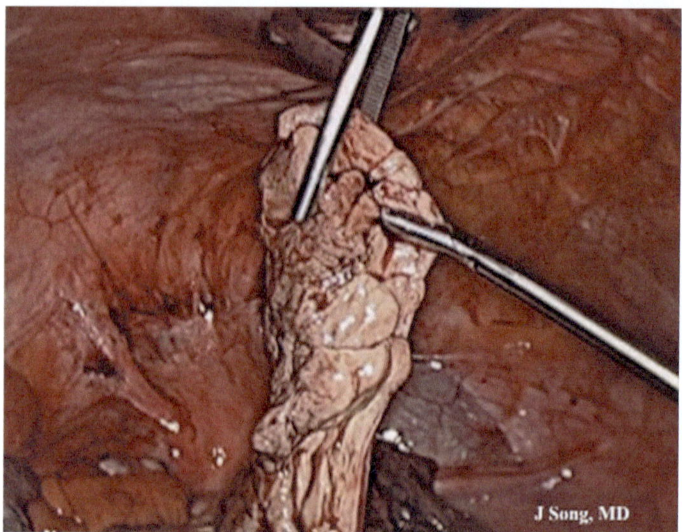

FIGURE 11.8 A Kocher clamp is introduced through the suprapubic incision to grasp the specimen

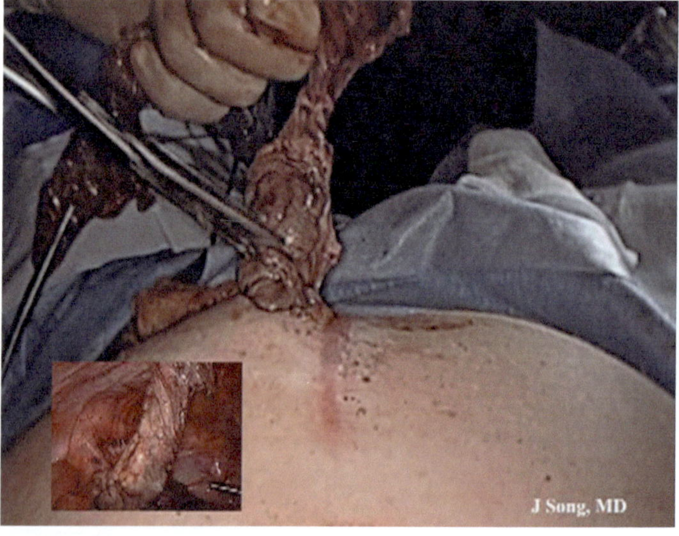

FIGURE 11.9 Specimen extraction shown here after the suprapubic incision is slightly extended

After all the counted specimen pieces are removed, the incision is copiously irrigated from the inside with the laparoscopic irrigator and again with the bulb-tip syringe from outside prior to the closure of the skin. This practice should be consistently observed to avoid potential inoculation of the incision, which can in rare circumstances lead to incisional implantation of pathology [48]. After confirming hemostasis and complete removal of the specimen, the fascial incision is re-approximated with a figure-of-eight stitch with 1-0 absorbable polyglactin suture, and the skin incision can be re-approximated with 4-0 absorbable suture. Various modifications of the SLAM technique exists around the world today, but the concept is still the same; large specimens can be removed quickly in a controlled and refined manner, without unwanted dissemination of tissue through a very cost-effective usage of a blade or two. The isthmic occlusion was repaired by performing a tubal anastomosis per patient's request [49].

Cases involving a large broad ligament fibroid such as this cannot be successfully managed in a conservative fashion. Given its large size, there is a significant mass effect that cannot be relieved by medical treatment. Uterine artery embolization will have little or no effect on the broad ligament leiomyoma due to the fact that this type of fibroid does not necessarily rely on the uterus for its blood supply, which is why it can exist outside the confines of the uterus. Although there have been numerous studies that have demonstrated decreased tumor volume with pretreatment with gonadotropin-releasing hormone agonists (GnRH agonists) prior to a myomectomy [50–53], most studies involve fibroids that are under 10 cm in size. In the authors' experience, GnRH agonists will soften the tumor and can at times impair the enucleation process since the capsule becomes compromised. Given the higher tendency of some degree of degeneration involving larger fibroids, presurgical treatment with GnRH agonists can increase risk of tearing and/or removing the fibroid specimen piece-meal due to its soft and weakened texture. Diluted vasopressin will work best to decrease blood loss during surgery compared to other medications or options, and establishing a clear plane with meticulous dissection and enucleation will further enhance the chances of a successful outcome.

Whether a robot-assisted laparoscopic myomectomy (RALM) or traditional laparoscopic myomectomy (LM) is performed is up to the preference of the surgeon. Based on the authors' experience, for difficult cases or for cases involving a large specimen, traditional LM is preferable for several reasons. Just as a blind-folded individual can sense the difference in cutting loose leaf paper vs. cardboard paper with scissors, tactile feedback allows the surgeon to "feel" what he/she is cutting, which is an invaluable asset to have in performing complex cases. Traditional LM also allows more flexibility due to the fact that nothing is fixated or docked and different angles and views can be assessed easily since the scope (and various different degrees of scopes) can be placed through different ports. This flexibility exists with the latest version of the robot (da Vinci Surgical System Xi), but the majority of hospitals may not possess the latest model. Limited range of motion where the robotic arms can come in contact with each other is also high when maneuvering large pathology in a confined space such as the pelvis. However, one noticeable advantage that RALM will offer is limited fatigue for the surgeon, since the robot is strong and allows comfort and ergonomically correct posturing for the surgeon. The approach is ultimately a matter of personal choice, a choice that comes with its associated advantages and disadvantages. RALM was discussed in detail in Chap. 5.

References

1. Sparic R, Mirkovic L, Malvasi A, Tinelli A. Epidemiology of uterine myomas: a review. Int J Fertil Steril. 2016;9(4):424–35.
2. Rein MS, Barbieri RL, Friedman AJ. Progesterone: a critical role in the pathogenesis of uterine myomas. Am J Obstet Gynecol. 1995;172(1 Pt 1):14–8.
3. Andersen J. Growth factors and cytokines in uterine leiomyomas. Semin Reprod Endocrinol. 1996;14(3):269–82.
4. Fields KR, Neinstein LS. Uterine myomas in adolescents: case reports and a review of the literature. J Pediatr Adolesc Gynecol. 1996;9(4):195–8.

5. Cramer SF, Patel A. The frequency of uterine leiomyomas. Am J Clin Pathol. 1990;94(4):435–8.
6. Ryan GL, Syrop CH, Van Voorhis BJ. Role, epidemiology, and natural history of benign uterine mass lesions. Clin Obstet Gynecol. 2005;48(2):312–24.
7. Lippman SA, Warner M, Samuels S, Olive D, Vercellini P, Eskenazi B. Uterine fibroids and gynecologic pain symptoms in a population-based study. Fertil Steril. 2003;80(6):1488–94.
8. Sparic R, Hudelist G, Berisavac M, Gudovic A, Buzadzic S. Hysterectomy throughout history. Acta Chir Iugosl. 2011;58(4):9–14.
9. Farquhar CM, Steiner CA. Hysterectomy rates in the United States 1990–1997. Obstet Gynecol. 2002;99(2):229–34.
10. Merrill RM. Hysterectomy surveillance in the United States, 1997 through 2005. Med Sci Monit. 2008;14(1):CR24–31.
11. Lurie S, Piper I, Woliovitch I, Glezerman M. Age-related prevalence of sonographically confirmed uterine myomas. J Obstet Gynaecol. 2005;25:42–8.
12. Laughlin SK, Baird DD, Savitz DA, Herring AH, Hartmann KE. Prevalence of uterine leiomyomas in the first trimester of pregnancy: an ultrasound-screening study. Obstet Gynecol. 2009;113(3):630–5.
13. Chen CR, Buck GM, Courey NG, Perez KM, Wactawski-Wende J. Risk factors for uterine fibroids among women undergoing tubal sterilization. Am J Epidemiol. 2001;153(1):20–6.
14. Borgfeldt C, Andolf E. Transvaginal ultrasonographic findings in the uterus and the endometrium: low prevalence of leiomyoma in a random sample of women age 25–40 years. Acta Obstet Gynecol Scand. 2000;79(3):202–7.
15. Marino JL, Eskenazi B, Warner M, Samuels S, Vercellini P, Gavoni N, Olive D. Uterine leiomyoma and menstrual cycle characteristics in a population-based cohort study. Hum Reprod. 2004;19(10):2350–5.
16. Wise LA, Palmer JR, Stewart EA, Rosenberg L. Age-specific incidence rates for self-reported uterine leiomyomata in the black Women's health study. Obstet Gynecol. 2005;105:563–8.
17. Kjerulff KH, Langenberg P, Seidman JD, Stolley PD, Guzinski GM. Uterine leiomyomas. Racial differences in severity, symptoms and age of diagnosis. J Reprod Med. 1996;41:483–90.
18. Ross RK, Pike MC, Vessey MP, Bull D, Yeates D, Casagrande JT. Risk factors for uterine fibroids: reduced risk associated with oral contraceptives [Published correction appears in Br Med

J (Clin Res Ed) 1986;293:1027]. Br Med J (Clin Res Ed). 1986;293:359–62.

19. Ligon AH, Morton CC. Leiomyomata: heritability and cytogenetic studies. Hum Reprod Update. 2001;7:8–14.

20. Chiaffarino F, Parazzini F, La Vecchia C, Marsico S, Surace M, Ricci E. Use of oral contraceptives and uterine fibroids: results from a case-control study. Br J Obstet Gynaecol. 1999;106:857–60.

21. Lumbiganon P, Rugpao S, Phandhu-fung S, Laopaiboon M, Vudhika-mraksa N, Werawatakul Y. Protective effect of depot-medroxyprogesterone acetate on surgically treated uterine leiomyomas: a multicentre case-control study. Br J Obstet Gynaecol. 1996;103:909–14.

22. Kurman RJ, editor. Blaustein's pathology of the female genital tract. 5th ed. New York: Springer; 2002.

23. Pallavee P, Ghose S, Begum J, et al. Fibroid after hysterectomy: diagnostic dilemma. J Clin Diagn Res. 2014;8:1–3.

24. Bhatla N. Tumours of the corpus uteri. Jeffcoats principles of gynaecology. 6th ed. London: Arnold Printers; 2001. p. 470.

25. Harrison BT, Berg RE, Mittal K. Massive ovarian edema associated with a broad ligament leiomyoma: a case report and review. Int J Gynecol Pathol. 2014;33:418–22.

26. Song JY. Laparoscopic resection of a rare, large broad ligament myoma. J Minim Invasive Gynecol. 2015;22(4):530–1.

27. Amant F, Coosemans A, Debiec-Rychter M, et al. Clinical management of uterine sarcomas. Lancet Oncol. 2009;10:1188.

28. Schwartz LB, Zawin M, Carcangiu ML, et al. Does pelvic magnetic resonance imaging differentiate among the histologic subtypes of uterine leiomyomata? Fertil Steril. 1998;70:580.

29. Goto A, Takeuchi S, Sugimura K, et al. Usefulness of Gd-DTPA contrast-enhanced dynamic MRI and serum determination of LDH and its isozymes in the differential diagnosis of leiomyosarcoma from degenerated leiomyoma of the uterus. Int J Gynecol Cancer. 2002;12:354.

30. Tanaka YO, Nishida M, Tsunoda H, et al. Smooth muscle tumors of uncertain malignant potential and leiomyosarcomas of the uterus: MR findings. J Magn Reson Imaging. 2004;20:998.

31. Baird DD, Dunson DB, Hill MC, et al. High cumulative incidence of uterine leiomyoma in black and white women: ultrasound evidence. Am J Obstet Gynecol. 2003;188:100.

32. Brooks SE, Zhan M, Cote T, Baquet CR. Surveillance, epidemiology, and end results analysis of 2677 cases of uterine sarcoma 1989–1999. Gynecol Oncol. 2004;93:204.

33. Fang Z, Matsumoto S, Ae K, et al. Postradiation soft tissue sarcoma: a multi-institutional analysis of 14 cases in Japan. J Orthop Sci. 2004;9(3):242.
34. Giuntoli RL 2nd, Metzinger DS, DiMarco CS, et al. Retrospective review of 208 patients with leiomyosarcoma of the uterus: prognostic indicators, surgical management, and adjuvant therapy. Gynecol Oncol. 2003;89(3):460.
35. Wickerham DL, Fisher B, Wolmark N, et al. Association of Tamoxifen and uterine sarcoma. J Clin Oncol. 2002;20:2758.
36. Wysowski DK, Honig SF, Beitz J. Uterine sarcoma associated with tamoxifen use. N Engl J Med. 2002;346:1832.
37. Moinfar F, Azodi M, Tavassoli FA. Uterine sarcomas. Pathology. 2007;39:55.
38. Launonen V, Vierimaa O, Kiuru M, et al. Inherited susceptibility to uterine leiomyomas and renal cell cancer. Proc Natl Acad Sci U S A. 2001;98(6):3387.
39. Toro JR, Nickerson ML, Wei MH, et al. Mutations in the fumarate hydratase gene cause hereditary leiomyomatosis and renal cell cancer in families in North America. Am J Hum Genet. 2003;73(1):95.
40. CL Y, Tucker MA, Abramson DH, et al. Cause-specific mortality in long-term survivors of retinoblastoma. J Natl Cancer Inst. 2009;101(8):581.
41. Sener AB, Seçkin NC, Ozmen S, et al. The effects of hormone replacement therapy on uterine fibroids in postmenopausal women. Fertil Steril. 1996;65(2):354.
42. Polatti F, Viazzo F, Colleoni R, et al. Uterine myoma in postmenopause: a comparison between two therapeutic schedules of HRT. Maturitas. 2000;37(1):27.
43. Ang WC, Farrell E, Vollenhoven B. Effect of hormone replacement therapies and selective estrogen receptor modulators in postmenopausal women with uterine leiomyomas: a literature review. Climacteric. 2001;4(4):284.
44. Yang CH, Lee JN, Hsu SC, et al. Effect of hormone replacement therapy on uterine fibroids in postmenopausal women—a 3-year study. Maturitas. 2002;43(1):35.
45. Song JY. Laparoscopic resection of the large broad ligament fibroid. Washington, D.C.: Surgical video session presented at the meeting of the American Association of Gynecologic Laparoscopists; 2013.
46. Hasson HM, Rotman C, Rana N, et al. Open laparoscopy: 29-year experience. Obstet Gynecol. 2000;96(5 P 1):763–6.

47. Hasson HM, Rotman C. Laparoscopic myomectomy. In: Sanfilippo JS, Levine RL, editors. Operative gynecologic endoscopy. 2nd ed. New York: Springer; 1996. p. 89–103.
48. Song JY, Borncamp E, Mehaffey P, Rotman C. Large abdominal wall endometrioma following laparoscopic hysterectomy. JSLS. 2011;15(2):261–3.
49. Rotman C, Rana N, Song JY, et al. Laparoscopic tubal anastomosis. In: Rizk B, Garcia-Velasco J, Sallam H, Makrigiannakis A, editors. Infertility and assisted reproduction. Cambridge: Cambridge University Press; 2008. p. 91–8.
50. Kashani BN, Centini G, Morelli S, et al. Role of medical management for uterine leiomyomas. Best Pract Res Clin Obstet Gynaecol. 2016;34:85–103.
51. Conforti A, Mollo A, Alviqqi C, et al. Techniques to reduce blood loss during open myomectomy: a qualitative review of literature. Eur J Obstet Gynecol Reprod Biol. 2015;192:90–5.
52. Zhang Y, Sun L, Guo Y, et al. The impact of preoperative gonadotropin-releasing hormone agonist treatment on women with uterine fibroids: a meta-analysis. Obstet Gynecol Surv. 2014;69(2):100–8.
53. Bassaw B, Mohammed N, Jaqqat A, et al. Experience with a gonadotropin-releasing hormone agonist prior to myomectomy-comparison of twice vs. thrice monthly doses and a control group. J Obstet Gynaecol. 2014;34(5):415–9.

Chapter 12
Asymptomatic Fibroids and Infertility

Alice Rhoton-Vlasak and Elizabeth Plasencia

Clinical Case

A 32-year-old nulligravida obese patient presents with oligomenorrhea and primary infertility of 2 years duration. She has 4–7 menstrual cycles a year and has had irregular cycles since menarche. Her last menstrual period was 4 months ago, and she has used no contraception. She tried to use ovulation kits to help time intercourse, but they never showed any LH surge. On further questioning, she states she has noticed her hair thinning in the last few years as well as poorly controlled acne. Her weight is stable and she has no galactorrhea. She rarely exercises. She denies ever having chlamydia or gonorrhea. She has no pelvic pain or pressure, dysmenorrhea, or menorrhagia. She has no

A. Rhoton-Vlasak, MD (✉) • E. Plasencia, MD
Department of Obstetrics and Gynecology, University of Florida College of Medicine, 1600 SW Archer Rd, Box 100294, Gainesville, FL 32610, USA
e-mail: rhotona@ufl.edu; eplasencia@ufl.edu

N.S. Moawad (ed.), *Uterine Fibroids*,
https://doi.org/10.1007/978-3-319-58780-6_12,
© Springer International Publishing AG 2018

significant past medical history, surgical history, or family history of malignancy. Her mother also had irregular cycles and had to take clomiphene citrate to be able to get pregnant with her. Her husband is a healthy 35-year-old male without any significant past medical or surgical history. He takes no medications, and they are able to have regular unprotected intercourse.

Exam Findings

On examination, she has a normal BP, pulse, respiratory rate, and temperature. She has a body mass index of 36 kg/m^2. She is overall a well-appearing pleasant female in no distress. There is dark facial hair on her chin and upper lip. There is no obvious balding or hair thinning. She has mild acne on her upper back. She has mild acanthosis in her cubital folds. No striae are noted. Pelvic examination revealed no clitoromegaly and normal female external genitalia. The vagina and cervix were normal appearing. The bimanual exam was limited due to her body habitus but a 10-week size enlarged mobile uterus was palpated, with no palpable adnexal masses.

Diagnostic Workup

Her initial infertility workup consisted of a hysterosalpingogram (HSG), which showed patent tubes and a normal intrauterine cavity (Fig. 12.1) and a normal semen analysis on her partner. A transvaginal ultrasound (TVUS) showed a 10-week size uterus with multiple small intramural fibroids ranging from 1–2.5 cm in diameter (Figs. 12.2 and 12.3) and bilateral ovaries with multiple subcapsular follicles (Fig. 12.4). None of the fibroids appeared to be in proximity to or within the endometrial cavity. The ovarian appearance is consistent with that of polycystic ovaries.

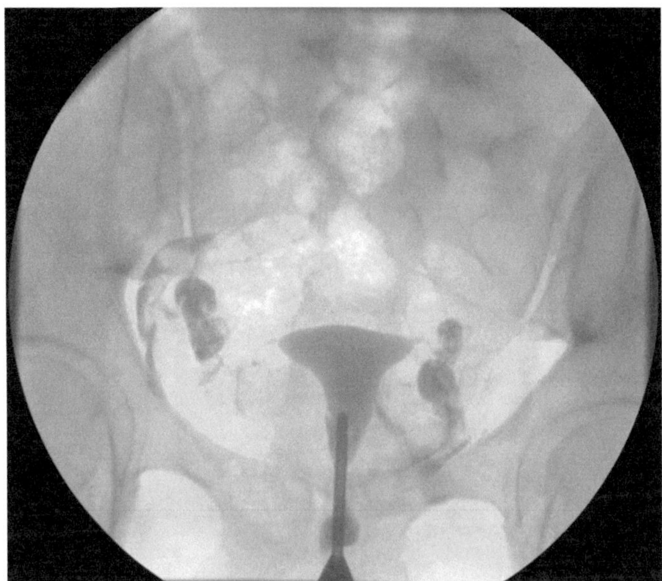

FIGURE 12.1 Hysterosalpingogram (HSG) showing normal uterine cavity without filling defects and free spill from bilateral patent fallopian tubes

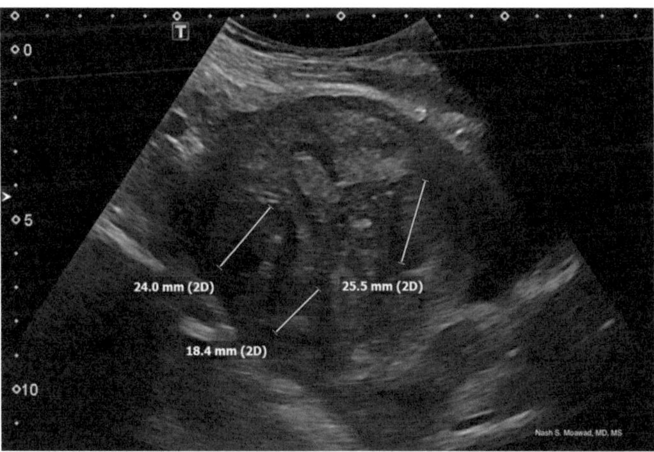

FIGURE 12.2 Transabdominal ultrasound showing a slightly enlarged uterus with multiple small intramural fibroids, not involving the uterine cavity

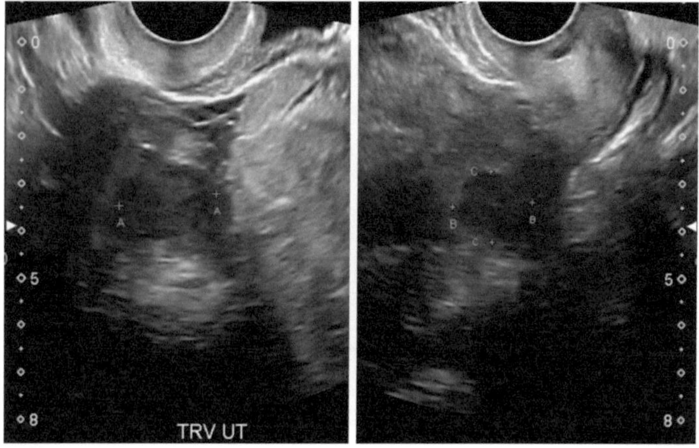

FIGURE 12.3 Transvaginal ultrasound (TVUS) showing an incidental finding of small intramural fibroids

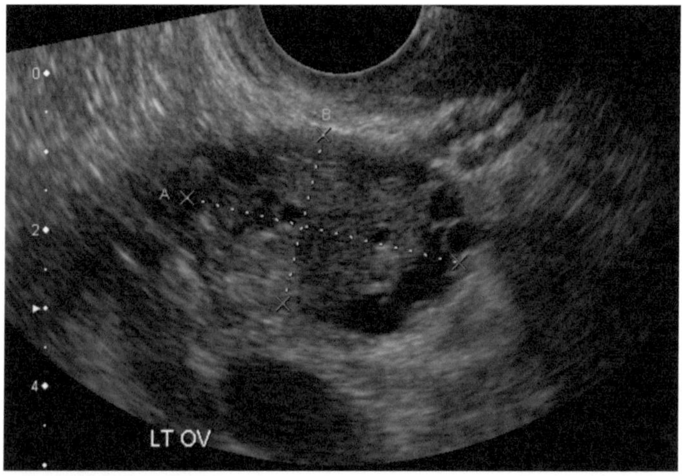

FIGURE 12.4 Transvaginal ultrasound (TVUS) showing the ovary with multiple sub-centimeter subcapsular follicles suggestive of polycystic ovaries syndrome (PCOS)

Treatment Options

This patient's history and physical exam findings are consistent with polycystic ovary syndrome (PCOS), but other causes of oligomenorrhea and anovulation should also be ruled out. Polycystic ovary syndrome is a well-recognized cause of infertility due to chronic anovulation, and it is not likely that her small fibroids that are asymptomatic are contributing to her infertility at this time. This case represents an example of where the underlying cause of infertility should be recognized as a separate medical issue from her fibroids. The next steps involve the laboratory evaluation of oligomenorrhea and androgen excess, then associated testing for metabolic disorders due to PCOS, followed by the treatments indicated to induce ovulation.

The revised 2003 criteria for PCOS diagnosis include having two out of three of the following: chronic anovulation and/or clinical or biochemical signs of hyper-androgenism and or polycystic ovaries with no evidence of related disorders [1]. This includes ruling out a thyroid disorder with thyroid function studies and prolactin level to rule out hyperprolactinemia. Other laboratory studies that may be indicated, depending on the severity of androgen excess symptoms, might include a 17-hydroxyprogesterone level, DHEA-S, and a total and free testosterone.

Women with PCOS need to be evaluated for metabolic syndrome before starting infertility treatment. Insulin resistance plays a crucial role in PCOS. As part of preconceptual health screening, this patient should be screened for hyperlipidemia, hypertension, and diabetes. A history looking for potential cardiac events and stroke should be obtained. In this patient, a hemoglobin A1c and a lipid panel would also be checked. The hemoglobin A1c will help guide therapy by determining if there is impaired glucose tolerance causing prediabetes or adult-onset type 2 diabetes. If this is found to be the case, metformin could be started in this patient. Lifestyle modification with diet, exercise, and weight loss would also be indicated.

For patients with PCOS, weight loss should be encouraged as this can regulate menstrual cycles and make fertility treatment more effective. Lifestyle modification with diet, exercise, and weight loss would also be indicated if she is overweight or obese.

For the incidental fibroids found in her exam and TVUS, their location (intramural), size (1–2 cm), and normal structure of her uterine cavity would result in a recommendation against a myomectomy. This patient's fibroids would be monitored throughout her pregnancy to assure that they are not significantly growing in size.

For ovulation induction, letrozole is now the first-line therapy, over clomiphene citrate. Because of the normal semen analysis, intrauterine insemination (IUI) is not the first-line therapy, but a discussion with the patient is vital in determining if they would like this procedure done as well. Other options include clomiphene citrate, gonadotropin therapy, and in vitro fertilization (IVF) to assist in reproduction.

Discussion

When a workup for infertility is completed, the most common causes for infertility should be considered. Ovulatory dysfunction, as seen in PCOS, makes up about 30% of the causes of female infertility [1]. Tubal factors are a growing cause of infertility due to the increased incidence of chlamydial and gonococcal salpingitis. Male factor as the cause of infertility makes up 20–30% of cases [2]. Peritoneal factor, particularly endometriosis, and advanced maternal age or diminished ovarian reserve should also be considered. In this case, this woman can clinically be diagnosed with PCOS, which is likely the cause of her primary infertility. Incidental fibroids were found on her clinical exam and confirmed by the TVUS.

Uterine fibroids are common benign tumors seen in up to 40% of women. Whether fibroids affect fertility is still a topic of debate and study with no definitive answer available for all types and location of uterine fibroids. Studying the exact effect of fibroids becomes complex due to the variation in size, location, number, and composition, in addition to several confounding factors. Fibroids are classified based on their location in the uterus as submucosal, intramural, and subserosal. Within these, the Federation of Gynecology and Obstetrics (FIGO) subdivided them based on percent within each of these locations [3]. The range is from type 0 where the submucosal fibroid is completely inside the uterine cavity to type 7 where the subserosal fibroid is completely inside the pelvis (Table 12.1).

TABLE 12.1 This categorization differentiates fibroids based on whether they are submucosal, intramural, or subserosal

Submucosal	0	Pedunculated intracavitary
	1	<50% intramural
	2	>50% intramural
Intramural	3	100% intramural with endometrium contact
	4	Intramural
Subserosal	5	Subserosal- >50% intramural
	6	Subserosal- <50% intramural
	7	Subserosal pedunculated
Others	8	Other site

This categorization differentiates fibroids based on whether they are submucosal, intramural, or subserosal. Fibroids completely in the uterine cavity on a stalk are classified as submucosal type 0. Types 1 and 2 are submucosal but have a portion that is intramural; the extent in myometrium determines if type 1 or 2, type 1 being <50% in the myometrium and type 2 being >50% intramural. Intramural fibroids are subdivided into types 3 and 4, type 3 with fibroid completely in myometrium but in contact with the endometrial surface. Type 4 is completely in myometrium without any involvement of endometrium or serosa. Subserosal fibroids extend toward the serosa, and the portion that remains intramural determines the type. Type 5 has >50% intramural, type 6 has <50% intramural, and type 7 has no intramural portion and is pedunculated subserosal. Any other location for a fibroid such as cervix is categorized as type 8
Adapted From Reference [3]

A meta-analysis of 18 studies by Pritt et al. was performed in 2009 to compile the data on the effects of fibroids on fertility [4]. When comparing women with myomas to control subjects, there was noted to be decreased implantation, ongoing pregnancies, and live birth rates. When fibroids were stratified by location, submucosal fibroids showed decreased clinical pregnancy rates, implantation rates, ongoing pregnancy/live birth rate, and increased spontaneous abortions compared to women without fibroids. There was no increase in preterm delivery in these women. When comparing women with fibroids with no intracavitary involvement to women with no fibroids, the data showed that implantation rates and ongoing pregnancy/live birth rates were lower and spontaneous abortion rates higher overall. Fibroids that did not distort the cavity did not seem to lower fertility. When non-distorting fibroids were split into subserosal and intramural fibroids, subserosal fibroids seemed to have no effect on fertility or pregnancy, while intramural fibroids did have negative effects on fertility and pregnancy. This conclusion is not definitive as many of these studies had poor evaluation of the uterine cavity. Most of the studies used hysterosalpingograms or transvaginal ultrasounds. Hysterosalpingograms can have sensitivities as low as 50% for intramural fibroids [5]. Transvaginal ultrasound has sensitivities a low as 69% when compared to hysteroscopy, which is the gold standard [6]. Currently sonohysterogram, hysteroscopy, and magnetic resonance imaging (MRI) are the best techniques available to diagnose the presence of intracavitary or submucosal fibroids [7]. Many of these studies also did not include the size of the fibroids, location of the intramural fibroid, or the proximity to the endometrium.

In 2010, Sunkara et al. performed another meta-analysis of 19 observational studies on infertility and fibroids. They concluded that subserosal myomas do not affect fertility and submucosal fibroids are detrimental to fertility [8]. They limited the size range of intramural fibroids from 0.7 to 5 cm and those not impinging on the intrauterine cavity. They did find significantly more adverse pregnancy outcomes and a reduced live birth rate in women with intramural non-distorting fibroids but called for well-designed randomized control trials.

It appears that size is an independent variable that determines the fertility and pregnancy outcomes in a woman. Some of the most recent studies show an association between size and pathogenesis, but they do not agree on the cutoff size for intramural fibroids. Recently Yan et al. found that patients with intramural fibroids greater than 3 cm did have lower delivery rates when compared to unaffected women [9]. Somigliana et al. found that intramural fibroids less than 5 cm had similar live birth rates to the control group [10]. Clearly, size may alter fertility and pregnancy outcomes. The size that appears to significantly decrease fertility rates and adversely alter pregnancy outcomes is not well established but appears to be around 3–4 cm.

The question remains: When is it reasonable to perform a myomectomy to improve fertility in the presence of intramural fibroids? If this patient had submucosal fibroids, it would be clear that she needed hysteroscopic myomectomy before undergoing ovulation induction to restore a normal cavity before pregnancy. The studies that have examined this include Bulletti et al. who found that delivery rates were significantly higher in patients with laparoscopic myomectomies (42%) compared to patients with fibroids that did not undergo myomectomy (11%, $p < 0.001$) [11]. Subsequent work by this group demonstrated that intramural-subserosal fibroids >5 cm that were excised had a pregnancy rate that was 25% higher in those with surgery compared to those without ($p < 0.01$) [12]. The 2009 meta-analysis on surgical management of fibroids found that surgical excision of submucosal fibroids improved fertility, but the data supporting this was limited, and they did not find it beneficial to excise intramural fibroids [4]. Gilliano et al. also found that mixed submucosal intramural fibroids can disrupt the endometrial cavity and result in poor results from IVF [13]. Whether removing intramural fibroids will normalize fertilization is not known, and there are many reasons to avoid unnecessary myomectomies. Abdominal and laparoscopic myomectomy have associated risks, including the risk of damage to internal organs, infection, blood loss, postoperative adhesions, and greater risk of a cesarean section and uterine rupture in pregnancy. Given the limited trials and significant risks associated with abdominal or laparoscopic myomectomies, at this time, it is not recommended to perform myomectomy for small intramural fibroids. This is especially true for fibroids less than 4 cm [9].

Polycystic ovary syndrome (PCOS) is the most common endocrine disorder in women of reproductive age. This condition occurs in 5–10% of women [14]. PCOS is a condition that causes anovulation or oligo-ovulation, which manifests as irregular periods. Levels of circulating androgens are often elevated which results in abnormal hair growth and hair thickening, acne, and male pattern balding. Women with this condition are often, but not always, overweight or obese. Insulin resistance is thought to play a critical role in the pathogenesis of this syndrome, but the mechanism by which insulin resistance or excess insulin results in anovulation or high androgen levels is not known [15]. It is thought to be partly due to insulin disrupting the hypothalamic-pituitary axis. During the menstrual cycle in women with PCOS, many small follicles ranging from 4 to 9 mm in size develop in the ovary, but these follicles are not capable of maturing to the point of ovulation. This therefore causes an imbalance in the levels of estrogen, progesterone, LH, and FSH. The high levels of LH and insulin are likely the reason for the androgen excess seen in women with PCOS.

Due to the association with insulin resistance, women with PCOS need to be screened for metabolic syndrome. Women with PCOS have a higher incidence of hypertension, diabetes, and hyperlipidemia. Progression from normal glucose tolerance to T2DM might be as high as 5–15% in 3 years [16]. A hemoglobin A1c or baseline glucose tolerance testing should be performed in any of these patients who will potentially undergo fertility treatment and every 1–2 years afterward [15]. It has also been shown that lean

PCOS women have higher low-density lipoprotein (LDL) and lower high-density lipoprotein (HDL) when compared to BMI and age-matched controls [17]. For this reason, a lipid panel should be obtained when evaluating PCOS patients. This also leads to a potentially higher risk of coronary disease and stroke prevalence, and women should be questioned about heart disease and stroke because of the added physical stress that comes with pregnancy. There is currently no genetic screen to diagnose PCOS, and it remains mostly a clinical diagnosis based on symptoms, physical exam findings, bloods tests and ovarian morphology on transvaginal ultrasound. Irregular menses caused by anovulation or irregular ovulation, elevated androgen levels or clinical signs of androgen excess, or polycystic ovaries on ultrasound are the three diagnostic criteria. Patients need at least two of the three criteria to be diagnosed with PCOS, and other conditions that cause similar symptoms may also need to be ruled out. Laboratory testing would often include a TSH, prolactin, FSH, and estradiol, as well as testing to rule out other causes of androgen excess including a DHEA-S, 17-OH-progesterone, and total and free testosterone.

Many women with PCOS do not ovulate regularly, and therefore are often subfertile or infertile. While an infertility evaluation is typically done after 1 year of infertility in women less than 35 years old, an infertility evaluation in women with PCOS could be started sooner. After determining patency of the tubes with an HSG, ruling out STIs, and confirming a normal semen analysis, other causes for anovulation should be explored. Thyroid function, adrenal function, and hyperprolactinemia should be excluded. The primary initial treatment for overweight or obese women with PCOS who are having difficulty becoming pregnant should undergo a lifestyle modification to help with weight loss including dietary changes and exercise. Even a 5% reduction in weight can result in regulation of ovulation [18]. Weight loss might also have the added benefit of improving the efficacy of fertility medications, but studies on this are limited.

Medications for ovulation induction are used with great frequency and this is the standard of care for PCOS patients, such as the patient described in this case. There are multiple ovulation induction medications used today. Clomiphene citrate is a selective estrogen receptor modulator that turns off the negative feedback estrogen has on the hypothalamus. This results in increased gonadotropins, which results in ovulation. This medication has been used for decades as the primary ovulation induction medication. Problems with clomiphene citrate include high multiple-pregnancy rates relative to unassisted conception, mood changes, poor efficacy, and rarely ovarian hyperstimulation syndrome (OHSS). Letrozole is a non-steroidal competitive aromatase inhibitor, which lowers the concentration of estrogen, therefore disinhibiting the feedback on the hypothalamus, which results in increased gonadotropins. In 2014, Legro et al. found that letrozole was more effective as a fertility treatment than clomiphene citrate (CC) in women with PCOS. It increased ovulation, conception, pregnancy, and live births [19]. This study has resulted in a push to use letrozole as first line in women with PCOS desiring fertility treatment. A few studies have also shown that taking metformin in addition to clomiphene can increase the rate of ovulation, but newer studies have not found this to be the case. Huang et al. performed a meta-analysis in 2015 on the effects of metformin on patients with polycystic ovary syndrome undergoing assisted reproductive technology [20]. They found that metformin does not improve assisted reproductive technology outcomes in patients with PCOS. The rates of pregnancy, spontaneous abortion, and live births between the metformin and placebo group had no significant difference. They did find that the risk of ovarian hyperstimulation syndrome was significantly reduced (RR 0.44, 0.26–0.77). Metformin would now primarily be used as an addition to improve impaired glucose tolerance or type 2 diabetes in women with PCOS, whether or not they are trying to conceive. Metformin would also be used to prevent OHSS in women with PCOS undergoing IVF [20].

If a woman with PCOS is CC or letrozole resistant, and does not ovulate on the medications after multiple cycles with escalating doses, then gonadotropin therapy with FSH injections may be considered. While this therapy is more effective, it is more expensive and has more associated risks of multiple gestation and OHSS. Ovarian drilling has also been used to improve fertility and spontaneous or medication-induced ovulation but has diminished in use likely because of the complications associated with surgery in general. In vitro fertilization (IVF) is also much more effective, but is more costly and time demanding.

The association between polycystic ovaries and fibroids has been studied. A prospective cohort study was done on 3631 new cases of uterine leiomyomata, to determine the incidence of PCOS. This study found that the incidence of fibroids was 65% higher in women with PCOS than women without PCOS, which indicates an association between the two [21]. The reason for this association is not known. It has been hypothesized that insulin-like growth factor (IGF-1), which is higher in women with PCOS, increases the risk of fibroids [22]. Other studies though have shown the opposite effect, with IGF-1 possibly playing a protective role against fibroids [23]. It is hypothesized that hyper-insulinemia results in poor vascularization for the fibroid decreasing the development [24]. Clearly, the effects of insulin on fibroids are not well known, and this is an area of ongoing and active research.

Recommendations

When determining whether to intervene surgically for fibroids, it is important to look at the entire clinical picture. The physician should determine the patient's age, previous pregnancies, and presence or absence of clinical symptoms attributable to the fibroids, in addition to the number, size, and location of fibroids. Other clinical factors should also be determined, as in this case, where a normal semen analysis, patent tubes, and a normal uterine cavity were found.

Our patient had clear evidence of anovulation and PCOS, which is a well-recognized, common, and very treatable cause of infertility.

Currently surgical removal of subserosal fibroids is not recommended if asymptomatic. Submucosal fibroids do affect fertility, and hysteroscopic resection has been shown to be beneficial, so it is reasonable to recommend removal in women desiring improved fertility. For intramural fibroids over 4 cm, even without involvement of the uterine cavity, it is reasonable to recommend a laparoscopic or abdominal myomectomy, for women who desire to improve their fertility. This corresponds with FIGO stages between 3 and 6. Removing multiple smaller fibroids that do not distort the cavity, such as in our case, should only be considered if there have been multiple IVF or reproductive failures that have no other identifiable cause.

In our patient with presumed anovulation and PCOS, different metabolic derangements should be explored. Weight loss, when appropriate, should be encouraged as a first-line therapeutic option to reduce anovulation and improve fertility. If weight loss does not occur or does not regulate the menstrual cycle, letrozole ovulation induction would currently be the first medical therapy prior the use of CC. If there is a male factor or multiple cycles of letrozole have been attempted without a resulting pregnancy, IUI can be considered. Gonadotropin ovulation induction carries a greater risk of multiple gestation and OHSS but is more effective than letrozole or clomiphene citrate. IVF is another potential option to discuss with the patient. Ultimately, all of the potential options need to be discussed with the patient, and the physician and the patient should come to an agreement on tailoring the best management strategy in her case. Our patient's fibroids could be observed, but no intervention would be recommended over those indicated for anovulation and PCOS. If she did conceive with therapy, she should be informed that her fibroids could grow under the influence of higher estradiol levels during any ovulation induction therapy, as well as during pregnancy itself. During therapy, and in any future pregnancy, any fibroid growth would be monitored via ultrasounds as indicated.

References

1. Rotterdam ESHRE/ASRM-Sponsored PCOS consensus workshop group. Revised 2003 consensus on diagnostic criteria and long-term health risks related to Polycystic Ovary Syndrome (PCOS). Hum Reprod. 2004;19(1):41–7.
2. WHO Technical Report Series. Recent advances in medically assisted conception. Report of a WHO Scientific Group. World Health Organ Tech Rep Ser. 1992;820:1–111.
3. Munro M, Critchley HOD, et al. The FIGO classification of causes of abnormal uterine bleeding in the reproductive years. Fertil Steril. 2011;95(7):2204–8.
4. Pritts EA, Parker WH, Olive DL. Fibroids and infertility: an updated systematic review of the evidence. Fertil Steril. 2009;91(4):1215–23.
5. Soares S, dos Reis MMB, Camargos A. Diagnostic accuracy of sonohysterogram, transvaginal sonography, and hysterosalpingography in patients with uterine cavity diseases. Fertil Steril. 2000;73:406–11.
6. Ayida G, Chamberlain P, Barlow D, Kennedy S. Uterine cavity assessment prior to in vitro fertilization: comparison of transvaginal scanning, saline contrast hysterosalpingogram and hysteroscopy. Ultrasound Obstet Gynecol. 1997;10:59–62.
7. Fukuda M, Shimizu T, Fukuda K, Yomura W, Shimizu S. Transvaginal hysterosonography for differential diagnosis between submucosal and intramural myoma. Gynecol Obstet Investig. 1993;35:236–9.
8. Sunkara SK, et al. The effect of intramural fibroids without uterine cavity involvement on the outcome of IVF treatment: a systematic review and meta-analysis. Hum Reprod. 2010;25(2):418–29. doi:10.1093/humrep/dep396.
9. Yan L, et al. Effect of fibroids not distorting the endometrial cavity on the outcome of in vitro fertilization treatment: a retrospective cohort study. Fertil Steril. 2014;1013:716–21.
10. Somigliana E, et al. Fibroids not encroaching the endometrial cavity and IVF success rate: a prospective study. Hum Reprod. 2011;26(4):834–9. doi:10.1093/humrep/der015.
11. Bulletti C, et al. The role of leiomyomas in infertility. J Am Assoc Gynecol Laparosc. 1999;6(4):441–5.
12. Bulletti C, et al. Myomas, pregnancy outcome, and in vitro fertilization. Ann N Y Acad Sci. 2004;1034:84–92.

13. Galliano D, et al. ART and uterine pathology: how relevant is the maternal side for implantation? Hum Reprod Update. 2015;21(1):13–38. doi:10.1093/humupd/dmu047.
14. Rotterdam ESHRE/ASRM-Sponsored PCOS Consensus Workshop Group. Revised 2003 consensus on diagnostic criteria and long-term health risks related to polycystic ovary syndrome. Fertil Steril. 2004;81:19–25.
15. Goodman NF, et al. American Association of Clinical Endocrinologists, American College of Endocrinology, and Andorgen excess and PCOS society disease state clinical review: guide to the best practices in the evaluation and treat, emt of polycystic ovary syndrome-part 2. Endocr Pract. 2015;21(12):1415–26.
16. Celik C, et al. Progression to impaired glucose tolerance or type 2 diabetes mellitus in polycystic ovary syndrome: a controlled follow-up study. Fertil Steril. 2014;101(4):1123–8.
17. Wild RA, et al. Assessment of cardiovascular risk and prevention of cardiovascular disease in women with the polycystic ovary syndrome: a consensus statement by the Androgen Excess and Polycystic Ovary Syndrome (AE-PCOS) Society. J Clin Endocrinol Metab. 2010;95(5):2038–49.
18. Clark AM, et al. Weight loss results in significant improvement in pregnancy and ovulation rates in anovulatory obese women. Hum Reprod. 1995;10(10):2705–12.
19. Legro RS, et al. Letrozole versus clomiphene for infertility in the polycystic ovary syndrome. N Engl J Med. 2014;371:119–29.
20. Huang X, et al. A systematic review and meta-analysis of metformin among patients with polycystic ovary syndrome undergoing assisted reproductive technology procedures. Int J Gynaecol Obstet. 2015;131(2):111–6.
21. Wise LA, et al. Polycystic ovary syndrome and risk of uterine leiomyomata. Fertil Steril. 2007;87(5):1108–15.
22. Ciarmela P, et al. Growth factors and myometrium: biological effects in uterine fibroid and possible clinical implications. Hum Reprod Update. 2011;17(6):772–90.
23. Baird DD, Travlos G, Wilson R, et al. Uterine leiomyomata in relation to insulin-like growth factor-I, insulin, and diabetes. Epidemiology. 2009;20(4):604–10.
24. Laughlin SK, Schroeder JC, Baird DD. New directions in the epidemiology of uterine fibroids. Semin Reprod Med. 2010;28(3):204–17. doi:10.1055/s-0030-1251477.

Chapter 13
Solitary Myoma: Laparo-Endoscopic Single Site (LESS) Surgery

Stacey Scheib

Twenty-seven year-old presents with menorrhagia and is found to have a 3.5 cm intramural fibroid. She desires fertility in the future. She elects medical management with oral contraceptive pills at this time. She returns 14 months later with significant pelvic pain, deep dyspareunia, and anemia with hemoglobin of 7.2 g/dL, and ultrasound reveals the fibroid has increased in size to 9 cm.

There are several questions that this case scenario brings up.

Electronic supplementary material The online version of this chapter (doi:10.1007/978-3-319-58780-6_13. contains supplementary material, which is available to authorized users.

S. Scheib, MD
Department of Gynecology and Obstetrics, Johns Hopkins University Hospital, 600 N. Wolfe Street, Phipps 249, Baltimore, MD 21287, USA
e-mail: stacey@scheib.com

N.S. Moawad (ed.), *Uterine Fibroids*,
https://doi.org/10.1007/978-3-319-58780-6_13,
© Springer International Publishing AG 2018

Is There a Concern for Malignancy?

This patient had a rapid growth of her fibroid with her fibroid growing from 3.5 to 9 cm in the course of 14 months. Rapid growth is considered to be when a uterus has increased by 6 weeks' gestational size within 1 year [1]. Historically, rapid growth of fibroids gave the suspicion for a leiomyosarcoma. In the premenopausal patient, there is wide variation in growth and that growth does not correlate with risk of leiomyosarcoma as it does in the postmenopausal patient [1–5]. Normal fibroids can demonstrate growth of up to 138% in 6 months [2]. If this patient was postmenopausal, a growing (slow or rapid) uterine mass should definitely be evaluated for a malignancy.

How do We Assess Her Risk
for a Leiomyosarcoma?

Screening markers are used to help identify leiomyosarcomas. This is important to minimize the need for surgery and especially a laparotomy due to the low incidence of leiomyosarcoma and the high incidence of fibroids. Nagai T et al. created a preoperative diagnostic scoring system to improve the identification of these patients [6]. They identified four predictive factors: preoperative age, serum lactate dehydrogenase (LDH) levels, endometrial cytology findings, and magnetic resonance imaging (MRI).

The first factor to consider is her age. This patient is 27 years old. Among myomectomy patients, age correlates with risk of a uterine cancer [7]. The risk of a hidden cancer in a patient <40 years old is 1 in 2337, in a 40-49 year old is 1 in 702, in a 50-59 year old is 1 in 154 and >/=60 year old is 1 in 31.

Serum levels of total LDH and its isoenzymes were evaluated in predicting leiomyosarcoma. Total has the highest sensitivity but diagnostic accuracy was only 88.6% [8]. LDH isoenzyme 3 has a sensitivity and specificity of >90% for predicting leiomyosarcoma [8], though both the total LDH and isoenzyme 3 can be elevated with leiomyoma, which is why it is not a good screen in isolation.

Preoperative endometrial sampling can suggest an invasive tumor 86% of the time and predict the correct histologic diagnosis in 64% [9].

MRI is the best imaging modality to predict for leiomyosarcoma preoperatively [10]. Diffusion weighted imaging can improve the sensitivity and specificity but is a technique that is not universally available [11].

Should We Proceed with Surgery Now or Resolve the Anemia First?

She is anemic at this point and how do we address it. There are two schools of thought here. One is to proceed with surgery now, but the patient is at increased risk for needing a blood transfusion at the time of surgery since her starting hemoglobin is 7.2 g/dL. Transfusions prior to pregnancy can increase the incidence of antibodies and can result in acquisition of viral disease, both of which can complicate any subsequent pregnancy. As a result, it is recommended for this patient population to request leuko-reduced packed red blood cells if transfusion is necessary.

The other option is to resolve the anemia first to allow for a larger potential blood loss reserve before a blood transfusion is necessary. To help resolve the anemia, iron supplementation is utilized to provide the building blocks for red cell production and hormonal suppression to decrease the blood loss related to her menses. Iron supplementation can be provided orally and through intravenous (IV) infusions. Oral iron supplementation can be associated with constipation and there is limitation in absorption. IV iron infusions work faster than the oral approach and can be helpful when a patient has side effects from the oral approach.

Hormonal suppression with combined oral contraception or progestins is usually first-line treatment. Depot Lupron can be used if the patient fails first-line treatment.

Depot Lupron usually will have 2–3 weeks of increased bleeding initially after the first injection before the bleeding improves. Per Cochran, it has not been shown to decrease blood loss at the time of myomectomy but may decrease operating time [12]. It does potentially increase the risk of resection of normal myometrium at the time of the myomectomy because it can blur the tissue planes between the fibroid and myometrium.

Is There an Optimal Approach to the Removal?

This is a solitary fibroid. Ideally, a minimally invasive approach is the best for myomectomy cases when feasible [13]. Myomectomies are notorious surgeries for adhesion formation. Adhesions can be a source for infertility [14]. A minimally invasive approach helps to decrease the risk of adhesion formation [15]. In addition, the use of fibrin gel and fibrin sheets helps minimize the risk of adhesion formation [16, 17]. Other aspects that influence the risk of adhesion formation include number of fibroids removed, number of incisions on the uterus, and size of the largest fibroid [18]. Febrile morbidity occurs half as often with a laparoscopic myomectomy versus via laparotomy [19].

A minimally invasive approach has no difference in pregnancy rates, abortion rates, or preterm delivery when compared to laparotomy [19–21]. But in a logistic regression model, it was shown that chance to conceive is significantly higher with young patients, larger removed fibroids, intramural localization, and laparoscopic surgery [22]. In women that had symptomatic fibroids, women who had their fibroids removed laparoscopically had a shorter time to pregnancy [21].

Higher blood losses and a more pronounced hemoglobin drop with laparotomy [13, 21, 23, 24]. And as stated before, transfusions prior to pregnancy can increase the incidence of antibodies and can result in acquisition of viral disease, both of which can complicate subsequent pregnancy.

There are a number of minimally invasive approaches that can be utilized for this patient, including laparo-endoscopic single site (LESS) surgery, traditional laparoscopy, robotic assisted laparoscopic, robotic laparo-endoscopic single site (R-LESS), and mini-laparotomy.

A LESS and R-LESS approach is an ideal when there is a solitary fundal or anterior fibroid and the uterus is no larger than 16 week sized. Currently, the da Vinci™ (Intuitive Surgical, Inc., Sunnyvale, CA, USA) single-site platform is not approved for myomectomy but there are studies that have demonstrated feasibility of the approach [25]. It is also feasible with the da Vinci Si Surgical System and the standard rigid instruments in conjunction with the GelPOINT Advanced Access Platform (Applied Medical, Rancho Santa Margarita, CA, USA) [26]. Incisions on the uterus should be vertical to help facilitate suturing with the LESS and R-LESS platform. For LESS myomectomy, any standard LESS port can be utilized. An articulating laparoscope helps facilitate the surgery but a tradition $30°$, $45°$, or $70°$ laparoscope can also be used. Articulating instruments are not necessary for this procedure and traditional rigid instrumentation seems to be superior for the dissection. A barbed suture helps eliminate the need for knot tying, helps create an even tension on the incision closure, and can reduce blood loss and operative time for laparoscopic myomectomies [27, 28]. The suturing portion is the most complicated portion of LESS and R-LESS, and an additional port may need to be placed during the learning curve. A benefit of LESS and R-LESS is the larger incision at the umbilicus that helps facilitate the removal of the fibroids.

Mini-laparotomy has the benefits of a classic laparotomy approach with its ease to perform and learn and the benefits of a laparoscopic approach with its lower blood loss, short hospitalization, reduced postoperative pain, and rapid return to routine activities [21]. A laparoscopic approach does seem to be superior to mini-laparotomy in regard to fertility outcomes [21]. A mini-laparotomy approach is an option for a patient who is not a candidate for a laparoscopic approach.

Whenever possible, surgery should be performed minimally invasively and that the patient should be referred to a surgeon when the primary gynecologist does not have the skill set to perform a minimally invasive approach.

References

1. Parker WH, YS F, Berek JS. Uterine sarcoma in patients operated on for presumed leiomyoma and rapidly growing leiomyoma. Obstet Gynecol. 1994;83(3):414.
2. Peddada SD, Laughlin SK, Miner K, Guyon JP, Haneke K, Vahdat HL, Semelka RC, Kowalik A, Armao D, Davis B, Baird DD. Growth of uterine leiomyomata among premenopausal black and white women. Proc Natl Acad Sci U S A. 2008;105(50):19887.
3. DeWaay DJ, Syrop CH, Nygaard IE, Davis WA, Van Voorhis BJ. Natural history of uterine polyps and leiomyomata. Obstet Gynecol. 2002;100(1):3.
4. Kawaura N, Ito F, Ichimura T, Shibata S, Tsujimura A, Minakuchi K, Ishiko O, Ogita S. Transient rapid growth of uterine leiomyoma in a postmenopausal woman. Oncol Rep. 1999;6(6):1289.
5. Baird DD, Garrett TA, Laughlin SK, Davis B, Semelka RC, Peddada SD. Short-term change in growth of uterine leiomyoma: tumor growth spurts. Fertil Steril. 2011;95(1):242.
6. Nagai T, Takai Y, Akahori T, et al. Highly improved accuracy of the revised PREoperative sarcoma score (rPRESS) in the decision of performing surgery for patients presenting with a uterine mass. Spring. 2015;4:520.
7. Wright JD, Tergas MD, Cui R, et al. Use of electric power morcellation and prevalence of underlying cancer in women who undergo myomectomy. JAMA Oncol. 2015;1(1):69–77. doi:10.1001/jamaoncol.2014.206.
8. Goto A, Takeuchi S, Sugimura K, Maruo T. Usefulness of Gd-DTPA contrast-enhanced dynamic MRI and serum determination of LDH and its isozymes in the differential diagnosis of leiomyosarcoma from degenerated leiomyoma of the uterus. Int J Gynecol Cancer. 2002;12(4):254–61.
9. Bansal N, Herzog TJ, Venkatraman E, et al. Uterine carcinosarcomas and grade 3 endometrioid cancers: evidence of distinct tumor behavior. Obstet Gynecol. 2008;112(1):64–70.
10. Skorstad M, Kent A, Lieng M. Preoperative evaluation in women with uterine leiomyosarcoma. A nation-wide cohort study. Acta Obstet Gynecol Scand. 2016;95(11):1228–34. doi:10.1111/aogs.13008.
11. Sato K, Yuasa N, Fujita M, Fukushima Y. Clinical application of diffusion-weighted imaging for preoperative differentiation

between uterine leiomyoma and leiomyosarcoma. Am J Obstet Gynecol. 2014;210(4):368.e1–8.
12. Kongnyuy EJ, Wiysonge CS. Interventions to reduce haemorrhage during myomectomy for fibroids. Cochrane Database Syst Rev. 2014;8:CD005355.
13. Iavazzo C, Mamais I, Gkegkes ID. Robotic assisted vs laparoscopic and/or open myomectomy: systematic review and meta-analysis of the clinical evidence. Arch Gynecol Obstet. 2016;294(1):5–17.
14. Diamond MP, Freeman ML. Clinical implications of postsurgical adhesions. Hum Reprod Update. 2001;7(6):567–76.
15. Tinelli A, Malvasi A, Guido M, et al. Adhesions formation after intracapsular myomectomy with or without adhesion barrier. Fertil Steril. 2011;95(5):1780–5.
16. Takeuchi H, Kitade M, Kikuchi I, Shimanuki H, Kumakiri J, Kinoshita K. Adhesion-prevention effects of fibrin sealants after laparoscopic myomectomy as determined by second-look laparoscopy: a prospective, randomized, controlled study. J Reprod Med. 2005;50(8):571–7.
17. Ahmad G, Duffy JM, Farquhar C, et al. Barrier agents for preventing adhesions after surgery fro subfertility. Cochrane Database Syst Rev. 2008;2:CD000475.
18. Kumakiri J, Kikuchi I, Kitade M, et al. Association between uterine repair at laparoscopic myomectomy and postoperative adhesions. Acta Obstet Gynecol Scand. 2012;91(3):331–7.
19. Seracchioli R, Rossi S, Govoni F, et al. Fertility and obstetric outcome after laparoscopic myomectomy of large myomata: a randomized comparison with abdominal myomectomy. Hum Reprod. 2000;15(12):2663–8.
20. Metwally M, Cheong YC, Horne AW. Surgical treatment of fibroids for subfertility. Cochrane Database Syst Rev. 2012;11:CD003857.
21. Palomba S, Zupi E, Falbo A, et al. A multicenter randomized, controlled study comparing laparoscopic versus minilaparotomic myomectomy: reproductive outcomes. Fertil Steril. 2007;88(4):933–41.
22. Campo S, Campo V, Gambadauro P. Reproductive outcome before and after laparoscopic or abdominal myomectomy for subserous or intramural myomas. Eur J Obstet Gynecol Reprod Biol. 2003;110(2):215–9.
23. Barakat EE, Bedaiwy MA, Zimberg S, Nutter B, Nosseir M, Falcone T. Robotic-assisted, laparoscopic, and abdominal myo-

mectomy: a comparison of surgical outcomes. Obstet Gynecol. 2011;117(2 Pt 1):256–65.
24. Advincula AP, Xu X, Goudeau S 4th, Ransom SB. Robotic-assisted laparoscopic myomectomy versus abdominal myomectomy: a comparison of short-term surgical outcomes and immediate costs. J Minim Invasive Gynecol. 2007;14(6):698–705.
25. Lewis EI, Srouji SS, Gargiulo AR. Robotic single-site myomectomy: an initial report and technique. Fertil Steril. 2015;103(5):1370–7.
26. Gargiulo AR, Choussein S, Srouji SS, Cedo LE, Escobar PF. Coaxial robot-assisted laparoendoscopic single-site myomectomy. J Robot Surg. 2017;11(1):27–35. doi:10.1007/s11701-016-0603-y.
27. Tulandi T, Einarsson JI. The use of barbed suture for laparoscopic hysterectomy and myomectomy: a systematic review and meta-analysis. J Minim Invasive Gynecol. 2014;21(2):210–6.
28. Zhang Y, Ma D, Zhang Q. Role of barbed suture in repairing uterine wall defects in laparoscopic myomectomy: a systematic review and meta-analysis. J Minim Invasive Gynecol. 2016;23(5):684–91.

Chapter 14
Massive Uterine Fibroids in an Anemic Patient

James Robinson

Case Description

The patient is a 28-year-old nulliparous African American female who is referred for evaluation and management of massive symptomatic uterine fibroids, heavy menstrual bleeding, and anemia. She desires fertility in the near future. She has known about her fibroids for 5 years but has been relatively asymptomatic until approximately 1 year ago.

Currently she can feel the fibroids through her abdomen and it has become uncomfortable to lie facedown. Interestingly, she denies other significant bulk symptoms including urinary

Electronic supplementary material The online version of this chapter (doi:10.1007/978-3-319-58780-6_14. contains supplementary material, which is available to authorized users.

J. Robinson, MD, MS, FACOG
Director, Minimally Invasive Gynecologic Surgery, National Center for Advanced Pelvic Surgery, Washington Hospital Center,
106 Irving Street, NW, Suite 405 South, Washington,
DC 20010, USA
e-mail: james.k.robinson@medstar.net

N.S. Moawad (ed.), *Uterine Fibroids*,
https://doi.org/10.1007/978-3-319-58780-6_14,
© Springer International Publishing AG 2018

frequency or urgency, constipation or pelvic pressure, or sexual dysfunction. Recently a number of people have inquired about a possible pregnancy.

Her menses are regular and heavy, occurring every 28 days, lasting 7 days, with 3 days of very heavy painful flow. They have been very heavy for 1 year, but in retrospect she notes they have been getting heavier and longer for a number of years. During her heaviest flow, she is changing both tampons and overnight pads hourly, often passing large clots of blood. She also complains of cramping which she rates 8/10 in severity. She uses Ibuprofen 800 mg three times daily for 3 days every period so she can make it to work. She craves ice, denies shortness of breath, palpitations, or chest pain, and is known to be anemic. She has never had a blood transfusion and only uses oral iron intermittently because it makes her nauseated.

Recent abdominal and transvaginal ultrasound showed an enlarged fibroid uterus measuring $19.3 \times 13.7 \times 12$ cm, described multiple fibroids the largest being fundal and 11.3 cm in diameter. The endometrial stripe was obscured by fibroids.

The patient had history of anemia. Her surgical history included a skin graft for a third degree burn, and she has had no intra-abdominal surgery. Her mother had a hysterectomy for fibroids in her 40s.

Physical Examination

Abdomen: Abdomen soft and non-tender, without hernias. She has a large grafted well-healed burn on her left flank. Her uterus is palpated 5–6 cm above the umbilicus and is mobile.

Genitourinary: Pelvic Exam:

External: normal female genitalia without lesions or masses

Vagina: normal without lesions or masses
Cervix: normal without lesions or masses, very high in the
   pelvis
Adnexa: normal bimanual exam without masses or
   fullness
Uterus: 28-week uterus, very high in the pelvis, good lateral mobility

Work-Up/Orders/Follow-Up

Imaging: MRI abdomen and pelvis with and without IV
contrast
   Labs: CBC, Iron Studies
   Return to clinic to review MRI images and plan most
appropriate management

Findings

Labs:

Hgb	7.9 g/dL
Hct	25.6%
Platelets	301 k/μL
MCV	55
MCHC	29.5
Iron sat	10%
Iron total	44 μg/dL
UIBC	404 μg/dL
Ferritin	10 mg/mL
TIBC	448

MRI (Figs. 14.1, 14.2, and 14.3):

Uterus	24.2 × 20.2 × 12 cm
Fibroid #1	Right fundal intramural 13 × 12.7 × 11.6 cm
Fibroid #2	Left fundal intramural 10.4 × 8.0 × 9.1 cm — degenerative
Fibroid #3	Left submucosal 5.4 cm

Multiple other small intramural and subserosal fibroids. Normal ovaries

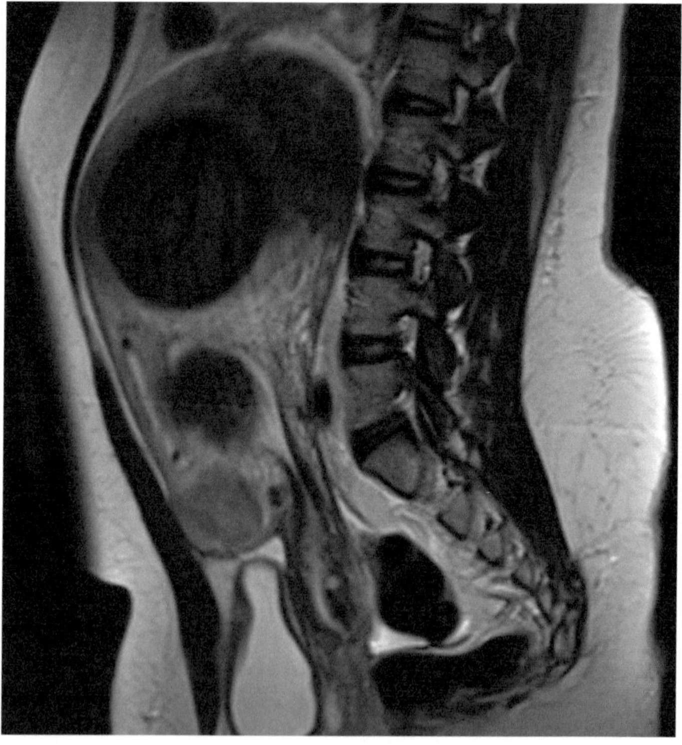

FIGURE 14.1 MRI; sagittal view: large fundal fibroid and a submucosal fibroid compressing the endometrial cavity anteriorly

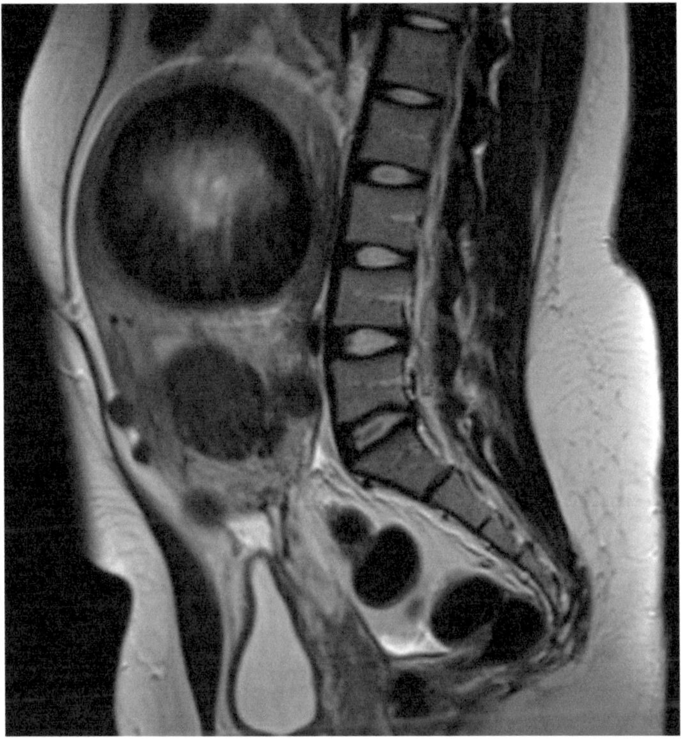

FIGURE 14.2 MRI; sagittal view: large fundal fibroid, submucosal fibroid, and multiple other intramural and Subserosal fibroids

Assessment

1. Massive symptomatic uterine fibroids causing bulk and bleeding symptoms in a patient desiring imminent fertility
2. Microcytic anemia of blood loss

Plan

1. Preoperative feraheme infusions with hematology
2. Continuous progestational therapy to suppress menses
3. Laparoscopic myomectomy with tourniquet, dilute vasopressin, and cell saver

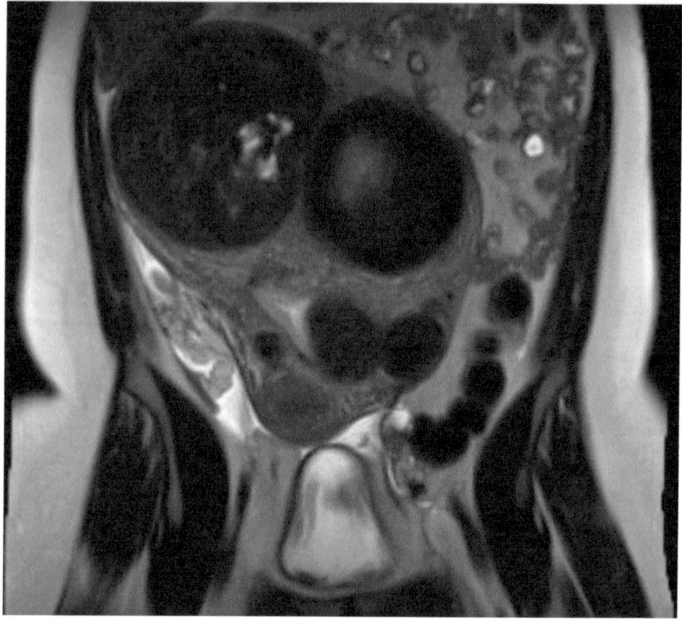

Figure 14.3 MRI; coronal view: two large fundal intramural myomas and multiple other smaller myomas displacing the uterine cavity to the right

Preoperative Considerations

In young patients with symptomatic fibroids who desire fertility preservation, myomectomy is currently the only appropriate intervention. Preoperative evaluation and work-up should be focused on identifying the appropriate route(s) of myomectomy and on mitigating and planning for potential complications. In the patient described above, two main preoperative issues stand out.

Initially the patient's fibroid burden is significant. Not only are her fibroids quite large. They are also deeply intramural and numerous. Each of these factors is a risk factor for bleeding and complications during myomectomy. A recent review of risk factors associated with complications at the time of laparoscopic myomectomy highlight uterine size, fibroid size, and fibroid number as independent risks factors for bleeding and transfusion [1].

In this patient's case, her large type 1-2 submucosal fibroid makes hysteroscopic myomectomy unreasonable. Given the complicating factors already identified, an open approach to myomectomy is reasonable in this case and is likely the most appropriate approach in the hands of all but the most experienced laparoscopic or robotic surgeons. Factors which make laparoscopy reasonable in the right hands include (1) uterine mobility and access to the lower uterine segment, (2) two large fibroids which once removed will make access to the uterus much easier, and (3) a discrete number of fibroids on MRI which will be identifiable at the time of laparoscopic surgery.

The second main preoperative issue in this patient is her significant iron deficiency anemia. In patients who report heavy menstrual bleeding and signs of anemia, assessment of a complete blood count and iron studies should occur following the initial visit. This allows time for preoperative treatment and decreases the operative risks of bleeding, transfusion, and associated postoperative complications.

Preoperative strategies to optimize blood count prior to surgery include starting the patient on a continuous progestational agent or initiation of GnRH therapy to stop preoperative menses for a period of time. Optimizing blood count and iron stores with preoperative intravenous iron infusions is a very effective approach to rapidly increase hemoglobin levels [2]. Of course preoperative blood transfusion is always an option in the most severe and refractory cases. We routinely attempt to stop menses preoperatively with continuous oral contraceptives and are quick to recommend iron infusions with a hematology group in all patients with a preoperative hemoglobin less than 10 g/dL. In patients with a religious objection to blood transfusion 6–8 weeks of GnRH agonist therapy in addition to iron infusions is often warranted.

This patient underwent infusions of feraheme spaced over a period of 9 days and was placed on continuous oral contraceptives. Her preoperative labs improved dramatically:

	Initial appointment	Preoperatively
Hgb (g/dL)	7.9	10.2
MCV	55	65
Ferritin (mg/mL)	10	710
Iron saturation (%)	10	52

Operative Considerations

Decreasing Blood Loss

Having stabilized the patient's anemia preoperatively, we scheduled a laparoscopic myomectomy. Again, recognizing the risk of increased blood loss, a number of mitigating steps were planned. Initially the surgery was scheduled in a hospital setting with access to a blood bank, and the patient was typed and crossed for two units of packed red blood cells. She was scheduled as a morning case to decrease preoperative dehydration, and a 23-h observational overnight stay was planned.

When the case was scheduled, we requested cell saver technology. Cell saver allows blood that is suctioned into the closed system to be collected, heparinized, spun down, and reinfused into the patient. Cell saver systems are designed for open surgery but are easily modified for use at the time of laparoscopy. To modify cell saver to laparoscopy, the end or the cell saver suction tubing, designed to fit a Yankauer suction tip, is cut off and fitted with a connector that has two male ends. Similarly, the suction tubing from a standard laparoscopic suction/irrigation unit is cut and merged with the cell saver suction tubing. As long as normal saline or lactated ringers is used as the irrigant, all blood and fluid collected by the laparoscopic suction/irrigation system will be recaptured by the cell saver. If significant bleeding occurs during the case, the patient can be transfused with her own red blood cells prior to utilization of the blood bank.

The preoperative examination demonstrated a large uterus "very high in the pelvis" with "good lateral mobility." This finding makes laparoscopic access to the broad ligament and uterine artery pedicles at the level of the internal cervical os possible. In this case, this access allowed us to place a laparoscopic tourniquet around the cervix, temporarily occluding the ascending branches of the uterine arteries. The use of similarly placed tourniquets at the time of open myomectomy has been shown to significantly decrease intraoperative blood loss [3].

Multiple other approaches are useful for occluding the uterine arteries at the time of laparoscopic myomectomy. When fibroids, endometriosis, or pelvic scarring make safe access to the board ligaments challenging or impossible, the advanced laparoscopic surgeon can develop the pararectal and paravesical spaces bilaterally identifying the uterine arteries at their origin where they bifurcate with the superior vesicle arteries. Once the uterine arteries have been isolated with good visualization of the ureters medially, a 5 mm liga-clip can be applied to the uterine artery temporarily. Following closure of the myomectomy defects, the clips can be easily pulled off the arteries with a fine grasper or needle driver.

Developing a strong collaborative relationship with interventional radiology can be useful in a number of complicated settings where intraoperative bleeding is a significant risk [4]. During laparoscopic myomectomy of massive pedunculated fibroids, there is an increased risk of parasitic blood supply to the fibroid. In these cases, it is possible for inferior mesenteric, superior mesenteric, or renal artery parasitic blood supply to exist. It is also possible that this blood supply enters the large fibroid posteriorly where it is not easily identified at the time of laparoscopic surgery. In these cases it is reasonable to schedule the patient for preoperative angiography (making sure to request angiography of uterine, ovarian, mesenteric, and renal vasculature) followed by gel foam embolization of the uterine arteries immediately followed by laparoscopic myomectomy. Arteries occluded with gel foam recanalize within 6 weeks making this a viable option for women desiring future fertility [5].

Even with temporary occlusion of uterine arterial blood flow, excess bleeding can still occur due to significant contribution from the ovarian arteries. Routine use of intraoperative dilute vasopressin injected subserosally causes local vasoconstriction, hydro-dissection, and decreases bleeding during surgery [6]. Due to the risk of coronary artery spasm, cardiac ischemia, severe hypotension, and pulmonary edema [7] vasopressin should always be used in a dilute form. We use 20 units in 200 mLs of injectable normal saline with care taken to avoid direct intravascular injection. Vasopressin use should be limited to no more than five units every 20 min.

Other medical approaches to decrease blood loss including preoperative rectal or vaginal misoprostol and intravenous or preoperative oral tranexamic acid administration have been suggested with less evidence of efficacy.

Laparoscopic Tourniquet (Video S1)

Tools:

1. #1 PDS suture (needle removed)
2. 5 mm right-angle dissector
3. 30° laparoscope
4. Monopolar or ultrasonic energy device
5. Laparoscopic needle drivers
6. Good uterine manipulator with vaginal fornix delineator (we use V Care—ConMed)

Technique (See Instructional Video S1):

- Pass a free end of the PDS suture into the pelvis through a low lateral port site.
- Introduce the right-angle dissector into the pelvis.

- Use the uterine manipulator to place the ipsilateral broad ligament on tension (by rotating the uterus to the contralateral side).
- Place the right-angle dissector under the ipsilateral utero-ovarian ligament and elevate the closed device into the posterior broad ligament. Performed correctly, the dissector should be placed in the avascular space between the ureter laterally and the uterine artery medially.
- While elevating the dissector into this space, retroflex the uterus with the manipulator and use the 30-degree laparoscope to visualize the anterior broad ligament. If the dissector is placed correctly, it will be visibly tenting the broad ligament anteriorly just cephalad from the uterine fornix delineator.
- Use the energy device to cut the broad ligament over the tip or the right-angle dissector and advance the dissector through the newly created broad ligament window.
- Grasp the end of the PDS suture in the right-angle dissector and pull the suture through the window from anterior to posterior.
- Pass the suture under the uterus (making sure not to capture intestine, epiploica, ovary, or fallopian tube between the suture and uterus/cervix).
- Reposition the uterus so the opposite broad ligament is now on tension.
- Pass the right-angle dissector through the opposite low lateral port site and grasp the end of the suture in the dissector.
- Repeat the process on the opposite side of the uterus, passing the PDS suture through a new window in the broad ligament this time from posterior to anterior.
- Pull the end of the suture through the port it was originally introduced through. At this point, the suture enters through a low lateral port, wraps around the cervix posteriorly, and exits the same port.
- Tie an extracorporeal Roeder slipknot.
- Cinch the knot over the anterior cervix while elevating the uterus cephalad. This is done to make sure the bladder does not get incorporated into the tourniquet.

- Use the needle drivers to tighten the cinch knot as much as possible.
- Finally throw a single intracorporeal overhand throw over the Roeder knot to lock it in place
- Trim the suture.

Surgical Approach

The patient was treated with preoperative oral Celebrex (400 mg) and Tylenol (1000 mg). After placement of the Foley catheter and uterine manipulator, laparoscopic ports were placed. Due to the size of the uterus, the camera port was placed approximately 5 cm cephalad to the umbilicus. Three ancillary lateral ports were also placed. In this case we placed our lower lateral ports at the level of the umbilicus and another lateral port approximately 10 cm cephalad to the lower port on the patient's left side.

After placement of the laparoscopic tourniquet, the serosa overlying the large fundal fibroids was injected with the dilute vasopressin, and a large transverse incision made with the ultrasonic scalpel. The fibroids were enucleated from the surrounding myometrium. With large intramural fibroids, enucleation of the fibroids is the most challenging portion of the case. The technique that works best follows a number of important rules.

1. Push the uterus off the fibroid into the pelvis as opposed to trying to pull the fibroid out of the uterus. This maintains the visual field and minimizes tearing of the fibroid.
2. Use a 10 mm tenaculum or myoma screw to stabilize the fibroid as close to the serosal edge you are working on as possible, regularly re-positioning the device as more and more of the fibroid is exposed.
3. Sweep tissue off the fibroid leaving myometrium, blood vessels, and endometrium with the uterus. It is generally possible to stay out of the endometrial cavity even with type 1 and 2 submucosal fibroids.

As fibroids were removed from the uterus, they were placed on a suture stringer. We use a 12-in. zero barbed suture for this purpose. The needle is passed through the first fibroid and the suture eyelet on the tail of the suture. Each subsequent fibroid is then placed sequentially on the stringer creating a string of fibroids. This allows for easy fibroid retrieval at the end of the case and decreases the risk of a fibroids being lost.

Following removal of the two largest transmural fibroids, the defect was closed in four layers with barbed zero delayed absorbable suture. The seromuscular layer was closed using an imbricating baseball stitch. Once the largest fibroids were removed, separate anterior and posterior transverse incisions were utilized to remove the remaining fibroids. The large submucosal fibroid was removed through the anterior incision without entering the endometrial cavity. The approach to fibroid enucleation, fibroid management, and defect closure was the same except that the myometrium was imbricated over the endometrium making sure not to place the deepest anterior throws through the endometrium into the endometrial cavity. A total of eight fibroids weighing 1342 g were removed.

We generally remove the laparoscopic tourniquet following uterine repair and prior to tissue extraction. This allows time for platelets and clotting factors to stop any serosal oozing which may occur immediately following tourniquet removal.

Our approach to tissue extraction utilizes the umbilicus whether the original optical trocar is placed there or not. By everting and vertically bivalving the umbilicus, the fascia can be extended vertically approximately 2.5 cm, and a small Alexis skin retractor can be placed (Alexis laparoscopic system with Kii Fios First Entry—Applied Medical). The 17 cm Alexis contained tissue extraction bag (Applied Medical) was then introduced through the umbilical incision and the pneumoperitoneum reestablished by placing the cap on the small Alexis retractor. The fibroids were now placed within the bag and the opening of the bag pulled up through the umbilical retractor using the drawstring on the retrieval bag. The fibroids were then removed utilizing a cold scalpel extraction technique.

At the conclusion of the case, the abdomen was suction irrigated and the uterus was treated with an adhesion barrier. The fascia under the umbilicus was closed in a running fashion with zero PDS suture (Ethicon). The fascia under the 12 mm part was closed with zero polysorb suture (Ethicon). The abdomen was suctioned of CO_2 and the skin incisions were closed subcuticularly with 4.0 monocryl suture (Ethicon).

The estimated blood loss was 450 mL. The patient was able to receive a 250 mL auto-transfusion utilizing the cell saver blood. She was hemodynamically stable through her observational hospitalization and was discharged the morning of postoperative day no. 1.

Discussion

This case highlights the importance of careful preoperative evaluation and surgical planning, as well as the importance of a well-rehearsed surgical approach when attempting laparoscopic removal of large transmural fibroids. In our experience there are no absolute limitations to the size or number of fibroids that can or should be removed laparoscopically. Each patient needs to be evaluated independently and a surgical approach planned well in advance of the day of surgery. Mastering the challenging techniques of tourniquet placement, myoma enucleation, defect closure, and tissue extraction should occur well in advance of attempting these challenging cases. With more and more success, progressively challenging cases can be completed safely and efficiently.

References

1. Vargas MV, Moawad GN, et al. Feasibility, safety, and prediction of complications for minimally invasive myomectomy in women with large and numerous myomata. J Minim Invasive Gynecol. 2017;24(2):315–22. doi:10.1016/j.jmig.2016.11.014.
2. Auerbach M, Deloughery T. Single dose intravenous iron for iron deficiency: a new paradigm. Hematology Am Soc Hematol Educ Program. 2016;1:57–66.
3. Alptekin H, Efe D. Effectiveness of pericervical tourniquet by Foley catheter reducing blood loss at abdominal myomectomy. Clin Exp Obstet Gynecol. 2014;41(4):440–4.
4. Hawa N, Robinson JK, Chahine B. Combined preoperative angiography with transient uterine artery embolization makes laparoscopic surgery for massive myomatous uteri a reasonable option: case reports. I Minim Invasive Gynecol. 2012;19(3):386–90.
5. Butori N, Tixier H, et al. Interest of uterine artery embolization with gelatin sponge particles prior to myomectomy for large and/ or multiple fibroids. Eur J Radiol. 2011;79(1):1–6.
6. Kongnyuy EJ, Wiysonge CS. Interventions to reduce haemorrhage during myomectomy for fibroids. Cochrane Database Syst Rev. 2014;15(8):CD005355.
7. Hobo R, Neto S, et al. Bradycardia and cardiac arrest caused by intramyometrial injection of vasopressin during laparoscopically assisted myomectomy. Obstet Gynecol. 2009;113(2 pt 2):484–6.

Chapter 15
Multiple Symptomatic Intramural Fibroids in a Patient Who Desires Fertility

Mona Omar, Paul C. Browne, Michael Diamond, and Ayman Al-Hendy

Case

This patient is an African American female aged 27 year-old G0 who complained of 9 months of heavy prolonged menstruation with flooding and clotting but no inter-menstrual bleeding or spotting. She also complained of dull-aching pain in her RLQ 2 weeks earlier, which was unrelated to food or menstrual cycle. She denied any pressure symptoms. She is nulliparous but she plans to have children in the next 3–4 years, as she just started postgraduate studies. She is sexually active with a stable partner and denied any dyspareunia, abnormal vaginal discharge, or history of sexually transmitted diseases. She uses

M. Omar, MD, PhD
OB/GYN, Augusta University, Augusta, GA, USA

OB/GYN, Tanta University, Tanta, Egypt

P.C. Browne, MD • A. Al-Hendy, MD, PhD (✉)
OB/GYN, Augusta University, Augusta, GA, USA
e-mail: aalhendy@augusta.edu

M. Diamond, MD
Research Department, Augusta University, Augusta, GA, USA

N.S. Moawad (ed.), *Uterine Fibroids*,
https://doi.org/10.1007/978-3-319-58780-6_15,
© Springer International Publishing AG 2018

male condoms for contraception. Her past medical and surgical history was unremarkable. She denied any use of medication, tobacco, or alcohol. Her last Pap was 2 years ago and was normal with no history of abnormal Pap smears. Her family history was significant as her mother had uterine fibroids. General physical examination was completely within normal limits. Vital signs were within normal levels; BMI was 32.

Speculum examination was within normal limits. Careful bimanual pelvic examination revealed: an enlarged non-tender uterus with irregular contour about 14–15 weeks size.

Laboratory studies showed a normal serum hormonal profile as progesterone was 9.5 ng/mL, estrogen 130 pg/mL, LH 2.33 mIU/mL, and FSH was 3.14 mIU/mL; a urine pregnancy test was negative. Serum 25 Hydroxy D vit was abnormal at 14 ng/mL (reference range 30–80 ng/mL). As for the complete blood count, Hemoglobin was 8 g/dL and the hematocrit value was 0.28I/L; the platelet and the white blood cell were within normal limits. Endometrial biopsy revealed proliferative endometrium, with no hyperplasia or malignancy. Transvaginal ultrasound examination of this patient showed five intramural fibroid all 2–3 cm in diameters. Endometrial thickness and adnexa were within normal limits (Fig. 15.1).

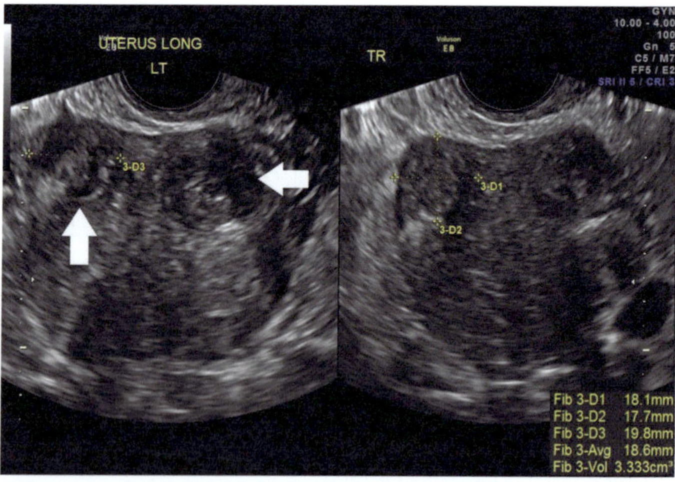

FIGURE 15.1 Transvaginal US showing three small intramural fibroid

Treatment Options

In this case we have a young patient with symptomatic multiple small intramural uterine fibroids who desires fertility preservation. The patient was counseled extensively regarding various treatment options ranging from medical, interventional radiology, and surgical treatment. In light of the patient's desire for future pregnancy, she elected to proceed with complementary medicine approach [Epigallocatechin Gallate (EGCG) and vitamin D] plus iron supplementation for 6 months followed by reevaluation of treatment success and develop potential additional treatment plans.

Medical Treatment

The challenge in the field is to develop an inexpensive oral medical treatment with the ability to safely and effectively shrink fibroid size, with minimal or no side effects, and ideally without interfering with the ovulatory cycles or future fertility potential. In this chapter we will summarize the state of the art of various available and under development compounds for effective and safe treatment of symptomatic uterine fibroids.

Complementary and Alternative Medicine

We could start with a natural treatment like green tea and if she is vitamin D deficient, we treat her with vitamin D. If she responses well, she can try to get pregnant while using this treatment.

Vitamin D

It is antifibrotic factor that inhibits growth and induces apoptosis in cultured human leiomyoma cells [1]. Recent studies have shown that 1,25 dihydroxyvitamin D3 and serum 25-hydroxyvitamin D3 are significantly lower in women with leiomyomas compared to normal healthy controls [1]. Also there are strong dose–response correlations between lower serum Vit D levels and increased severity of uterine leiomyomas [2]. From all of the above, Vit D or its potent analogues can be considered as novel treatment options or as a preventive measure for uterine fibroid; till now no clinical trial has been proven. So we recommend screening women with symptomatic uterine fibroids for serum level of 25-hydroxy vitamin D. If the level is deficient ($\leq$20 ng/mL) or insufficient (20–30 ng/mL), we recommend treating the hypo-vitamin D by oral 50,000 IU/W $\times$ 12 weeks followed by retesting of the serum level, and retreat as needed. This dose is recommended by the Endocrine Society [3].

Epigallocatechin Gallate (Green Tea Extract)

The main ingredient in green tea is Epigallocatechin gallate (EGCG) [4]. The results of the papers suggest that EGCG may be a potential antifibroid agent acting through multiple signal transduction pathways as it has potent antioxidant and anti-inflammation capacity, and promotes apoptosis [5]. From our previous study we show that by the end of 4 months of treatment with 800 mg/day of EGCG, we identified a significant decline in the average menstrual blood loss in the treatment group (a decrease from 71 to 45 mL/month), while mean hemoglobin levels increased in the treatment group from 11.7 to 12.4 g/dL in the same group. We also showed significant reduction in total fibroid volume (32.6%) compared to placebo. In addition, EGCG treatment significantly reduced fibroid-specific symptom severity (32.4%) and induced significant improvement in quality of life score by (18.53%) [6].

Hormonal Treatment

If these natural treatments show no benefit, and she is in a country where selective progesterone receptor modulators

(SPRM) are available (e.g., ulipristal (UPA), she can use UPA until ready to attempt pregnancy. If she is in a country where UPA is not available, she can use Lupron for 3–6 months with add-back therapy until she is ready to pursue pregnancy.

Receptor Modulators

Selective Estrogen Receptor Modulator (SERMs)

They are nonsteroidal estrogen receptor ligands that display tissue-specific agonist-antagonist estrogenic actions which result in differential expression of specific estrogen-regulated genes in different tissues [7].

Tamoxifen is one of the oldest known SERMs. It showed a significant improvement in menstrual blood loss but no improvement in fibroid size or uterine volume after 6 months of treatment [8]. The study also reported many side effects, including hot flushes, dizziness, and benign endometrial thickening. This endometrial thickening occurs due to the ER agonist effect of tamoxifen on the endometrium; other studies have suggested that it actually increases leiomyoma growth [9]. Because of this side effect, its use is not recommended for the treatment of symptomatic leiomyomas. Raloxifene is a second-generation SERM, with no agonist effect on the endometrium and only subtle antiestrogenic effects on mammary tissue, so it was considered to be a candidate therapeutic option for uterine fibroids [10, 11]. Walker et al. showed that administration of SERMs over a 2- to 4-month course of treatment to Eker rats reduced tumor incidence by more than 50% [12]. Another prospective randomized single-blind placebo-controlled clinical trial was performed to evaluate the effects of raloxifene administration for 6 months on uterine and leiomyoma sizes in premenopausal women. It showed that raloxifene has no significant effect on uterine and leiomyoma size or on menstrual cycle in premenopausal women [13].

Selective Progesterone Receptor Modulators (SPRMS)

Progesterone is a major enhancer of fibroid growth and fibroids typically demonstrate overexpression of progesterone receptor A and B. SPRMs are effective in the treatment of fibroids by reducing uterine volume and fibroid size through blockage of progesterone receptor signaling causing tumor shrinking and control of bleeding [14, 15]. It also may block ovulation especially with continuous administration [16].

1. **Mifepristone (RU-486)**
   Mifepristone (RU-486) is an antiprogesterone agent. Although it was used as an abortifacient, it also exhibits inhibitory effects on myoma growth [17]. A systematic review of six trials demonstrated that daily treatment with mifepristone (5–50 mg/day) for 3–6 months resulted in a 26:75% reduction in leiomyoma volume with decreasing of the severity of dysmenorrhea, menorrhagia, and pelvic pain, as well as amenorrhea during the treatment period [14, 18]. It also reported side effects, e.g., hot flushes in approximately 38% of women, and endometrial hyperplasia in 28% of the women [14]. So the authors recommended treatment-free intervals to decrease the risk of these endometrial changes.

2. **Asoprisnil (J-867)**
   A randomized controlled trial that used asoprisnil in three doses (5, 10, or 25 mg) for 12 weeks showed a significant decrease in fibroid size, reduction in pressure symptoms, and decreased menstrual bleeding, and up to 80% of the women experienced amenorrhea in a dose-related manner [19]. As for the side effects, 10% of women reported vasomotor side effects but it was considered minimal. Also when asoprisnil was administered daily for longer than 3–4 months, significant endometrial thickening and unusual histological appearance of the endometrial glands occurred [20]. Potential deleterious effects of asoprisnil on the endometrium and safety concerns derailed further clinical development of this compound [21].

3. **Telapristone (CDB-4124)**
   It is a pure progesterone antagonist. It showed some adverse liver effects but it is still being evaluated at an adjusted dose regimen to address its safety and dose effectiveness in the treatment of uterine fibroids [22].

4. **Ulipristal acetate (UPA, CDB-2914/VA2914)**
   It is the most recent drug that had been studied for many years; these studies showed that it is the most effective drug in the treatment of the bleeding symptoms of uterine fibroids. It has recently been approved in Europe (2012) and Canada (2014) for the preoperative and short-term treatment of symptomatic fibroids [23, 24–26]. However, in the USA, it is only approved by the FDA as an emergency contraceptive at a different dose range (30 mg). It has the advantages of oral availability, rapid onset of action, and minimal vasomotor symptoms with prolonged fibroid volume reduction after treatment discontinuation if compared to GnRH agonists [27]. The side effects of UPA treatment include headaches and breast tenderness; there have also been some reversible benign effects on the endometrium called progesterone receptor modulator-associated endometrial changes (PAECs) [15, 27, 28].

   In Europe, there have been multiple serial studies of UPA. In PERAL I and II [28, 29], they studied the short-term therapy of UPA (13 weeks). They concluded that 5 and 10 mg treatment was able to control myoma-associated bleeding in 90% of cases; patients developed amenorrhea in 5–7 days. They also reported 50% reduction in the fibroid volume in 50% of patients. Furthermore, this reduction is maintained for 6 months after stopping of the UPA in the patients that didn't undergo surgery.

   In PERAL III [27], the trial was extended to show the efficacy of long-term intermittent treatment. They used four 3-month courses of UPA 10 mg daily, immediately followed by 10-day double-blind treatment with NETA (10 mg daily) or placebo. They demonstrated that more than one course of UPA is able to maximize its potential benefits in terms of control of bleeding and fibroid volume reduction. Seventy-nine percent of the females will develop amenorrhea with the rate increasing to 89%, 88%, and 90% in the next 2, 3, and 4 treatment cycles respectively. The reduction of the fibroid size was 49.9%, 63.2%, 67%, and 72.1% after 1, 2, 3, and 4 treatment courses respectively. And in PERAL IV [30], the safety profile of long-term ulipristal acetate was confirmed, and repeated treatment courses did not increase the occurrence of adverse reactions. The percentage of subjects with endometrial thickness >16 mm was 7.4% after the first treatment course, and returned to below screening levels (4.9%) in subsequent treatment courses. The frequency of non-physiological changes did not increase with repeated treatment.

Another paper reported the first pregnancies achieved after UPA treatment; they show that 21 patients attempted to get pregnant; among whom 15 (71%) succeeded. Twelve resulted in the birth of 13 healthy babies and three ended in early miscarriage. No regrowth of fibroids was observed during pregnancy. They also describe pregnancies obtained after UPA treatment for fibroids in women who did not undergo surgery. There were no maternal complications related to myomas during pregnancy. All the babies were healthy [31].

Combination Oral Contraceptive Pills

Studies have demonstrated that the ovarian steroids estradiol and progesterone stimulate leiomyoma growth [32, 33]. This has led to the advent of various forms of hormonal medical management to block the stimulatory effects of ovarian steroids, decrease fibroid growth, and alleviate symptoms in women with leiomyomas. COCs can be used to improve heavy menstrual bleeding associated with fibroids without expected reduction in the leiomyoma volume or uterine size [23, 34]. The advantages of COCs are the ease of accessibility, oral administration, low cost, and minimal side effect profile [24]. However, overall COCs are not recommended for the treatment of leiomyomas.

Levonorgestrel Intrauterine System (LNG-IUS)

It effectively improves the menstrual bleeding and hemoglobin levels in women with leiomyomas, but they do not demonstrate any change in fibroid volume. It consists of a 32-mm T shaped polyethylene frame with reservoir containing 52 mg of levonorgestrel (LNG) coated with a silicone membrane. It releases LNG into the uterine cavity. After a few weeks, the plasma concentration of LNG reaches plateau level (150–200 pg/mL). LNG released from the device leads to atrophy of the endometrial gland and devascularization of the stroma that suppresses endometrial growth and desensitization of the endometrium to estrogen. Once inserted, the LNG-IUS is effective for up to 5 years, thus potentially providing women with a long-term treatment option [24]. In 2009, the FDA approved the levonorgestrel-intrauterine system (LNG-IUS) as a method of contraception in women with heavy menstrual bleeding [35]. Because it is not administered systemically, minimal side effects are reported, and patient compliance is not required after insertion. However, given the increased risk of expulsion, the LNG-IUS is contraindicated in patients with severe uterine cavity distortion [24, 25, 36].

Danazol

It is an isoxazole derivative of 17α-ethinyl testosterone. It causes hypo-estrogenemia by inhibition of pituitary gonadotropin secretion and ovarian steroid production [25, 32]. When 100 mg of danazol per day for a 4:6-month duration was used it showed reduction in both fibroid size by $37.6\% \pm 10\%$ and uterine volume by $29\% \pm 6.8\%$ ($p < 0.05$ for both) alone with improvement in hemoglobin concentrations [37]. It has a lot of side effects, e.g., endometrial atrophy weight gain, muscle cramps, edema, hot flushes, headaches, depression, skin rash, acne, and/or androgenic effects, such as deepening of the voice and hirsutism [38]. Because danazol is less effective than GnRH agonists, and because of its many associated side effects, its use in women with symptomatic leiomyomas is generally discouraged.

Gestrinone

Gestrinone is a synthetic steroid derived from ethinyl nortestosterone that has both antiestrogenic and antiprogestogenic properties in the endometrium [38, 39]. Women given gestrinone 2.5 mg twice a week for 6 months showed a 32% reduction in uterine volume. Also there was a relatively slow reactivation, i.e., benefits of treatment lasted 18 months following a 6-month treatment course [40]. The reported side effects include weight gain, edema, decreased breast size, hirsutism, hot flushes, acne, and/or headaches [32, 36, 38, 40]. This medication is not recommended until more data are obtained via larger, randomized controlled trials.

GnRH Agonists

GnRH agonists are synthetic peptides that are structurally related to endogenous GnRH; however, they exhibit longer half-lives, greater receptor affinity, and greater potency [35, 38, 41]. GnRH agonists were one of the first medical therapies to be used in the treatment of leiomyomas (FDA approved in 1999) [35]. Continuous (not pulsatile as occurs with endogenous pituitary GnRh) administration of GnRH agonists causes downregulation of pituitary GnRH receptors resulting in a decrease in the production of FSH and LH and a hypoestrogenic state [24, 38, 41] (Table 15.1).

Within the first 3:6 months of treatment, most women show a 30:65% reduction in fibroid volume and significant improvement of their symptoms, while preserving the option for fertility [24, 35]. Also it had been used 3 months

TABLE 15.1 GnRh agonists, route of administration, and the dose regimen

	Route of administration	Dose regimen
Leuprolide (Lupron)	Subcutaneous injection	500–1000 mg/day
		400 mg 4 days
	Intranasal	3.75–7.5 mg/month
	Intramuscular depot	11.25 mg/3 months
Buserelin (Suprefact, CinnaFact)	Subcutaneous injection	200 mg/day
		300–344 mg 4 days
	Intranasal	
Nafarelin (Synarel)	Intranasal	3 mg/month
	Intramuscular depot	Depot2-4 mg/month
Goserelin (Zoladex)	Subcutaneous implant	3.6 mg/month
		10.8 mg/3 months
Triptorelin (Decapeptyl, Diphereline, Gonapeptyl, Trelstar)	Intramuscular depot	3 mg/month
Histrelin (Vantas, Supprelin LA)	Subcutaneous injection	100 mg/day

preoperatively before hysterectomy or myomectomy, which helps to reduce uterine volume and fibroid size, control intraoperative bleeding, and correct preoperative anemia [42–44].

The most commonly reported side effects of GnRH agonists are related to the hypoestrogenic state which include distressing hot flushes, mood changes, vaginal dryness, and bone demineralization [24, 36, 42, 45, 46]. Moreover, treatment is associated with changes within the leiomyoma that may complicate surgical intervention. Other disadvantages to treatment include the relatively high cost of therapy and rapid regrowth of leiomyomas within 3 months after cessation of treatment [21, 42].

GnRH Antagonists

GnRH antagonists act by competing with endogenous GnRH for pituitary-binding sites, resulting in suppression of the secretion of FSH and LH and creation of a hypo-estrogen state [36, 38]. The subsequent reduction in estradiol levels leads to improvement in bleeding patterns and reduction in leiomyoma size as early as 3 weeks after initiation of treatment. Because of its rapid onset of action, and avoidance of a gonadotropin flare phase, patients experience faster symptom relief [32]. In the United States, cetrorelix and ganirelix (the two available injectable GnRH antagonists) are US FDA approved, but they are rarely used to treat fibroids due to the cost of GnRH antagonists [47]. The requirement for daily injections is another major factor further limiting their use. Elagolix is the frontrunner among an emerging class of GnRH antagonists, which unlike their peptide predecessors has a nonpeptide structure resulting in its oral bioavailability [48]. Elagolix is a short-acting agent which is administered orally so that unlike injectable depot GnRH agonists and antagonists, produces a dose-dependent suppression of ovarian estrogen production (partial suppression at lower doses to full suppression at higher doses). These properties provide an opportunity to minimize the hypoestrogenic side effects that limit long-term treatment with GnRH agonists. In addition, oral administration and a short half-life (~6 h) allow for rapid elimination of elagolix from the body, if treatment needs to be stopped [49].

Inhibitors

A lot of these inhibitors like thiazolidinediones, TGF-B receptor inhibitors, EGF receptor inhibitor, and Catechol-O-methyl transferase inhibitor are still under laboratory investigation.

Retinoic acid is the active metabolic form of Vit A. It can be used to suppress the proliferation of fibroid cell, but it has high teratogenic effect [50]. This is why it cannot be used in long-term treatment of the uterine fibroid [51].

Aromatase inhibitors act by inhibition of the aromatase enzyme, which is the enzyme that catalyzes the conversion of androgenic substances into estrogens resulting in significant blocking of both ovarian and peripheral estrogen production within 1 day of treatment [52]. Two third-generation agents, letrozole (2.5 mg daily) and anastrozole (1 mg daily), have been studied for the treatment of symptomatic leiomyomas [53]. The benefits of these third-generation agents are their rapid absorption. When 1 mg/day anastrozole was taken over 3 months, it resulted in decreases in the size of the fibroids by 32% [54]. The main side effects associated with the use of the Aromatase inhibitor are menopausal symptoms, (e.g., hot flushes, vaginal dryness, and bone loss) [55]. However other authors suggested that letrozole did not affect bone density [56]. Actually this side effect is mild in comparison with that which results from the use of GnRHa. So aromatase inhibitor can be used in women with fibroids on a short-term basis, or in women who want to avoid surgical intervention to preserve their potential fertility [57].

Nonhormonal Medical Management

(a) **Tranexamic acid**
Tranexamic acid is a synthetic lysine derivative that reversibly blocks the lysine-binding site on plasminogen, thereby preventing fibrin degradation. It competitively inhibits the activation of plasminogen to plasmin, which subsequently inhibits endometrial plasminogen activator [58]. Its effects are to decrease fibrinolysis and clot breakdown, and thus to decrease menstrual blood loss. Also tranexamic acid causes thrombosis of the fibroid vessels which results in ischemic necrosis of the fibroid with subsequent reduction in size [58]. Tranexamic acid was approved by the FDA in 2009, and it is used globally for the treatment of heavy menstrual bleeding in women with and without fibroids [32, 59]. The recommended dose is a 1:1.5 g three times daily for 3:4 days [60]. Generally it is well tolerated, and the risk of venous

thromboembolism is not increased. The more commonly reported side effects are gastrointestinal complaints, such as nausea, vomiting, or diarrhea and dysmenorrhea, which may be attributable to the development of necrosis within the myoma [61].

(b) **Nonsteroidal anti-inflammatory drugs (NSAIDs):**
They inhibit the prostaglandin synthesis reducing menstrual bleeding. NSAIDs appear to be effective only for symptom relief, without affecting fibroid size or uterine volume [62].

Surgical and Radiological Treatment

If the symptoms of the fibroid show no improvement on the medical treatment or result in complications such as severe anemia, we should shift to interventional options such as surgery or radiological options. Radiological options include Uterine Artery Embolization (UAE) and MRI-guided focused ultrasound (MRg/US). Myomectomy is the commonly used option for women who wish to retain their uterus and their fertility [63]. This is discussed in detail in other chapters. One study showed that laparoscopic myomectomy has a longer operating time but it remains a preferable method due to less blood loss and less hospital stay [64]. The major disadvantages of the myomectomy operation are adhesions and blood loss. The adhesions affect future fertility of the patient. Also good hemostasis is important for controlling the blood loss and the prevention of the adhesion [65]. It should be noted that inadequate approximation of the uterine incision can progress to uterine rupture in subsequent pregnancy. Another disadvantage is that 50–60% of patients will present with new myomas within 5 years following the procedure [66, 67]. Also they have an increased risk of placenta previa and postpartum hemorrhage. The risk of uterine rupture at the site of previous myomectomy is high during pregnancy [68]. Hysterectomy, which is the definitive treatment, has no role here as the patient desired to preserve her fertility. Myolysis is the laparoscopic thermal coagulation or cryoablation of fibroid tissues [69, 70]. Because of several reported cases of uterine rupture and severe adhesion after myolysis, this method is considered an inappropriate option. Although pregnancy is possible after UAE despite the synechiae and premature ovarian failure, there are increased incidence of several obstetric complications, such as miscarriage, preterm labor, placenta previa, and postpartum hemorrhage [52, 71]. ACOG considers the UAE procedure relatively contraindicated for women who desire future fertility [72].

References

1. Sharan C, et al. Vitamin D inhibits proliferation of human uterine leiomyoma cells via catechol-O-methyltransferase. Fertil Steril. 2011;95(1):247–53.
2. Abdelraheem MS, Al-Hendy A. Serum vitamin D3 level inversely correlates with total fibroid tumor burden in women with symptomatic uterine fibroid. Fertil Steril. 2010;94(4):S74.
3. Holick MF, et al. Evaluation, treatment, and prevention of vitamin D deficiency: an Endocrine Society clinical practice guideline. J Clin Endocrinol Metab. 2011;96(7):1911–30.
4. Lin JK, Liang YC, Lin-Shiau SY. Cancer chemoprevention by tea polyphenols through mitotic signal transduction blockade. Biochem Pharmacol. 1999;58(6):911–5.
5. Mukhtar H, Ahmad N. Green tea in chemoprevention of cancer. Toxicol Sci. 1999;52(2 Suppl):111–7.
6. Roshdy E, et al. Treatment of symptomatic uterine fibroids with green tea extract: a pilot randomized controlled clinical study. Int J Womens Health. 2013;5:477–86.
7. Mitlak BH, Cohen FJ. In search of optimal long-term female hormone replacement: the potential of selective estrogen receptor modulators. Horm Res. 1997;48(4):155–63.
8. Sadan O, et al. The role of tamoxifen in the treatment of symptomatic uterine leiomyomata—a pilot study. Eur J Obstet Gynecol Reprod Biol. 2001;96(2):183–6.
9. Lethaby AE, Vollenhoven BJ. An evidence-based approach to hormonal therapies for premenopausal women with fibroids. Best Pract Res Clin Obstet Gynaecol. 2008;22(2):307–31.

10. Premkumar A, et al. Gynecologic and hormonal effects of raloxifene in premenopausal women. Fertil Steril. 2007;88(6):1637–44.
11. Lingxia X, Taixiang W, Xiaoyan C. Selective estrogen receptor modulators (SERMs) for uterine leiomyomas. Cochrane Database Syst Rev. 2007;2:CD005287.
12. Walker CL. Role of hormonal and reproductive factors in the etiology and treatment of uterine leiomyoma. Recent Prog Horm Res. 2002;57:277–94.
13. Palomba S, et al. Raloxifene administration in premenopausal women with uterine leiomyomas: a pilot study. J Clin Endocrinol Metab. 2002;87(8):3603–8.
14. Steinauer J, et al. Systematic review of mifepristone for the treatment of uterine leiomyomata. Obstet Gynecol. 2004;103(6):1331–6.
15. Nieman LK, et al. Efficacy and tolerability of CDB-2914 treatment for symptomatic uterine fibroids: a randomized, double-blind, placebo-controlled, phase IIb study. Fertil Steril. 2011;95(2):767–72.e1–2.
16. Pei K, et al. Weekly contraception with mifepristone. Contraception. 2007;75(1):40–4.
17. Duhan N. Current and emerging treatments for uterine myoma — an update. Int J Womens Health. 2011;3:231–41.
18. Murphy AA, et al. Regression of uterine leiomyomata in response to the antiprogesterone RU 486. J Clin Endocrinol Metab. 1993;76(2):513–7.
19. Chwalisz K, et al. A randomized, controlled trial of asoprisnil, a novel selective progesterone receptor modulator, in women with uterine leiomyomata. Fertil Steril. 2007;87(6):1399–412.
20. Spitz IM. Clinical utility of progesterone receptor modulators and their effect on the endometrium. Curr Opin Obstet Gynecol. 2009;21(4):318–24.
21. Talaulikar VS, Manyonda I. Progesterone and progesterone receptor modulators in the management of symptomatic uterine fibroids. Eur J Obstet Gynecol Reprod Biol. 2012;165(2):135–40.
22. Roeder H, et al. CDB-4124 does not cause apoptosis in cultured fibroid cells. Reprod Sci. 2011;18(9):850–7.
23. Guo XC, Segars JH. The impact and management of fibroids for fertility. An evidence-based approach. Obstet Gynecol Clin North Am. 2012;39(4):521–33.
24. Singh SS, Belland L. Contemporary management of uterine fibroids: focus on emerging medical treatments. Curr Med Res Opin. 2015;31(1):1–12.

25. Biglia N, et al. Ulipristal acetate: a novel pharmacological approach for the treatment of uterine fibroids. Drug Des Devel Ther. 2014;8:285–92.
26. Talaulikar VS, Manyonda IT. Ulipristal acetate: a novel option for the medical management of symptomatic uterine fibroids. Adv Ther. 2012;29(8):655–63.
27. Donnez J, et al. Long-term treatment of uterine fibroids with ulipristal acetate. Fertil Steril. 2014;101(6):1565–73.e1–18.
28. Donnez J, et al. Ulipristal acetate versus leuprolide acetate for uterine fibroids. N Engl J Med. 2012;366(5):421–32.
29. Donnez J, et al. Ulipristal acetate versus placebo for fibroid treatment before surgery. N Engl J Med. 2012;366(5):409–20.
30. Donnez J, et al. Efficacy and safety of repeated use of ulipristal acetate in uterine fibroids. Fertil Steril. 2015;103(2):519–27. e3
31. Luyckx M, et al. First series of 18 pregnancies after ulipristal acetate treatment for uterine fibroids. Fertil Steril. 2014;102(5):1404–9.
32. Doherty L, et al. Uterine fibroids: clinical manifestations and contemporary management. Reprod Sci. 2014;21(9):1067–92.
33. Chwalisz K, et al. Selective progesterone receptor modulator development and use in the treatment of leiomyomata and endometriosis. Endocr Rev. 2005;26(3):423–38.
34. Rackow BW, Arici A. Options for medical treatment of myomas. Obstet Gynecol Clin North Am. 2006;33(1):97–113.
35. Islam MS, et al. Uterine leiomyoma: available medical treatments and new possible therapeutic options. J Clin Endocrinol Metab. 2013;98(3):921–34.
36. Sabry M, Al-Hendy A. Medical treatment of uterine leiomyoma. Reprod Sci. 2012;19(4):339–53.
37. La Marca A, et al. Hemodynamic effect of danazol therapy in women with uterine leiomyomata. Fertil Steril. 2003;79(5):1240–2.
38. Sankaran S, Manyonda IT. Medical management of fibroids. Best Pract Res Clin Obstet Gynaecol. 2008;22(4):655–76.
39. Sabry M, Al-Hendy A. Innovative oral treatments of uterine leiomyoma. Obstet Gynecol Int. 2012;2012:943635.
40. La Marca A, et al. Gestrinone in the treatment of uterine leiomyomata: effects on uterine blood supply. Fertil Steril. 2004;82(6):1694–6.
41. De Leo V, et al. A benefit-risk assessment of medical treatment for uterine leiomyomas. Drug Saf. 2002;25(11):759–79.
42. Owen C, Armstrong AY. Clinical management of leiomyoma. Obstet Gynecol Clin North Am. 2015;42(1):67–85.

43. Segars JH, et al. Proceedings from the third National Institutes of Health international congress on advances in uterine leiomyoma research: comprehensive review, conference summary and future recommendations. Hum Reprod Update. 2014;20(3):309–33.
44. Lethaby A, Vollenhoven B, Sowter M. Pre-operative GnRH analogue therapy before hysterectomy or myomectomy for uterine fibroids. Cochrane Database Syst Rev. 2000;2:CD000547.
45. Stovall TG, et al. GnRH agonist and iron versus placebo and iron in the anemic patient before surgery for leiomyomas: a randomized controlled trial. Leuprolide acetate study group. Obstet Gynecol. 1995;86(1):65–71.
46. Khan AT, Shehmar M, Gupta JK. Uterine fibroids: current perspectives. Int J Womens Health. 2014;6:95–114.
47. Gonzalez-Barcena D, et al. Treatment of uterine leiomyomas with luteinizing hormone-releasing hormone antagonist Cetrorelix. Hum Reprod. 1997;12(9):2028–35.
48. Struthers RS, et al. Suppression of gonadotropins and estradiol in premenopausal women by oral administration of the nonpeptide gonadotropin-releasing hormone antagonist elagolix. J Clin Endocrinol Metab. 2009;94(2):545–51.
49. Carr B, et al. Elagolix, an oral GnRH antagonist, versus subcutaneous depot medroxyprogesterone acetate for the treatment of endometriosis: effects on bone mineral density. Reprod Sci. 2014;21(11):1341–51.
50. Boettger-Tong H, et al. Cultured human uterine smooth muscle cells are retinoid responsive. Proc Soc Exp Biol Med. 1997;215(1):59–65.
51. Toma S, et al. 13-cis retinoic acid in head and neck cancer chemoprevention: results of a randomized trial from the Italian Head and Neck Chemoprevention Study Group. Oncol Rep. 2004;11(6):1297–305.
52. American College of Obstetricians and Gynecologists. ACOG practice bulletin. Alternatives to hysterectomy in the management of leiomyomas. Obstet Gynecol. 2008;112(2 Pt 1):387–400.
53. Song H, et al. Aromatase inhibitors for uterine fibroids. Cochrane Database Syst Rev. 2013;10:CD009505.
54. Hilario SG, et al. Action of aromatase inhibitor for treatment of uterine leiomyoma in perimenopausal patients. Fertil Steril. 2009;91(1):240–3.

55. Bedaiwy MA, Liu J. Long-term management of endometriosis: medical therapy and treatment of infertility. Sexuality Reprod Menopause. 2010;8(3):10–4.
56. Shozu M, et al. Successful treatment of a symptomatic uterine leiomyoma in a perimenopausal woman with a nonsteroidal aromatase inhibitor. Fertil Steril. 2003;79(3):628–31.
57. Parsanezhad ME, et al. A randomized, controlled clinical trial comparing the effects of aromatase inhibitor (letrozole) and gonadotropin-releasing hormone agonist (triptorelin) on uterine leiomyoma volume and hormonal status. Fertil Steril. 2010;93(1):192–8.
58. Ip PP, et al. Tranexamic acid-associated necrosis and intralesional thrombosis of uterine leiomyomas: a clinicopathologic study of 147 cases emphasizing the importance of drug-induced necrosis and early infarcts in leiomyomas. Am J Surg Pathol. 2007;31(8):1215–24.
59. Wellington K, Wagstaff AJ. Tranexamic acid: a review of its use in the management of menorrhagia. Drugs. 2003;63(13):1417–33.
60. Lukes AS, et al. Tranexamic acid treatment for heavy menstrual bleeding: a randomized controlled trial. Obstet Gynecol. 2010;116(4):865–75.
61. Khaund A, et al. Evaluation of the effect of uterine artery embolisation on menstrual blood loss and uterine volume. BJOG. 2004;111(7):700–5.
62. Pinkerton JV. Pharmacological therapy for abnormal uterine bleeding. Menopause. 2011;18(4):453–61.
63. Matchar DB, et al. Management of uterine fibroids. Evid Rep Technol Assess (Summ). 2001;34:1–6.
64. Nisolle M, et al. Laparoscopic myolysis with the Nd:YAG laser. J Gynecol Surg. 1993;9(2):95–9.
65. Jin C, et al. Laparoscopic versus open myomectomy—a meta-analysis of randomized controlled trials. Eur J Obstet Gynecol Reprod Biol. 2009;145(1):14–21.
66. Fedele L, et al. Recurrence of fibroids after myomectomy: a transvaginal ultrasonographic study. Hum Reprod. 1995;10(7):1795–6.
67. Hanafi M. Predictors of leiomyoma recurrence after myomectomy. Obstet Gynecol. 2005;105(4):877–81.
68. Parker WH, et al. Risk factors for uterine rupture after laparoscopic myomectomy. J Minim Invasive Gynecol. 2010;17(5):551–4.

69. Zupi E, et al. Directed laparoscopic cryomyolysis: a possible alternative to myomectomy and/or hysterectomy for symptomatic leiomyomas. Am J Obstet Gynecol. 2004;190(3):639–43.
70. Visvanathan D, et al. Interstitial laser photocoagulation for uterine myomas. Am J Obstet Gynecol. 2002;187(2):382–4.
71. Tse G, Spies JB. Radiation exposure and uterine artery embolization: current risks and risk reduction. Tech Vasc Interv Radiol. 2010;13(3):148–53.
72. Chan AH, et al. An image-guided high intensity focused ultrasound device for uterine fibroids treatment. Med Phys. 2002;29(11):2611–20.

Chapter 16
The Cervical Fibroid

Grace Liu

Clinical Case Presentation

A 37-year-old nulligravida patient with a cervical fibroid presents with dysfunctional uterine bleeding and anemia. She notes that over the course of the past one and a half years, her periods, while still regular, have slowly increased in amount. Her cycles are 33 days in length, and last for a total of 5 days. Days one through three are heavy, and she will change both a super tampon and overnight pad every 2 h on these days. She is otherwise completely healthy. She has no preexisting conditions and has not had any previous surgeries. She is on no medications and has no known drug allergies. Her last pap smear was 2 years ago and

Electronic supplementary material The online version of this chapter (doi:10.1007/978-3-319-58780-6_16. contains supplementary material, which is available to authorized users.

G. Liu, MD
Department of Obstetrics and Gynaecology, Sunnybrook Health Sciences Centre, Suite B627, 2075 Bayview Avenue, Toronto, ON, Canada, M4N 3M5
e-mail: grace.liu@sunnybrook.ca

N.S. Moawad (ed.), *Uterine Fibroids*,
https://doi.org/10.1007/978-3-319-58780-6_16,
© Springer International Publishing AG 2018

was normal. She has never had any history of abnormal pap smears or sexually transmitted infections. There is no family history of breast, ovarian, or colon cancer.

Two years prior to presentation, the patient had an ultrasound showing a single, dominant, posterior, low body/cervical fibroid measuring 5 cm in diameter. Her symptoms at that time included vaginal pressure, and some mild discomfort with deep penetration during intercourse. Her periods were manageable, but just started to become heavier. Six months following this ultrasound, a follow-up scan did not show any change in the size of her fibroid, nor were there any other abnormalities. Options were discussed with the patient at this time, including hormonal management and surgery. Because the patient was desirous of pregnancy and she felt that her symptoms were completely manageable, she was not keen to have any hormonal medical treatment. As well, surgery, with its risks to surrounding structures, possible adhesion formation, and even possible hysterectomy, was not an option that she was willing to entertain. Therefore, the patient opted to attempt pregnancy.

One year prior to presentation, the patient started to have unprotected intercourse, and in the last 7 months prior to presentation, she has been actively trying to conceive with each cycle. Despite these attempts, she has been unable to achieve spontaneous pregnancy despite actively trying. The patient also reports increasing urinary frequency, abdominal tenderness, vaginal pressure, and menorrhagia. A repeat ultrasound is performed by her family physician at an outside laboratory and now shows a marked change in the size of her low uterine body/cervical fibroid. Her fibroid is now 11 cm in diameter.

She is understandably concerned about the growth of the fibroid over the past 2 years and is worried about her chances to conceive, given the fibroid's size and her increasing maternal age. She would like to know what her options are.

Exam Findings

Clinical examination reveals a healthy Caucasian woman in no apparent distress. Her vital signs are completely stable. Head and neck examination is unremarkable. Her abdominal exam, however, reveals the presence of an 18–20 week size uterus extending up to her umbilicus. Bimanual examination reveals that the uterus is quite mobile and there is no evidence of any scarring posteriorly involving the uterosacral ligaments. The adnexa are not palpable. A speculum examination is performed, and her cervix is normal. A routine pap smear is performed as well as an endometrial biopsy.

Diagnostic Workup

Despite her reported heavy bleeding, her hemoglobin is 140 g/L and her serum ferritin is 60 μg/L. Her TSH is 2.03 mIU/L, and her beta hcg is negative.

Her pap smear is normal, and her endometrial biopsy shows normal proliferative endometrium with no evidence of malignancy.

A repeat ultrasound is performed, as the last ultrasound done by her family physician was approximately 3 months ago.

This pelvic and transvaginal ultrasound reveals the following:

The uterus measures 19.0 cm × 10.0 cm × 11.5 cm, and has a large cervical fibroid displacing the endometrium fundally and anteriorly. The fibroid measures 13.5 cm × 7.0 cm × 12.0 cm. The endometrial lining measures 0.5 cm in thickness. Both ovaries are seen transvesically and are normal. Both kidneys are also evaluated for obstructive uropathy, and mild right pelviectasis is noted.

Images

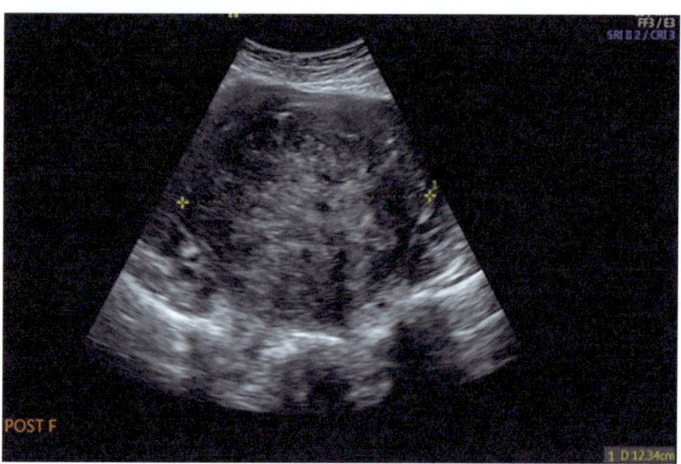

FIGURE 16.1 Transvaginal ultrasound: transverse view: posterior fibroid

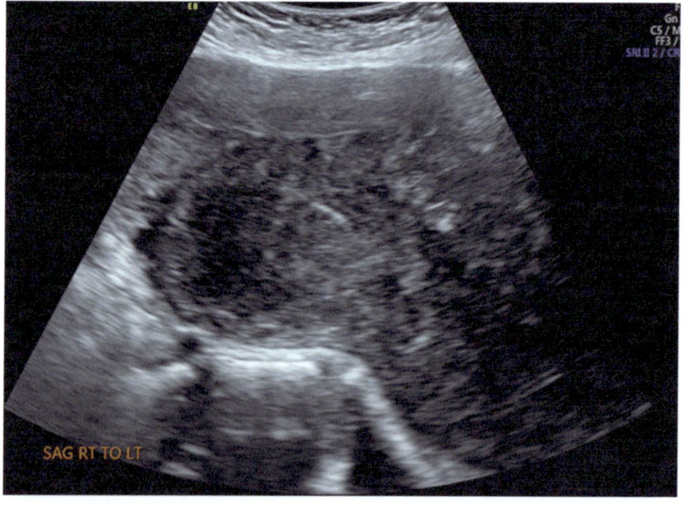

FIGURE 16.2 Transvaginal ultrasound: sagittal view: cervical fibroid

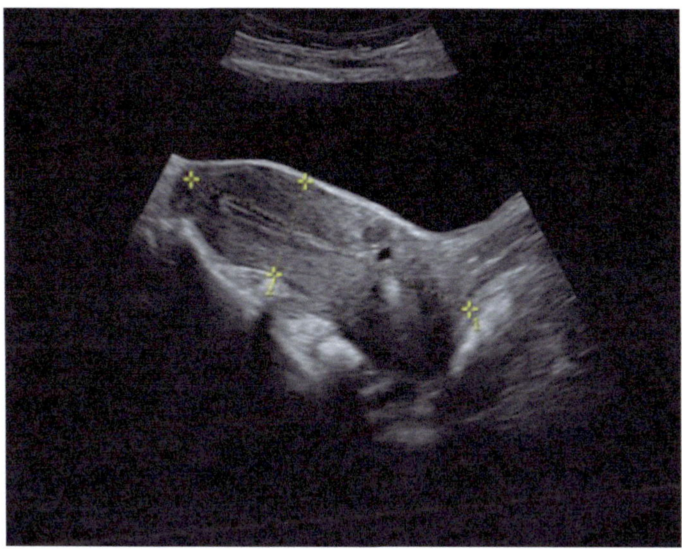

Figure 16.3 Transabdominal ultrasound: sagittal view: postoperative

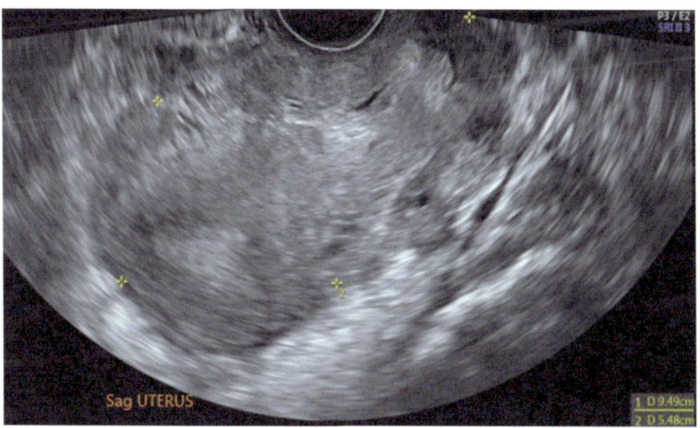

Figure 16.4 Transvaginal ultrasound: sagittal view: postoperative

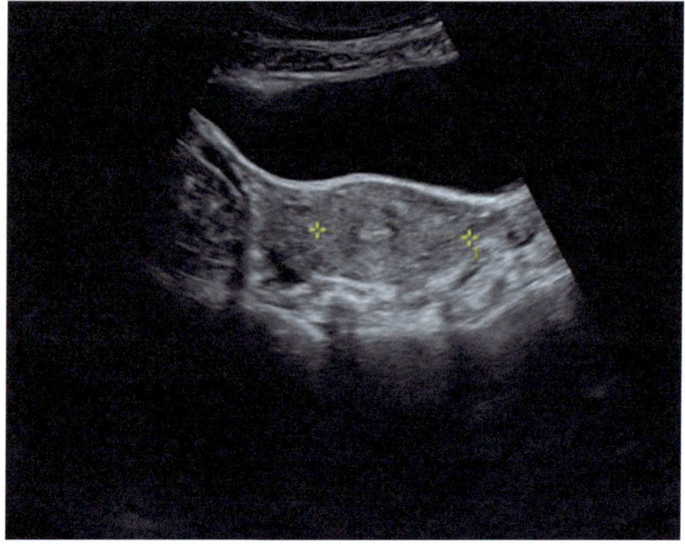

FIGURE 16.5 Transvaginal ultrasound: transverse view: postoperative

Treatment Options

The following treatment options are presented to her at this time (from least invasive to most invasive):

Lifestyle and dietary modifications: There have been numerous studies looking at the epidemiology of uterine fibroids, and different lifestyle modifications to help treat the symptoms of uterine fibroids. These include decreasing exposure to plastics and chemicals, preservatives, pesticides, foods with additives such as hormones, soybeans, dairy, caffeine, and alcohol [1–4]. All of these options are discussed with the patient as an initial step to try to help with some symptom control and as a path towards a healthier lifestyle, especially given her desire to pursue pregnancy.

Medication (nonhormonal): Following a discussion of lifestyle modification, medications are discussed with this patient. She has already tried nonsteroidal analgesics that had been recommended to her by her family physician; however, she has not really found any change in her symptomatology. Her flow did not decrease with the NSAID, and she was not experiencing much cramping with her menses to begin with. One older randomized controlled trial in the literature has demonstrated that while Naprosyn might help with idiopathic heavy menses, it does not necessarily have an effect on fibroid-induced menses [5]. A more recent Cochrane database review of nonsteroidal anti-inflammatory drugs for heavy menses also demonstrated that while it is more effective than placebo, other medications, such as tranexamic acid and hormonal medications, might be more efficacious [6].

Tranexamic acid is also a widely used nonhormonal medication for treatment of symptomatic uterine fibroids in the setting of heavy menses [7–9]. By inhibiting fibrinolysis, it can be a useful treatment for women who do not wish to take a daily medication and who still want to get pregnant. It is safe and generally well tolerated [9]. This medication is one which the patient is amenable to trying, particularly because she is not keen on taking daily medication.

Medication (hormonal): Hormonal medications are also discussed with the patient, and these include combined oral contraceptives, oral and injectable progestins, progesterone-releasing intrauterine devices, selective progesterone receptor modulators (SPRMs), and gonadotropin releasing hormone (GnRH) agonists. Several studies have shown significant reduction in bleeding with these hormonal agents, and that GnRH agonists are likely to be the most effective with respect to both bleeding and reduction in fibroid size [10–12]. Europe and Canada have also seen some effect with SPRMs for management of bleeding secondary to fibroids and for reduction in fibroid volume, particularly for smaller uterine fibroids [13–15]. In this patient's case, however, none of these medications would allow her the option to attempt pregnancy, except for perhaps the gonadotropin releasing hormone agonists combined with concomitant in vitro fertilization. This regimen, however, is something that the patient is not prepared to undertake at this point in time. She expresses her desire to consider further non-medicinal options.

Radiologic procedures: Uterine artery embolization (UAE) is discussed with the patient. This procedure has been shown to be an effective minimally invasive nonsurgical treatment option for women with uterine fibroids, treating both abnormal uterine bleeding, and fibroid volume or "bulk" symptoms by shrinking fibroids by up to 50% [16–18]. The placement of her cervical fibroid is not expected to adversely affect the success of the procedure, and interventional radiology feels that she would be a good candidate for the procedure, based on her initial ultrasound results. Risks of serious complications such as postembolization syndrome, premature ovarian failure, vaginal discharge/expulsion of infarcted fibroid, infection, and sepsis are felt to be quite low in her case as per radiology. The patient wonders, however, what the long-term implications on her fertility following UAE would be. Several recent studies have looked at the impact of uterine artery embolization on ovarian reserve in the young reproductive-aged woman, such as this patient [19–23]. The results of these studies are mixed. While one of the established risks of UAE is premature ovarian failure, there is no consistent evidence that there is clinical or subclinical reduction in ovarian function in women below the age of 40. Traditionally, however, UAE has been a treatment choice for women who do not desire surgery and are also not anxious for pregnancy. MRI guided high intensity focused ultrasound (HiFU) treatment of the fibroid is also discussed with the patient. However, after discussion with the interventional radiologists, they feel that the fibroid is too large to consider this option. Furthermore, they are concerned that treatment of this large cervical fibroid with HiFU might damage the adjacent bowel. UAE, as far as they are concerned, is the better of the two options for this patient.

Surgery: The discussion then turns to surgery. The patient is interested in uterine preserving surgery and makes it clear that she absolutely does not want a hysterectomy. Her main surgical option at this point is either laparoscopic or abdominal myomectomy. The patient would prefer a laparoscopic approach as opposed to the abdominal approach, as a shorter length of stay in the hospital and a quicker postoperative recovery are appealing to her. She understands, however, that there is always the possibility that it would need to be converted to a laparotomy. Furthermore, risks of power morcellation are discussed with the patient. The risk of a leiomyosarcoma (LMS) is discussed and while it is unlikely, the chance of upstaging, spreading concern, and worsening prognosis not only with power morcellation but also with any form of myomectomy are clearly and openly discussed. If she is truly worried about a LMS, then the only procedure that could be safely offered would be an abdominal hysterectomy.

The patient decides she would like to have a laparoscopic myomectomy. Her surgery is scheduled for 4 months later. In the interim, medications to help control her bleeding and raise her preoperative hemoglobin prior to surgery are again discussed, with the goal being short term preoperative use only. These medications include tranexamic acid, ulipristal acetate, levonorgestrel-releasing IUD, and GnRH agonists. The benefit of GnRH agonists on decreasing risk of even intraoperative bleeding and fibroid volume [24] is specifically emphasized. The patient decides to try only tranexamic acid during her menses for symptom control. As her hemoglobin is 140 g/L, it is felt that this decision is reasonable.

During her surgery, after induction of the general anesthetic, the patient is given an examination under anesthesia. This examination confirms that her uterus extends to her umbilicus, and bimanual examination confirms that there is a mass filling her pelvis, but that the entire uterus is quite mobile. After this examination, port placement is decided. The camera is placed through Palmer's point, and all ports are moved up so that all laparoscopic instruments can work "down" on the uterus. One port is placed on the patient's left, and two ports are placed on the patient's right side. This is to facilitate the laparoscopic suturing anticipated with the laparoscopic myomectomy. The posterior cervical fibroid is noted to distort her entire pelvis. Vasopressin is then injected into serosa and myometrium overlying the fibroid to help decrease blood loss. A solution of 20 U in 20 mL of normal saline is used, and a total of 7 mL is used for the entire case. Vasopressin injection has been shown in several studies to help decrease blood loss during myomectomy [25–27]. Newer therapies such as transient occlusion of the uterine arteries with clips or suture have also been shown to be effective for decreasing intraoperative blood loss [28, 29]. Unfortunately the cervical fibroid resulted in too great of a distortion of the uterine arteries to make this feasible.

A horizontal incision is made overlying the fibroid. Surgeon preference often dictates the direction of the incision, although other concerns such as extension into the uterine arteries and other surrounding structures such as major vessels and ureters can influence this decision. Horizontal incisions, however, are more in keeping with the direction of the uterine smooth muscle fibers, possibly decreasing risk of uterine rupture concerns postoperatively, rather than performing a large vertical uterine incision. A recent analysis of arterial vessels around uterine fibroids suggests that with respect to blood loss, direction of the incision does not impact damage to arterial vessels, which travel diagonally on the surface of uterine fibroids [30]. After examining this patient's pelvis and fibroid, the decision is made to continue with a horizontal incision. The ureters, major vessels, and uterine arteries are deemed to be far enough away from the site of the incision.

Monopolar energy with the laparoscopic Metzenbaum scissors on a cutting current (30–35 W) is used to make the incision. This makes the incision rapidly and with the least amount of smoke, as compared to a LASER, which often generates plume which can interfere with visualization. Minimal cautery of the incision is performed, as the most effective method to ultimately stop the bleeding is to quickly enucleate the fibroid and commence suturing of the defect. As well, minimal bipolar cautery is used, so that there is minimal thermal damage to the tissue around the incision. This will aid in postoperative healing of the uterus. The incision is quickly continued down to the level of the fibroid. It is often helpful to actually incise the fibroid to ensure that the correct depth is achieved and that the layer between the myometrium and the fibroid has been reached. This layer can often be deceptive if one is not careful, and dissecting the fibroid when this layer is not reached, even if the surgeon is a few cell layers too superficial, can result in more bleeding.

Once this layer is identified, the key to fibroid enucleation is adequate traction and countertraction. Often, a 10 mm single or double toothed tenaculum is used to grasp the fibroid, and traction is applied. The other two 5 mm ports are used to give counter traction, and slowly, the fibroid is enucleated. Care is taken to ensure that laparoscopic graspers do not dig into tissue without good visualization so as to avoid accidentally piercing into the uterine cavity. Care is also taken not to apply so much traction with the tenaculum on the fibroid so that the fibroid is not "ripped" away from the myometrium resulting in inadvertent damage to the endometrium, particularly during the dissection at the base of the uterine fibroid.

After the fibroid is shelled out, one gram of tranexamic acid is given intravenously by anesthesia to help decrease intraoperative blood loss while the myometrial defect is being sutured laparoscopically. While there is more experience with intraoperative tranexamic acid in the orthopedic and cardiovascular literature, it is also felt to be effective and safe in the setting of uterine fibroids [9, 31, 32]. Had the patient opted for abdominal myomectomy, another blood conserving measure in addition to vasopressin and tranexamic acid would be to place a tourniquet around the uterus, thereby compressing the uterine arteries bilaterally. This can be achieved with the use of either a foley catheter or penrose drain. The resulting decrease in blood loss can often be dramatic, particularly for patients with multiple large uterine fibroids [26, 33, 34]. Other measures have also been described to reduce intraoperative blood loss during myomectomy, such as intravenous oxytocin, misoprostol, intramyometrial bupivacaine, sodium-2-mercaptoethane sulfonate, and gelatin-thrombin matrix [25]. More research is needed, however, to establish clinical effectiveness.

Once the fibroid is enucleated, it is stored in the upper abdomen while the uterine defect is sutured. The base of the defect must be carefully identified, and care also must be taken to ensure that the uterine cavity has not been damaged or entered. If it has been, it is sutured separately and carefully to ensure good re-approximation. Fortunately, this patient's cavity has not been entered, and the defect is sutured in multiple layers to ensure a sound closure. Interrupted #1 Biosyn stitches are used, and these stitches are tied extracorporeally using Roeder's knots. The defect could be sutured in many different ways, using continuous suture or using barbed suture. The mode of suturing is often surgeon preference. In this case, the interrupted sutures were strong and easy to place. Care was taken to ensure that there was no dead space left, where a hematoma could form. The serosa of the defect was closed using 2–0 Biosyn in a continuous manner using a baseball stitch. This is to try to decrease the amount of exposed suture, thereby decreasing postoperative adhesion formation.

Removal of the fibroid is then performed using laparoscopic power morcellation. At the time of the surgery, concerns regarding power morcellation and inadvertent spread of leiomyosarcoma were just starting to reach the public. The hospital did not yet have any closed morcellation system. The patient was carefully counseled with respect to risk of leiomyosarcoma and spread with the myomectomy and the power morcellation technique. She had consented without reservation. Care is taken during her procedure, and care is also taken to ensure that all "chips" are removed. Once the morcellation is finished, intercede is placed overlying her uterine incision to help decrease adhesion formation.

The patient's surgery is completed successfully, and she is admitted overnight and discharged the next day. Her postoperative course is unremarkable. A follow-up ultrasound is performed 3 months postoperatively and reveals a new small anterior fibroid 1.9 cm in size, but otherwise normal uterus and adnexa. She is keen to attempt pregnancy as soon as possible.

References

1. Shen Y, Xu Q, Xu J, Ren ML, Cai YL. Environmental exposure and risk of uterine leiomyoma: an epidemiologic surgery. Eur Rev Med Pharmacol Sci. 2013;17(23):3249–56.
2. Sparic R, Mirkovic L, Malvasi A, Tinelli A. Epidemiology of uterine myomas: a review. Int J Fertil Steril. 2016;9(4):424–35.
3. Shen Y, Wu Y, Lu Q, Ren M. Vegetarian diet and reduced uterine fibroids risk: a case-control study in Nanjing. China J Obstet Gynaecol Res. 2016;42(1):87–94. doi:10.1111/jog. 12834.
4. Parazzini F, Di Martino M, Candiani M, Vigano P. Nutr Cancer. 2015;67(4):569–79. doi:10.1080/01635581.2015.1015746.
5. Ylikorkala O, Pekonen F. Obstet Gynecol. 1986;68(1):10–2.
6. Lethaby A, Duckitt K, Farquhar C. Non-steroidal anti-inflammatory drugs for heavy menstrual bleeding. Cochrane Database Syst Rev. 2013;(1):CD000400. doi:10.1002/14651858. CD000400. PII: S1521-6934(15)00230-8.
7. Kashani BN, Centini G, Morelli SS, Weiss G, Petraglia F. Role of medical management for uterine leiomyomas. Best Pract Res Clin Obstet Gynaecol. 2016;34:85–103. doi:10.1016/j. bpobgyn.2015.11.016.
8. Bradley LD, Gueye NA. The medical management of abnormal uterine bleeding in reproductive-aged women. Am J Obstet Gynecol. 2016;214(1):31–44. doi:10.1016/j.ajog.2015.07.044.
9. Peitsidis P, Koukoulomati A. Tranexamic acid for the management of uterine fibroid tumors: a systematic review of the current evidence. World J Clin Cases. 2014;2(12):893–8. doi:10.12998/ wjcc.v2.i12.893.
10. Sangkomkamhang US, Lumbiganon P, Laopaiboon M, Mol BW. Progestogens or progestogen-releasing intrauterine systems for uterine fibroids. Cochrane Database Syst Rev. 2013;(2):CD008994. doi:10.1002/14651858.CD008994.
11. Moroni RM, Martins WP, Ferriani RA, Vieira CS, Nastri CO, Candido Dos Reis FJ, Brito LG. Add-back therapy with GnRH

analogues for uterine fibroids. Cochrane Database Syst Rev. 2015;(3):CD010854. doi:10.1002/14651858. CD010854.

12. Gurusamy KS, Vaughan J, Fraser IS, Best LMJ, Richards T. Medical therapies for uterine fibroids—a systematic review and network meta-analysis of randomized controlled trials. PLoS ONE. 11(2):e0149631. doi:10.1371/journal.pone.0149631.

13. Arendas K, Leyland NA. Use of ulipristal acetate for the management of fibroid-related acute abnormal uterine bleeding. J Obstet Gyneaecol Can. 2016;38(1):80–3. doi:10.1016/j.jogc.2015.11.005.

14. Donnez J, Tatarchuk TF, Bouchard P, Pascasiu L, Zakharenko NF, Ivanova T, Ugocsai G, Mara M, Jilla MP, Bestel E, Terrill P, Osterloh I, Loumaye E, PEARL 1 Study Group. Ulipristal acetate versus placebo for fibroid treatment before surgery. New Engl J Med. 2012;366(2):409–20. doi:10.1056/NEJMoa1103182.

15. Donnez J, Tomaszewski J, Vazquez F, Bouchard P, Lemieszczuk B, Baro F, Nouri K, Selvaggi L, Sodowski K, Bestel E, Terrill P, Osterloh I, Loumaye E, PEARL II Study Group. N Engl J Med. 2012;366(5):421–32. doi:10.1056/NEJMoa1103180.

16. Czuczwar P, Wozniak S, Szkodziak P, Wozniakowska E, Paszkowki M, Wrona W, Milart P, Paszkowski T, Popajewki M. Predicting the results of uterine artery embolization: correlation between initial intramural fibroid volume and percentage volume decrease. Prz Menopauzalny. 2014;13(4):247–52. doi:10.5114/pm.2014.45001.

17. Firouznia K, Ghanaati H, Sanaati M, Jalali AH, Shakiba M. Uterine artery embolization in 101 cases of uterine fibroids: do size, location, and number of fibroids affect therapeutic success and complications? Cardiovasc Intervent Radiol. 2008;31(3):521–6. doi:10.1007/s00270–007-9288-y.

18. Wang X, Zhang Z, Pan J, Zhang W. Effects of embolic agents with different particle sizes on interventional treatment of uterine fibroids. Pak J Med Sci. 2015;31(6):1490–5. doi:10.12669/pjms.316.7955.

19. Kaump GR, Spies JB. The impact of uterine artery embolization on ovarian function. J Vasc Interv Radiol. 2013;24(4):459–67. doi:10.1016/j.jvir.2012.12.002.

20. Tropeano G, Di Stasi C, Litwicka K, Romano D, Draisci G, Mancuso S. Uterine artery embolization for fibroids does not

have adverse effects on ovarian reserve in regularly cycling women younger than 40 years. Fertil Steril. 2004;81(4):1055–61.

21. McLucas B, Danzer H, Wambach C, Lee C. Ovarian reserve following uterine artery embolization in women in reproductive age: a preliminary report. Minim Invasive Ther Allied Technol. 2013;22(1):45–9. doi:10.3109/13645706.2012.743918.

22. McLucas B, Voorhees WD, Chua KJ. Anti Mullerian hormone levels before and after uterine artery embolization: a preliminary report. Minim Invasive Ther Allied Technol. 2015;24(4):242–5. doi:10.3109/13645706.2015.1012084.

23. Arthur R, Kachura J, Liu G, Chan C, Shapiro H. Laparoscopic myomectomy versus uterine artery embolization: long-term impact on markers of ovarian reserve. J Obstet Gynaeol Can. 2014;36(3):240–7.

24. Lethaby A, Vollenhoven B, Sowter M. Pre-operative GnRH analogue therapy before hysterectomy or myomectomy for uterine fibroids. Cochrane Database Syst Rev. 2001;(2):CD000547.

25. Kongnyuy EJ, Wiysonge CS. Interventions to reduce haemorrhage during myomectomy for fibroids. Cochrane Database Syst Rev. 2011;11:CD005355. doi:10.1002/14651858.CD005355.

26. Fletcher H, Frederick J, Hardie M, Simeon D. A randomized comparison of vasopressin and tourniquet as hemostatic agents during myomectomy. Obstet Gynaecol. 1996;87(6):1014–8.

27. Frederick J, Fletcher H, Simeon D, Mullings A, Hardie M. Intramyometrial vasopressin as a hemostatic agent during myomectomy. Br J Obstet Gynaecol. 1994;101(5):435–7.

28. Kwon YS, Jung DY, Lee SH, Ahn JW, Roh HJ, Im KS. Transient occlusion of uterine arteries with endoscopic vascular clip preceding laparoscopic myomectomy. J Laparoendosc Adv Surg Tech A. 2013;23(8):679–83. doi:10.1089/lap.2012.0540.

29. Kwon YS, Roh HJ, Ahn JW, Lee SH, Im KS. Transient occlusion of uterine arteries in laparoscopic uterine surgery. JSLS. 2015;19(1):e2014.00189. doi:10.4294/JSLS.2014.00189.

30. Discepola F, Valenti DA, Reinhold C, Tulandi T. Analysis of arterial blood vessels surrounding the myoma: relevance to myomectomy. Obstet Gynecol. 2007;110(6):1301–3.

31. Ngichabe S, Obura T, Stones W. Intravenous tranexamic acid as an adjunct haemostat to ornipressin during open myomectomy. A randomized double blind placebo controlled trial. Ann Surg Innov Res. 2015;9:10. doi:10.1186/s13022-015-0017-y.

32. Shaaban MM, Ahmed MR, Farhan RE, Dardeer HH. Efficacy of tranexamic acid on myomectomy-associated blood loss in patients with multiple myomas: a randomized controlled clinical trial. Reprod Sci. 2016;23(7):908–12. doi:10.1177/1933719115623646.
33. Ikechebelu JI, Ezeama CO, Obiechina NJ. The use of tourniquet to reduce blood loss at myomectomy. Niger J Clin Pract. 2010;13(2):154–8.
34. Alptekin H, Efe D. Effectiveness of pericervical tourniquet by foley catheter reducing blood loss at abdominal myomectomy. Clin Exp Obstet Gynecol. 2014;41(4):440–4.

Chapter 17
Uterine Fibroids and Recurrent Pregnancy Loss

Mohamed A. Bedaiwy, Christa Lepik, and Sukinah Alfaraj

Abbreviations

APH	Antepartum haemorrhage
APS	Antiphospholipid syndrome
FDA	Food and Drug Administration
FSH	Follicular stimulating hormone
GA	Gestational age
GDM	Gestational diabetes mellitus
HSG	Hysterosalpingogram
MRgFUS	Magnetic resonance-guided focused ultrasound surgery
MRI	Magnetic resonance imagine
PPH	Postpartum hemorrhage
PROM	Premature rupture of membranes
RCT	Randomized control trial
RFVTA	Radiofrequency volumetric thermal ablation

M.A. Bedaiwy, MD, PhD (✉) • C. Lepik, MD • S. Alfaraj, MD
Division of Reproductive Endocrinology and Infertility,
Department of Obstetrics and Gynecology, The University of
British Columbia, D415A-4500 Oak Street,
Vancouver, BC V6H 3N1, Canada
e-mail: mohamed.bedaiwy@cw.bc.ca

N.S. Moawad (ed.), *Uterine Fibroids*,
https://doi.org/10.1007/978-3-319-58780-6_17,
© Springer International Publishing AG 2018

RPL	Recurrent pregnancy loss
SIS	Saline infusion sonography
UAE	Uterine artery embolization

Introduction

An estimated 20–40% of woman will develop uterine fibroids in their reproductive years (ASRM 2011). Fibroids are observed in 3.3–10.7% of pregnant women and may impact pregnancy outcomes [1, 2]. The prevalence of uterine fibroids in women with recurrent pregnancy loss was estimated to be 4.08% in a recent meta-analysis published by Russo et al. [3]. Approximately, 10–40% of patients with fibroids develop pregnancy complications [4, 5]. The mechanism by which fibroids cause obstetrical complications is not known.

Most women with uterine fibroids are asymptomatic in pregnancy. However, the most common complication is pain associated with large fibroids (>5 cm) in the second and third trimesters. Smaller fibroids are less likely to result in admissions for pain (5% 4–7 cm vs. 23% 7–10 cm vs. 21% >10 cm; $P = 0.01$) [6]. Severe abdominal pain can occur when a fibroid undergoes "red degeneration" torsion (most common with subserosal fibroids) or impaction. Three theories exist to explain the pain associated with red degeneration. One theory is that the accelerated growth of fibroids leads to outgrowth of blood supply resulting in ischemia, necrosis, and infarction. The second is that the growing uterus distorts anatomy and affects blood supply to fibroids leading to ischemia and necrosis even if the fibroid size remains stable. The third theory is that prostaglandins are released from damaged cells within the fibroid causing pain [4, 7, 8].

Besides pain, fibroids have been associated with increased risk of miscarriage, caesarean section, fetal malpresentation, preterm birth, placental abruption, and postpartum hemorrhage [9]. However, the impact of fibroids on pregnancy differs depending on the characteristics such as size, anatomical location, and number.

A review published in 1981 by Buttram et al. was the first to establish a relationship between fibroids and miscarriage noting a decrease in miscarriage rates from 41 to 19% following myomectomy [10]. However, many studies included in this review were small case studies without controls and used different methodology. A more recently published review article by Klatsky et al. calculated the cumulative risk of miscarriage when intramural fibroids are noted in the first trimester via ultrasound to be 20.4% vs. 12.9% in women without a fibroid (OR 1.6) [9].

In the Klatsky review 13.3% of women without fibroids and 48.8% of those with fibroids delivered via C-section. This increased rate was attributed to fetal malpresentation (13%) rather than labor dystocia.

Preterm birth is the most commonly reported poor neonatal outcome associated with fibroids with rates of 16.0% vs. 8.0% without fibroids. The exact process by which fibroids cause preterm labor is unknown; however there are several theories. One possibility is that fibroid uteri are less distensible than nonfibroid uteri resulting in preterm uterine contractions and cervical dilation [11]. At the molecular level, decreased oxytocinase activity has been noted in the fibroid gravid uterus and results in higher levels of oxytocin, predisposing to premature contractions [12]. On the other side, there is no conclusive data to support higher rates of preterm premature rupture of membranes (PPROM) or intrauterine growth restriction (IUGR). Fibroids have been shown to be associated with placental abruption with the strongest correlation between submucosal and retroplacental fibroids.

Fibroid volume change during pregnancy is controversial. In one series, 60–78% of fibroids do not demonstrate any significant change in volume during pregnancy. Of the 22–32% of fibroids which increase, the majority do so in the first trimester prior to 10 weeks' gestational age [13]. Lam et al. determined that although fibroid size did not impact birth weight, rate of preterm delivery, or mode of delivery there was a significant impact on estimated blood loss and rates of postpartum hemorrhage (PPH). Rates of PPH were 11% for fibroids sized 4–7 cm vs. 13% for those sized 7–10 cm vs. 36% for those >10 cm ($P = 0.04$). Estimated blood loss also increased significantly depending on size:

567 cm^3 (4–7 cm) vs. 643 cm^3 (7–10 cm) vs. 961 cm (>100 cm); $P = 0.01$) [6].

Although fibroids have the potential to negatively affect pregnancy, their association with recurrent pregnancy loss and impact of treatment on future pregnancy is not entirely clear, especially in the context of noncavity-distorting intramural location.

Clinical Case Presentation

We present a 19-year-old G2 T0 P0 A2 L0 with an incidental finding of a 12 cm intramural mass during her second pregnancy that was complicated by a second trimester loss at 18 weeks' gestation.

The patient describes her second pregnancy as uncomplicated until the diagnosis of a second trimester miscarriage was made. All of her prenatal blood work was within normal limits. She declined genetic screening. During her dating ultrasound at 7 weeks' gestational age there was an incidental finding of a 10 cm mass consistent with intramural fibroid. At her 18-week detailed ultrasound intrauterine fetal demise was diagnosed due to absent fetal cardiac activity. Biometry estimated the fetal size to be consistent with 16 weeks' gestational age. The intramural mass had increased in size to 12 cm diameter. She decided to have evacuation of the pregnancy in the operating room under general anesthetic. The procedure was uncomplicated.

In terms of her obstetrical history the patient has had two pregnancies. Both of which she conceived spontaneously after 2–3 months of actively trying. Her first pregnancy resulted in a spontaneous miscarriage at 7 weeks' gestational age and passed spontaneously. She denies any previous gynecological concerns and was previously unaware that she had a fibroid. There is no history of any prior sexually transmitted infections and she has never had a pap smear. She describes her menstrual cycles as regular, occurring every 28–30 days and lasting 5 days. There is no history of abnormal uterine bleeding. She uses condoms and has never used any other type of contraception. She does not endorse a history of any abdominal or pelvic pain, pressure symptoms, or change in bladder or bowel function.

Her medical history is otherwise unremarkable and she has undergone no other surgeries besides the dilation and evacuation. She denies a history of smoking and recreational drug use and drinks 3 oz of alcohol per week. In terms of family history, she believes that her mother had a hysterectomy at the age of 35 but is not entirely sure of the reason. She is unaware of any family history of recurrent pregnancy loss, autoimmune disease, or congenital malformations. She does not take any medications besides a prenatal vitamin and has no known drug allergies.

Exam Findings

On examination, the patient appears well and has a BMI of 21 kg/m^2. Vital signs are stable. Palpation of the head and neck is negative for any nodules or areas of fullness including the thyroid. There are no signs of clinical hyper-androgenism or insulin resistance. Cardiovascular and respiratory examinations are both within normal limits. On inspection of the abdomen there are no surgical scars although her abdomen is slightly distended. On palpation, there is no organomegaly; however a mobile mass in the midline of the lower abdomen is palpable.

On pelvic examination, the patient has normal external female genitalia. Speculum examination revealed normal vaginal mucosa and a nulliparous cervical os. On bimanual examination the ovaries were nonpalpable; however there was a large midline mass noted that seemed to be associated with the uterus. It was nontender and mobile.

Diagnostic Workup

As the patient's second miscarriage occurred at 18 weeks the fetus was sent to pathology. No congenital anomalies were noted and karyotype revealed euploid 46XY on the pathology report.

Because this patient has had two consecutive clinical miscarriages, she warrants investigation for recurrent pregnancy loss (RPL), defined by two or more spontaneous pregnancy losses [14]. Investigations for thyroid disease, hyperprolactinemia, APS, and glucose intolerance were all within normal limits. Parental karyotyping was euploid for both the male and female (Table 17.1).

As per ASRM guidelines (2012), suggested investigations for RPL assess potential contributing factors related to genetics, antiphospholipid syndrome (APS), anatomic uterine anomalies, and hormonal and metabolic factors.

Parental karyotyping is recommended to detect any balanced translocations that are present in an estimated 2–5% of cases of recurrent pregnancy loss.

As well, APS should be ruled out by testing for lupus anticoagulant, anti-beta-2-glycoprotein, and anticardiolipin IgG/IgM. 5–20% of women with recurrent pregnancy loss will test

TABLE 17.1 Investigations: results of patient's initial laboratory investigations for recurrent pregnancy loss

Lab value	Result
Female parent karyotype	46XX
Male parent karyotype	46XY
Prolactin	8 ng/mL
TSH	1.5 µU/mL
HgA1C	5.2%
Lupus anticoagulant	Not detected
Anti-beta-2-glycoprotein 1	Not detected
Anti-cardiolipin IgG	Not detected

positive for APS antibodies. As per the International Consensus Classification criteria for the antiphospholipid syndrome APS is present if one of the following clinical and laboratory criteria are met [15].

1. Clinical Criteria:

   (a) Vascular thrombus
   (b) Pregnancy morbidity

       • One or more unexplained losses of morphologically normal fetus >10 weeks' gestational age
       • One or more unexplained losses of morphologically normal fetus before 34 weeks' gestational age due to severe preeclampsia or eclampsia as per standard definitions or placental insufficiency
       • Three or more consecutive unexplained losses of morphologically normal fetuses <10 weeks' gestational age

2. Laboratory Criteria:

   (a) Lupus anticoagulant in plasma on two or more occasions at least 12 weeks apart
   (b) Anticardiolipin IgG and/or IgM in serum or plasma present in medium or high titer (>40 GPL or MPL or greater than the 99th percentile) on two or more occasions at least 12 weeks apart
   (c) Anti-beta-2-glycoprotein-1 IgG and/or IgM on 2 or more occasions at least 12 weeks apart

Maternal endocrine disorders should also be ruled out. If TSH levels are within normal range (i.e., <2.5 µU/mL) there is no indication to check thyroxine (T4) levels or antithyroid antibodies [16]. Uncontrolled diabetes is also a risk factor; therefore HgA1C or fasting glucose should also be included in initial investigation for RPL [17]. Prolactin is also measured because hyperprolactinemia affects the hypothalamic-pituitary axis and may cause RPL.

Imaging

The patient's incidental diagnosis of the intramural mass was made during her dating ultrasound at 7 weeks' gestational age. Appearance was most consistent with an intramural fibroid and it was estimated to be 10 cm in diameter (Fig. 17.1).

Transvaginal ultrasound has been shown to be accurate, efficient, safe, and cost-effective method of detecting the presence of fibroids (sensitivity: 99%; specificity: 91%) [18]. However, this level of accuracy is dependent on uterine volumes <375 cm^3 and when the number of fibroids is between 1 and 4.

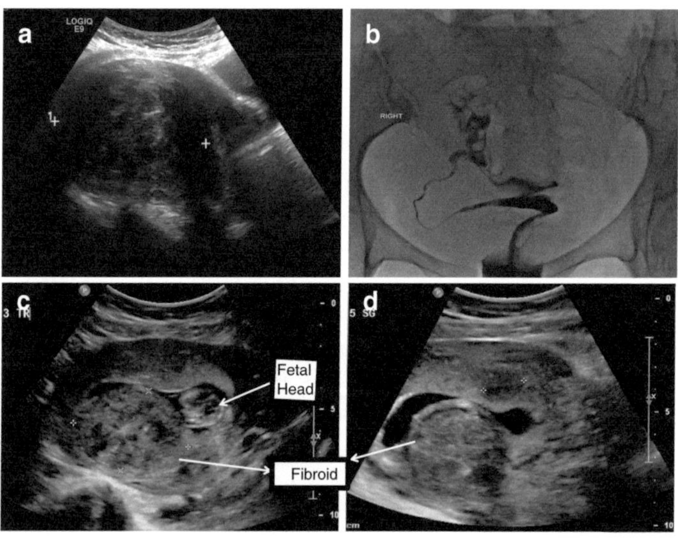

FIGURE 17.1 (a) Sagittal view of intramural fibroid on detailed ultrasound estimated to be 11.9 cm × 12.1 cm × 8.86 cm on transabdominal ultrasound. (b) Hysterosalpingogram confirming patency of fallopian tubes bilaterally and normal uterine cavity contour with no lesions detected. (c) Transabdominal ultrasound showing large intramural fibroid and fetal head. (d) Transabdominal ultrasound showing large intramural fibroid

There has been substantial research of the use of magnetic resonance imaging (MRI) in the evaluation of fibroids. In the double-blind study by Dueholm et al. [19] the accuracy of detecting the presence of fibroids was comparable to transvaginal ultrasound with sensitivity of 99% and specificity of 86% with pathological examination the gold standard. However, MRI is superior to transvaginal ultrasound when uterine volumes are greater than 375 cm^3 and the number of fibroids exceeds 4. MRI is also superior in determining location and correct uterine wall embedment (i.e., intramural component). Of course, the drawbacks of MRI for evaluation of intramural fibroid are accessibility and cost. However, MRI should be obtained when fibroid mapping is critical, for example when planning an advanced surgical procedure.

Saline infusion sonography (SIS) uses saline injected into the uterine cavity as contrast to enable improved definition of submucosal fibroids, endometrial polyps, endometrial hyperplasia, or carcinomas. SIS is noted to have 83% sensitivity and 90% specificity for submucosal fibroid detection; however it is not considered to be as efficient at assessing intramural fibroids [19].

Hysterosalpingogram (HSG) is classically useful in evaluating patency of the fallopian tubes, excluding intrauterine pathology, and evaluates the contour of the endometrial cavity. However, this imaging modality has a sensitivity of 50% and positive predictive value of 28.6% for intrauterine lesions such as polyps and submucosal fibroids [20]. It is not considered a useful technique for assessing the myometrium or detecting intramural fibroids.

Treatment Options

Currently there is no medical management of fibroids available that is considered curative. It is generally agreeable that submucous fibroids and intramural fibroids distorting the endometrial cavity should be removed particularly in the context of reproductive complications. In the context of a large intramural fibroid and desire to conceive the patient has two options including expectant vs. surgical management.

In our practice, patients with large fibroids are advised to pursue surgical management, typically a preconception myomectomy. The decision to follow a laparoscopic versus open approach depends on the number and diameter of the fibroids. The criteria used when recommending a laparoscopic myomectomy is as follows:

1. One fibroid <15 cm in diameter
2. Two fibroids <7.5 cm in diameter
3. Three fibroids <5 cm in diameter

If the previously mentioned criteria are not met, then an open approach is advised. For noncavity-distorting intramural fibroids, less than 5 cm surgical management is not advised unless there is distortion of the endometrial cavity or the patient is symptomatic.

For this patient, although she is asymptomatic, because the fibroid is 12 cm in diameter preconception surgical management is recommended. As she has a single fibroid less than 15 cm in diameter she is eligible for a laparoscopic approach. We typically advise the patients to postpone conception for 3–6 months postoperatively to allow for healing of the myoma bed.

The patient had a laparoscopic myomectomy. For detailed techniques of laparoscopic myomectomy, please refer to Chaps. 4, 8, 13, 14, and 16. The patient's postoperative course was unremarkable. She conceived spontaneously 12 months later. She then delivered a live newborn female via elective caesarean section at 39 weeks' GA.

Medical Management

Medical management of fibroids is based on the role that estrogen and progesterone may play in regard to growth. Currently, there is no pharmacological treatment available that is considered curative. Contemporary medical treatment is considered an option for symptom control. Available medical therapy is associated with ovulation suppression, reduction of estrogen, and inhibition of estrogen and progesterone at the level of receptors. Theoretically it has the potential to inhibit ovulation, endometrium development, and implantation and should not be used in women wishing to conceive or who are pregnant.

Ulipristal is a relatively new medication, which is a selective progesterone receptor modulator that suppresses neovascularization and cell proliferation while inducing apoptosis of fibroids [21]. Ulipristal's ability to reduce fibroid volume and symptoms has been well established in clinical trials [22–24]; however its effect on fertility and pregnancy outcomes is not known. Case studies and series have reported successful term pregnancies in the context of ulipristal use with surgical resection [25–27]. Recently, a case report was published reporting a term pregnancy following ulipristal use without surgery [28]. These studies suggest the potential utility of ulipristal for the reduction of fibroid size in women wishing to conceive but avoid surgical intervention.

However, now there is no recommended medical management for fibroids in the context of women who are planning to conceive or pregnant.

Myomectomy

Myomectomy for intramural fibroids may be completed via laparoscopy or laparotomy depending on surgeon preference. Hysteroscopic myomectomy is reserved for fibroids with a submucosal component.

Several, noncontrolled studies suggest a decrease in miscarriage rate after myomectomy. Saravelos et al. found that women undergoing myomectomy demonstrated a decrease in miscarriage rates from 21.7 to 0% and live birth rate increased from 23.3 to 52.0% ($p < 0.05$), however, only when the fibroid distorted the cavity. Women with fibroids that did not distort the cavity achieved live birth rates of 70.4% without intervention [29].

Another study demonstrated marked reduction in miscarriage rates following laparoscopic myomectomy from 43 to 24%. Fifty-one percent of these fibroids were partially intramural and 28% completely intramural [30].

However, a Cochrane review by Metwally et al. included one RCT that investigated the effects of myomectomy on obstetrical outcomes. This review demonstrated that myomectomy of intramural fibroids had no significant effect on clinical pregnancy rates or miscarriages. In those women that underwent myomectomy (via laparotomy or laparoscopy), this did not result in significant difference for live birth rate, clinical pregnancy rate, miscarriage rate, caesarean section, or preterm delivery [31].

To date, there have been no studies examining the effect of myomectomy on RPL.

Clearly, there is disagreement in the literature that brings up the issue if asymptomatic intramural fibroids should be treated. Myomectomy has unique risks besides the general surgical complications of bleeding, infection, damage to viscous, and postoperative thrombus that also need to be considered when recommending surgical management.

Postoperative adhesions have been noted following myomectomy, with an incidence of 94% when the incision is made on the posterior uterine wall and 55% when anterior [32]. The rate of uterine rupture in pregnancy is 0.002%. Even though the incidence is lower than the risk following previous caesarean section (0.1%), delivery via caesarean section is recommended following transmural incision for abdominal or laparoscopic myomectomy [33].

Two randomized controlled trials (RCTs) have been published comparing outcomes of laparoscopic vs. abdominal myomectomy [34, 35]. Besides time to first live birth (14 vs. 15 months, $p = 0.003$) and time to first pregnancy (5 vs. 6 months, $p = 0.008$) there were no other significant differences in reproductive outcomes.

In the literature, myomectomy during pregnancy has not been recommended because of presumed increased risk of bleeding. However, case series have been published with positive outcomes associated with myomectomy performed during pregnancy or C-section [36–39].

Uterine Artery Embolization

Uterine artery embolization (UAE) was first introduced in 1995 as a noninvasive technique for treating uterine fibroids [40]. Current contraindications to UAE include pregnancy or desire for future pregnancy.

An RCT published by Mara et al. includes 121 patients with intramural fibroids >4 cm and plans for future pregnancy. Patients were randomized to UAE or abdominal (open or laparoscopic based on surgeon preference) myomectomy [41]. Fifty percent of the UAE group vs. 78% of the myomectomy group conceived. Relative risk of UAE patients for spontaneous miscarriage was 2.79 in comparison to myomectomy.

Another finding in the aforementioned RCT is the significantly elevated FSH levels >10 IU/L 6 months following UAE compared to myomectomy (13.8% vs. 3.2%, $p < 0.05$). Various other studies have also noted loss of ovarian reserve and increase in ovarian failure in women undergoing UAE.

As well, the incidences of caesarean section and postpartum hemorrhage were also noted to be elevated following UAE (66% vs. 48.5% and 13.9% vs. 2.5%, respectively) compared to control pregnancies [42].

There is also concern about the formation of uterine synechiae following UAE secondary to small particles. Small particles from the embolic material used can enter endometrial arteries causing ischemia, synechiae, or ovarian failure if they pass into the utero-ovarian anastomoses [43].

There are lower pregnancy rates, higher spontaneous miscarriage rates, and greater obstetrical complications such as PPH in women who have had uterine fibroids treated with

UAE. At this time, this method of treatment is not recommended in patients with large intramural fibroids who wish to conceive in the future.

Magnetic Resonance-Guided Focused Ultrasound Surgery

Magnetic resonance-guided focused ultrasound surgery (MRgFUS) is a noninvasive, thermal ablation technique approved by the US Food and Drug Administration (FDA) in 2004. This technique uses MRI to direct ultrasound energy to a focal point within the fibroid which causes tissue necrosis of the tumor with limited damage to surrounding structures. The platform used in the United States, Canada, Europe, Asia, and Australia is the ExAblate 2000 (InSightec), ExAblate 2100 (InSightec), and Sonalleve MR-HIFU (Philips Medical System). One treatment lasts up to 3 h and recovery time is 24–48 h.

Patient selection depends on various criteria including fibroid imaging characteristics and location, number, size, and proximity to critical structures. Exclusion criteria included weight exceeding 115 kg, serious health complications, contraindications to MRI, abdominal scarring, uterine size greater than 24 weeks, and pedunculated, nonenhancing or heavily calcified fibroids [44]. The exclusion of patients planning future pregnancies is now questioned due to multiple uncomplicated pregnancies post-MRgFUS.

Although selection criteria for MRgFUS includes women with no desire for future fertility there have been multiple anecdotal pregnancies. A case series published in 2010 by Rabinovici et al. reports on 54 pregnancies in 51 women who had been treated with MRgFUS for symptomatic uterine fibroids and/or focal adenomyosis. Twenty-seven out of 51 of women had fibroids described as intramural [45]. Forty-one percent of pregnancies resulted in live births and 20% of pregnancies were ongoing at the time of publication.

Twenty-six percent ended in spontaneous abortion, 93% of which occurred at 13 weeks' GA or earlier. Thirteen percent ended secondary to elective termination.

To date, there are no studies comparing MRgFUS to myomectomy; however the series by Rabinovici is reassuring that term pregnancies can be achieved following this relatively novel method of fibroid treatment. However, this case series was underpowered to detect rare but serious outcomes such as uterine rupture or placenta accrete. Until further studies are available, this treatment should not be offered to women desiring future fertility but may be a potential option in the future.

Laparoscopic Cryomyolysis

Laparoscopic cryomyolysis is another alternative treatment for women wishing to conserve their uterus in the context of uterine fibroids. This procedure involves cooling the fibroid to temperatures $-20\ ^{\circ}C$ or lower which causes necrosis and ablation.

There are few studies assessing pregnancy outcomes after myolysis. However a case series of nine cases of unexpected pregnancies following laparoscopic myolysis was published in 2006 by Ciavattini et al. [46]. Eleven fibroids underwent treatment: one subserosal, three subserosal-intramural, and seven intramural. Average time to pregnancy following the procedure was 18.6 months. Nine of 11 fibroids increased in size during the pregnancy; the mean average increase was 71.1%. Two miscarriages occurred, one at 9 and one at 11 weeks' GA. Otherwise, the remaining seven pregnancies were uncomplicated. In particular, there were no increased rates of preterm labor, placental abruption, PROM, preeclampsia, congenital malformations, APH, GDM, uterine rupture, or postpartum complications including PPH.

In the literature there are concerns over the risk of uterine dehiscence, fibroid recurrence, and obstetrical outcomes following laparoscopic myolysis. In the previously described case series seven of the nine pregnancies had uneventful outcomes and two of the nine resulted in first-trimester miscarriage. However, there are reports of three cases of uterine rupture in the literature, one of which resulted in a catastrophic impact on the fetus [47].

At this time, the integrity and tensile strength of the uterus have not been determined following laparoscopic myolysis; therefore pregnancy is not recommended in women who have undergone this procedure. However, there are no RCTs or large studies comparing laparoscopic myolysis to classical surgical methods for treating fibroids in women wishing to conserve the uterus.

Overall, this case series suggested that pregnancy had a negative effect on fibroids treated with cryomyolysis as there was a significant increase in volume in the first 20 weeks of pregnancy. However, there were seven uneventful term pregnancies following laparoscopic cryomyolysis suggesting that successful pregnancy is possible.

Laparoscopic cryomyolysis remains an alternative only for women wishing to conserve their uterus, but do not desire future fertility.

Radiofrequency Ablation

Radiofrequency volumetric thermal ablation (RFVTA: the Acessa procedure; Halt Medical, Inc., Brentwood, CA, USA) uses heat produced by oscillations of high frequency alternating with an electric field which causes tissue damage and localized coagulation necrosis [48]. Typically this procedure is done under ultrasound or laparoscopic camera guidance, an ablation needle is inserted into the center of the fibroid, and ablation temperatures reach anywhere from 85 to 100 °C. The efficacy and safety of this procedure need to be validated in larger populations. Its safety in the context of future fertility and pregnancy outcomes has not been determined.

Berman et al. published a retrospective analysis of pregnancy outcomes for six unexpected pregnancies following radiofrequency volumetric thermal ablation from three different trials [49]. Of the 202 women enrolled 6 became spontaneously pregnant despite the studies' requirement to continue contraception and to have complete childbearing. Number of fibroids ranged from 1 to 7 and size from 1.0 to 7.6 cm. The subjects conceived 3.5 to 15 months posttreatment. One patient had a spontaneous miscarriage at 10 weeks and the five other pregnancies were uncomplicated term deliveries. The only complication was expulsion of a degenerated fibroid 48 h after delivery for one of the patients that resulted in the need for blood products due to excessive bleeding. Otherwise, besides the one miscarriage there were no obstetrical complications including uterine rupture.

At this point, pregnancy is not recommended following RFVTA; however the aforementioned study is encouraging. Until there are more robust studies assessing pregnancy outcomes after RFTVA it remains contraindicated.

Laparoscopic and Vaginal Occlusion of Uterine Arteries

Temporary transvaginal occlusion of uterine arteries is an emerging noninvasive technique for fibroid treatment. This technique causes temporary occlusion of uterine vessels, causing myoma ischemia leading to infarcts, necrosis, and reduction in myoma volume [50]. There is one case in the literature of an uneventful pregnancy following this procedure; however this procedure remains contraindicated in those seeking future fertility [51].

Laparoscopic occlusion of the uterine arteries involves occlusion at the level of the internal iliac artery and coagulation of collateral arteries between the uterus and ovaries. There are no studies involving this technique and effects on fertility; therefore it is contraindicated.

Conclusion

The exact relationship of cavity-distorting uterine fibroids and recurrent pregnancy loss is well established. However, the same relationship to noncavity-distorting uterine fibroids is yet to be determined. The presented case illustrates that surgical correction of the latter improved the live birth outcome in this case. In another patient who is 35 years old with infertility a 9-cm intramural noncavity-distorting fibroid was diagnosed. MRI confirmed the absence of intracavitary component; however the lining was intended (Fig. 17.2a, b). She conceived via in vitro fertilization. Unfortunately, she has a second-trimester loss at 19 weeks' gestation. She elected to undergo myomectomy prior to any further fertility treatment (Fig. 17.2c, d). This case further illustrates the relationship between noncavity-distorting fibroids and pregnancy loss.

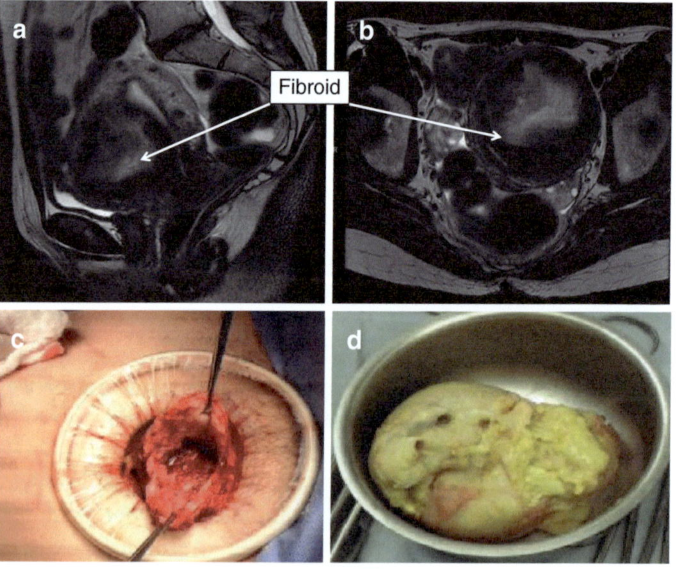

FIGURE 17.2 MRI sagittal view (**a**) and coronal view (**b**) indicating intramural fibroid impinging the endometrial cavity. Myoma Bed on the left lateral uterine wall (**c**). Excised degenerated myoma (**d**)

Given the available evidence, it seems that myomectomy is the treatment of choice for cavity-distorting and noncavity-distorting fibroids in the context of recurrent pregnancy loss.

References

1. Stout MJ, Odibo AO, Graseck AS, Macones GA, Crane JP, Cahill AG. Leiomyomas at routine second-trimester ultrasound examination and adverse obstetric outcomes. Obstet Gynecol. 2010;116(5):1056–63.
2. Laughlin SK, Baird DD, Savitz DA, Herring AH, Hartmann KE. Prevalence of uterine leiomyomas in the first trimester of pregnancy: an ultrasound-screening study. Obstet Gynecol. 2009;113(3):630–5.
3. Russo M, Suen M, Bedaiwy M, Chen I. Prevalence of uterine myomas among women with 2 or more recurrent pregnancy losses: a systematic review. J Minim Invasive Gynecol. 2016;23(5):702–6.
4. Katz VL, Dotters DJ, Droegemeuller W. Complications of uterine leiomyomas in pregnancy. Obstet Gynecol. 1989;73(4):593–6.
5. Coronado GD, Marshall LM, Schwartz SM. Complications in pregnancy, labor, and delivery with uterine leiomyomas: a population-based study. Obstet Gynecol. 2000;95(5):764–9.
6. Lam SJ, Best S, Kumar S. The impact of fibroid characteristics on pregnancy outcome. Am J Obstet Gynecol. 2014;211(4):395.e1–5.
7. De Carolis S, Fatigante G, Ferrazzani S, Trivellini C, De Santis L, Mancuso S, et al. Uterine myomectomy in pregnant women. Fetal Diagn Ther. 2001;16(2):116–9.
8. Parker WH. Etiology, symptomatology, and diagnosis of uterine myomas. Fertil Steril. 2007;87(4):725–36.
9. Klatsky PC, Tran ND, Caughey AB, Fujimoto VY. Fibroids and reproductive outcomes: a systematic literature review from conception to delivery. Am J Obstet Gynecol. 2008;198(4):357–66.
10. Buttram VC Jr. Uterine leiomyomata—aetiology, symptomatology and management. Prog Clin Biol Res. 1986;225:275–96.
11. Rice JP, Kay HH, Mahony BS. The clinical significance of uterine leiomyomas in pregnancy. Am J Obstet Gynecol. 1989;160(5 Pt 1):1212–6.
12. Blum M. Comparative study of serum CAP activity during pregnancy in malformed and normal uterus. J Perinat Med. 1978;6(3):165–8.

13. Lee HJ, Norwitz ER, Shaw J. Contemporary management of fibroids in pregnancy. Rev Obstet Gynecol. 2010;3(1):20–7.

14. Kolte AM, Bernardi LA, Christiansen OB, Quenby S, Farquharson RG, Goddijn M, et al. Terminology for pregnancy loss prior to viability: a consensus statement from the ESHRE early pregnancy special interest group. Hum Reprod (Oxford, England). 2015;30(3):495–8.

15. Miyakis S, Lockshin MD, Atsumi T, Branch DW, Brey RL, Cervera R, et al. International consensus statement on an update of the classification criteria for definite antiphospholipid syndrome (APS). J Thromb Haemost. 2006;4(2):295–306.

16. Management of thyroid dysfunction during pregnancy and postpartum: an Endocrine Society Clinical Practice Guideline. Thyroid. 2007;17(11):1159–67.

17. Jovanovic L, Knopp RH, Kim H, Cefalu WT, Zhu XD, Lee YJ, et al. Elevated pregnancy losses at high and low extremes of maternal glucose in early normal and diabetic pregnancy: evidence for a protective adaptation in diabetes. Diabetes Care. 2005;28(5):1113–7.

18. Dueholm M, Lundorf E, Hansen ES, Ledertoug S, Olesen F. Accuracy of magnetic resonance imaging and transvaginal ultrasonography in the diagnosis, mapping, and measurement of uterine myomas. Am J Obstet Gynecol. 2002;186(3):409–15.

19. Dueholm M, Lundorf E, Hansen ES, Ledertoug S, Olesen F. Evaluation of the uterine cavity with magnetic resonance imaging, transvaginal sonography, hysterosonographic examination, and diagnostic hysteroscopy. Fertil Steril. 2001;76(2):350–7.

20. Soares SR, Barbosa dos Reis MM, Camargos AF. Diagnostic accuracy of sonohysterography, transvaginal sonography, and hysterosalpingography in patients with uterine cavity diseases. Fertil Steril. 2000;73(2):406–11.

21. Talaulikar VS, Manyonda IT. Ulipristal acetate: a novel option for the medical management of symptomatic uterine fibroids. Adv Ther. 2012;29(8):655–63.

22. Donnez J, Tatarchuk TF, Bouchard P, Puscasiu L, Zakharenko NF, Ivanova T, et al. Ulipristal acetate versus placebo for fibroid treatment before surgery. N Engl J Med. 2012;366(5):409–20.

23. Donnez J, Tomaszewski J, Vazquez F, Bouchard P, Lemieszczuk B, Baro F, et al. Ulipristal acetate versus leuprolide acetate for uterine fibroids N Engl J Med. 2012;366(5):421–32.

24. Donnez J, Vazquez F, Tomaszewski J, Nouri K, Bouchard P, Fauser BC, et al. Long-term treatment of uterine fibroids with ulipristal acetate. Fertil Steril. 2014;101(6):1565–73.e1–18.
25. Luyckx M, Squifflet JL, Jadoul P, Votino R, Dolmans MM, Donnez J. First series of 18 pregnancies after ulipristal acetate treatment for uterine fibroids. Fertil Steril. 2014;102(5):1404–9.
26. Monleon J, Martinez-Varea A, Galliano D, Pellicer A. Successful pregnancy after treatment with ulipristal acetate for uterine fibroids. Case Rep Obstet Gynecol. 2014;2014:314587.
27. Wdowiak A. Commentary on the article "Pre-treatment with ulipristal acetate before ICSI procedure: a case report" published in Menopause Review 6/2013 (Przeglad Menopauzalny 2013; 6: 496-500). Menopause Rev. 2014;13(2):150–1.
28. Murad K. Spontaneous pregnancy following ulipristal acetate treatment in a woman with a symptomatic uterine fibroid. J Obstet Gynaecol Canada. 2016;38(1):75–9.
29. Saravelos SH, Yan J, Rehmani H, Li TC. The prevalence and impact of fibroids and their treatment on the outcome of pregnancy in women with recurrent miscarriage. Hum Reprod. 2011;26(12):3274–9.
30. Bernardi TS, Radosa MP, Weisheit A, Diebolder H, Schneider U, Schleussner E, et al. Laparoscopic myomectomy: a 6-year follow-up single-center cohort analysis of fertility and obstetric outcome measures. Arch Gynecol Obstet. 2014;290(1):87–91.
31. Metwally M, Cheong YC, Horne AW. Surgical treatment of fibroids for subfertility. Cochrane Database Syst Rev. 2012;(11):CD003857.
32. Tulandi T, Murray C, Guralnick M. Adhesion formation and reproductive outcome after myomectomy and second-look laparoscopy. Obstet Gynecol. 1993;82(2):213–5.
33. Stewart EA, Laughlin-Tommaso SK, Catherino WH, Lalitkumar S, Gupta D, Vollenhoven B. Uterine fibroids. Nat Rev Dis Primers. 2016;2:16043.
34. Seracchioli R, Rossi S, Govoni F, Rossi E, Venturoli S, Bulletti C, et al. Fertility and obstetric outcome after laparoscopic myomectomy of large myomata: a randomized comparison with abdominal myomectomy. Hum Reprod. 2000;15(12):2663–8.
35. Palomba S, Zupi E, Falbo A, Russo T, Marconi D, Tolino A, et al. A multicenter randomized, controlled study comparing laparoscopic versus minilaparotomic myomectomy: reproductive outcomes. Fertil Steril. 2007;88(4):933–41.

36. Lolis DE, Kalantaridou SN, Makrydimas G, Sotiriadis A, Navrozoglou I, Zikopoulos K, et al. Successful myomectomy during pregnancy. Hum Reprod. 2003;18(8):1699–702.
37. YL M, Wang S, Hao J, Shi M, Yelian FD, Wang XT. Successful pregnancies with uterine leiomyomas and myomectomy at the time of caesarean section. Postgrad Med J. 2011;87(1031):601–4.
38. Gbadebo AA, Charles AA, Austin O. Myomectomy at caesarean section: descriptive study of clinical outcome in a tropical setting. J Ayub Med Coll Abbottabad. 2009;21(4):7–9.
39. Park BJ, Kim YW. Safety of cesarean myomectomy. J Obstet Gynaecol Res. 2009;35(5):906–11.
40. Ravina JH, Herbreteau D, Ciraru-Vigneron N, Bouret JM, Houdart E, Aymard A, et al. Arterial embolisation to treat uterine myomata. Lancet. 1995;346(8976):671–2.
41. Mara M, Maskova J, Fucikova Z, Kuzel D, Belsan T, Sosna O. Midterm clinical and first reproductive results of a randomized controlled trial comparing uterine fibroid embolization and myomectomy. Cardiovasc Intervent Radiol. 2008;31(1):73–85.
42. Homer H, Saridogan E. Uterine artery embolization for fibroids is associated with an increased risk of miscarriage. Fertil Steril. 2010;94(1):324–30.
43. Berkane N, Moutafoff-Borie C. Impact of previous uterine artery embolization on fertility. Curr Opin Obstet Gynecol. 2010;22(3):242–7.
44. Behera MA, Leong M, Johnson L, Brown H. Eligibility and accessibility of magnetic resonance-guided focused ultrasound (MRgFUS) for the treatment of uterine leiomyomas. Fertil Steril. 2010;94(5):1864–8.
45. Rabinovici J, David M, Fukunishi H, Morita Y, Gostout BS, Stewart EA. Pregnancy outcome after magnetic resonance-guided focused ultrasound surgery (MRgFUS) for conservative treatment of uterine fibroids. Fertil Steril. 2010;93(1):199–209.
46. Ciavattini A, Tsiroglou D, Litta P, Vichi M, Tranquilli AL. Pregnancy outcome after laparoscopic cryomyolysis of uterine myomas: report of nine cases. J Minim Invasive Gynecol. 2006;13(2):141–4.
47. Vilos GA, Daly LJ, Tse BM. Pregnancy outcome after laparoscopic electromyolysis. J Am Assoc Gynecol Laparosc. 1998;5(3):289–92.
48. Shen SH, Fennessy F, McDannold N, Jolesz F, Tempany C. Image-guided thermal therapy of uterine fibroids. Semin Ultrasound CT MR. 2009;30(2):91–104.

49. Berman JM, Bolnick JM, Pemueller RR, Garza Leal JG. Reproductive outcomes in women following radiofrequency volumetric thermal ablation of symptomatic fibroids. A retrospective case series analysis. J Reprod Med. 2015;60(5-6):194–8.
50. Patel A, Malik M, Britten J, Cox J, Catherino WH. Alternative therapies in management of leiomyomas. Fertil Steril. 2014;102(3):649–55.
51. Hald K, Klow NE, Qvigstad E, Istre O. Treatment of uterine myomas with transvaginal uterine artery occlusion: possibilities and limitations. J Minim Invasive Gynecol. 2008;15(5):631–5.

Chapter 18
Asymptomatic Type 1 Submucosal Myoma in the Setting of Tubal Factor Infertility Requiring IVF

Gregory M. Christman and Cyra Cottrell

Clinical Case Presentation

A 29-year-old nulligravid woman presents with a chief complaint of a 5-year history of infertility and a 2-year history of progressively heavier periods. She has been married for 5 years and she and her partner have never used contraception during their marriage. Her menses occur every 27–33 days, with heavy flow requiring up to 8–10 pads per 24 h on the first 2 days of flow and her menstrual flow duration lasts for 7 days. The patient also occasionally reports 1–3 days of light spotting between her periods. Her partner has a normal semen analysis and her workup for

G.M. Christman, MD (✉)
Division of Reproductive Endocrinology and Infertility, University of Florida College of Medicine, PO Box 100294, Gainesville, FL 32611-0294, USA
e-mail: gchristman@ufl.edu

C. Cottrell
University of Florida College of Medicine, Gainesville, FL, USA

N.S. Moawad (ed.), *Uterine Fibroids*,
https://doi.org/10.1007/978-3-319-58780-6_18,
© Springer International Publishing AG 2018

primary infertility showed evidence of bilateral distal tubal blockage without evidence of a hydrosalpinx on her hysterosalpingogram with a filling defect in the cavity protruding from the left lateral margin of the uterus. Her thyroid function testing (TSH and total T4) is normal and her ovarian reserve testing is reassuring with an anti-mullerian hormone (AMH) level of 5.8 ng/mL and a cycle day 3 FSH level of 5 mIU/mL and an estradiol level of 49 pg/mL. Her past medical, surgical, and social histories are unremarkable with the exception of a prior chlamydia infection treated as an outpatient in college and mild anemia for the last 2 years recently corrected with oral ferrous sulfate.

Exam Findings

On physical examination, her blood pressure is 127/82 and her BMI is 33 kg/m^2. Her speculum exam shows a normal-appearing cervix and the bimanual exam reveals a mobile nontender 8–10 weeks' size uterus with no adnexal masses or tenderness. Her general exam is unremarkable with the exception for mild hirsutism and acne, obesity, and acanthosis nigricans.

Diagnostic Workup

Her laboratory evaluation included a hemoglobin level of 12 g/dL and a hemoglobin A1c level of 6.2%. A transvaginal ultrasound was performed and located a single 6 cm × 5 cm × 4 cm posterior myoma in the middle of a retroflexed uterus projecting to the left parasagittal side of the uterus. The ovaries appeared consistent with polycystic ovarian morphology bilaterally. The patient was then evaluated with a flexible office hysteroscopy study which was consistent with a submucous myoma projecting into the uterine cavity (Fig. 18.1). Evaluation via hysteroscopy allows direct inspection of the cavity since ultrasound for smaller intracavitary lesions may be difficult to discriminate between a polyp and a submucous leiomyoma [1]. A saline infusion sonogram showed only a single leiomyoma within the uterus with 4 cm projecting into the cavity and 2 cm extending into the myometrium which classifies this lesion as a type I submucous myoma (Fig. 18.2).

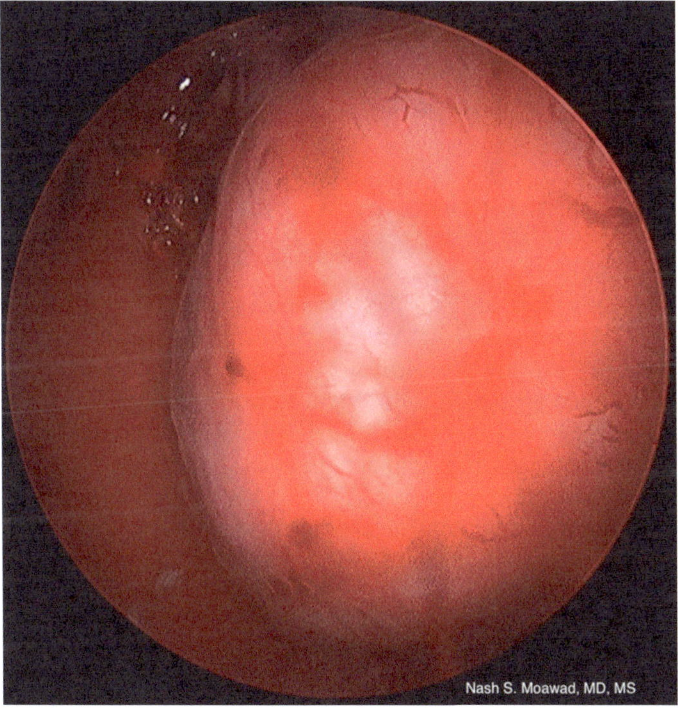

FIGURE 18.1 Large type 1 submucosal myoma

Type 0

Entirely within endometrial cavity

No Myometrial extension (pedunculated)

Type I

<50% myometrial extension (sessile)

<90-degree angle of myoma surface to uterine wall

Type II

≥50% myometrial extension (sessile)

Modified from Wamsteker et al. Obstet Gynecol. 1993;82:736-740.

FIGURE 18.2 Classification of submucous myomas

Treatment Options and Considerations

Currently there are four therapies recognized or approved by the US Food and Drug Administration (FDA) for the treatment of uterine fibroids: (1) preoperative therapy with Leuprolide acetate (Lupron) and ferrous sulfate; (2) various embolic agents for uterine artery embolization; (3) hardware for magnetic resonance imaging-guided high-energy focused ultrasound; and (4) surgery [2].

Uterine leiomyomas are believed to influence reproduction in several ways. The incidence of infertility and uterine leiomyomas increases with advancing maternal age, and no specific data exist to ascertain if the proportion of infertile women with leiomyomas is greater than the proportion of fertile women with leiomyomas. Yet the indirect evidence is substantial. In one review, annual pregnancy rates among women with leiomyomas distorting and not distorting the uterine cavity were 9% and 35%, respectively, as compared to 40% among age-matched controls with no leiomyomas [3].

Furthermore, multiple reports of successful pregnancies among infertile women following myomectomy strongly suggest a connection [4–6].

Though the exact physiologic mechanisms for reproductive dysfunction from leiomyomas are unclear, many plausible theories exist. There is a potential for reduced fecundity if a myoma occurs in the cornual region of the uterus due to mechanical occlusion of a fallopian tube [7]. It is also possible that large leiomyomas may impair the rhythmic uterine contractions that facilitate sperm motility [8]. It has further been documented that endometrial histology may vary in relation to the location of the leiomyoma. Submucosal leiomyomas may be associated with localized endometrial atrophy as well as alterations in the vascular blood flow, which may impede the implantation of an embryo; delivery of hormones or growth factors involved in implantation such as HOXA10, HOXA11, leukemia inhibitory factor (LIF), and BTEB1 protein; or interference with the normal immune response to pregnancy [9–11]. Submucosal leiomyomas, which distort the uterine cavity, are associated with first-trimester pregnancy loss, preterm delivery, abruption, abnormal presentations in labor, and postpartum hemorrhage [12].

In regard to the effectiveness of assisted reproductive technology, the presence of submucous or intramural leiomyomas is generally thought to reduce the effectiveness of assisted reproductive procedures. Early evidence demonstrated that both pregnancy and implantation rates were significantly lower in patients with intramural or submucosal leiomyomas [13, 14]. In one study, the presence of an intramural leiomyoma decreased the chances of an ongoing pregnancy by 50% following in vitro fertilization [15]. Evidence however suggests that patients with subserosal leiomyomas generally have assisted reproductive technology outcomes consistent with patients without leiomyomas [14–16]. The standard of care worldwide is to perform a removal of any submucous leiomyoma prior to the performance of in vitro fertilization (IVF).

	Pregnant
Hysteroscopy – diagnostic only	**29/103 (28.2%)**
Hysteroscopy with fibroid resection	**64/101 (63.4%)**

RR = 2.1 (95% CI 1.5-2.9), NNT =3

Note: There was no significant difference in fertility rate for those with Type II submucous myomas

FIGURE 18.3 RCT of hysteroscopic myomectomy for submucosal fibroids shows the impact of hysteroscopic myomectomy on fertility. Source: Modified from Shokeir T, El-Shafei M, Yousef H, Allam AF, Sadek E. Submucous myomas and their implications in the pregnancy rates of patients with otherwise unexplained primary infertility undergoing hysteroscopic myomectomy: a randomized matched control study. Fertil Steril. 94(2):724–9, 2010

Treatment planning about how to best treat patient's uterine fibroids depends on the patient's symptoms, the precise size and location of the fibroids, and the patient's immediate and future fertility plans. For women who want to preserve their fertility, myomectomy is always clearly indicated when fibroids result in any distortion of the endometrial cavity (Fig. 18.3) and should be strongly considered with the presence of large ($\geq$4 cm diameter) intramural fibroids. In the case described above, this woman has tubal factor infertility as the primary reason for her infertility along with a type 1 submucous leiomyoma resulting in heavy vaginal bleeding and mild anemia which should be removed to best promote her fertility with IVF therapy, reduce potential future pregnancy complications, and assist in the immediate correction of her symptomatic heavy uterine bleeding.

In patients who unlike our case have patent fallopian tubes, the removal of submucosal fibroids clearly increases the chance of spontaneous and assisted conception [17]. The universal recommendation to remove any submucous leiomyoma prior to assisted reproductive technology has been linked to early studies and initial clinical experience demonstrating that submucosal fibroids that distort the uterine cavity have been found to carry a relative risk of 0.3 for pregnancy and 0.28 for implantation after ART [18]. Women with submucous leiomyomas or large uterine fibroids in any location within the uterus >5 cm in pregnancy are at significantly increased risk for delivery at an earlier gestational age as compared to women with small or no fibroids, as well as obstetric complications including excess blood loss and increased frequency of postpartum blood transfusion [19].

In the case presented above, due to the significantly enlarged size of the submucous leiomyoma, this patient was prepared for surgery with a 3 months' preoperative treatment with leuprolide acetate (Lupron, Abbvie Pharmaceuticals). GnRH agonist (GnRHa) therapy induces apoptosis in leiomyoma cells and stops angiogenesis [20, 21]. GnRHa therapy also facilitates hysteroscopic resection of large submucous myomas via less operative blood loss due to decreased vascularity of the leiomyoma, decreased blood flow to the uterus, and a smaller lesion for resection [22]. The disadvantages of GnRHa include the cost of the medication, menopausal symptoms during administration, and bone demineralization with prolonged therapy for periods over 6 months [22]. Short-term preoperative treatment with letrozole 2.5 mg daily for 3 months used as an alternative to GnRHa has been shown to decrease hysteroscopic operative time and the volume of fluid absorbed during hysteroscopic resection of uterine submucosal myomas [22].

Surgical resection of this submucous leiomyoma was performed with a hysteroscopic resectoscope using a bipolar loop electrode and normal saline as the distending medium (Fig. 18.4). The use of a bipolar loop electrode and the use of isotonic fluid virtually eliminate the risk of hyponatremia associated with the use of nonionic solutions such as glycine required for unipolar cutting electrodes, thus greatly increasing the safety of the procedure. The submucous myoma is resected in strips with tissue fragments removed piece by piece through the scope, via periodic aspiration using a straight suction D&C curette or via a hysteroscopic morcellation device (Fig. 18.5). Care must be taken to keep track of fluid intake and output carefully so that any excess fluid absorption can be detected. Any suspicion that an imbalance exists suggesting that the patient

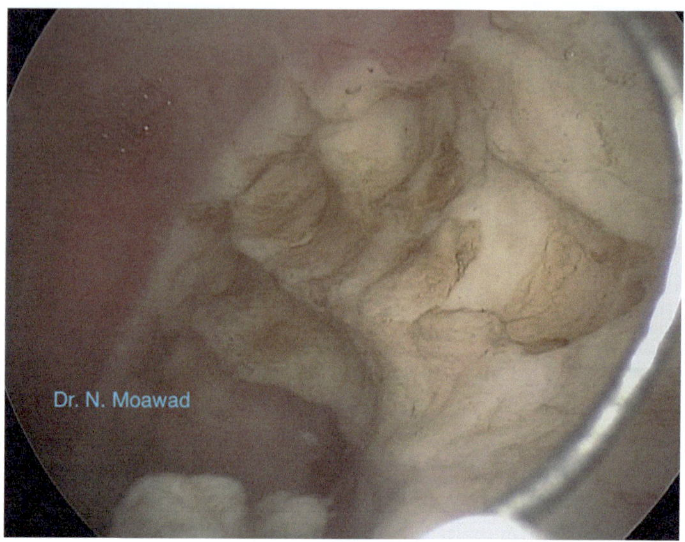

FIGURE 18.4 Bipolar loop electrode used for hysteroscopic myomectomy of large type 1 submucosal myoma

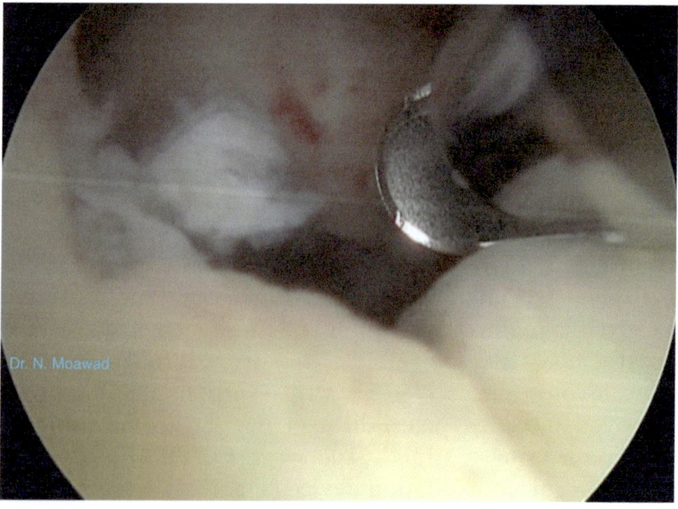

FIGURE 18.5 Hysteroscopic morcellators are the most recent advances in hysteroscopic myomectomy

may have absorbed 2.5 L of normal saline should prompt immediate cessation of the procedure and evaluation of the patient with the assistance of anesthesia for any clinical evidence of fluid overload or compromise. In healthy reproductive-age women, placement of a Foley catheter to monitor urinary output and the prompt use of diuretics such as Lasix can manage most cases of mild fluid overload with a rapid return to baseline. Resection of large fibroids may need to be stopped if significant fluid overload is noted in the middle of the case and staged with a return to the OR at a later date to complete the resection of the leiomyoma.

After complete resection of a submucous leiomyoma it is generally advised that patients should wait for 4–6 months before starting IVF treatment. The cavity should be reassessed prior to IVF with another office hysteroscopy procedure to assure normal healing as visualized by a normal cavity without uterine adhesions. This patient clearly appears to have evidence of polycystic disorder as noted by the polycystic morphology of her ovaries on ultrasound, clinical signs of elevated androgens (acne and hirsutism), and slight menstrual irregularity. This is further supported by the elevated anti-mullerian hormone level, acanthosis nigricans, and metabolic evidence of insulin resistance and prediabetes in this patient. In such cases, metformin should be instituted prior to IVF to further reduce the hemoglobin A1c level and to reduce the potential to develop ovarian hyperstimulation syndrome during superovulation therapy required for in vitro fertilization. In vitro fertilization can now be performed in the standard fashion but patients should be counselled about the advantages of electively transferring only a single embryo to eliminate the increased pregnancy risks associated with a multiple gestation. If this patient has a successful pregnancy, she should also be counselled regarding the increased risk of future leiomyoma recurrence after her myomectomy which is associated with a higher BMI, weight gain, and insulin resistance and diabetes.

Hysteroscopic myomectomy remains the standard treatment for women with symptomatic submucous fibroids who wish to retain their fertility. Although many submucosal fibroids can be removed hysteroscopically, an abdominal approach may occasionally be required for very large type 1 or type 2 submucosal leiomyomas. Myomectomy in these cases can be performed laparoscopically (with or without robotic assistance) or via laparotomy. Extreme care needs to be taken in the laparoscopic removal of large leiomyomas with a known submucous component so that the endometrium is not accidentally removed if there should be entry into the uterine cavity. For more details on the techniques of laparoscopic myomectomy, please refer to Chaps. 4, 8, 13, 14, and 16; for robot-assisted myomectomy technique, please refer to Chap. 5; and for hysteroscopic myomectomy technique, please refer to Chap. 7.

References

1. Wilde S, Scott-Barrett S. Radiological appearances of uterine fibroids. Indian J Radiol Imaging. 2009;19(3):222.
2. Segars JH, Parrott EC, Nagel JD, et al. Proceedings from the Third National Institutes of Health International Congress on Advances in Uterine Leiomyoma Research: comprehensive review, conference summary and future recommendations. Hum Reprod Update. 2014;20(3):309–33.
3. Donnez J, Jadoul P. What are the implications of myomas on fertility? A need for debate? Hum Reprod. 2002;17:1424–30.
4. Bulletti C, De Zieger D, Polli V, Flamigni C. The role of leiomyomas in infertility. J Am Assoc Gynecol Laparosc. 1999;6:441.
5. Vercellini P, Maddalena S, De Giorgi O, Pesole A, Ferrari L, Crosignani PG. Determinants of reproductive outcome after abdominal myomectomy for infertility. Fertil Steril. 1999;72:109–14.
6. Dubuisson J-B, Chapron C, Chalet X, Gregorakis SS. Infertility after laparoscopic myomectomy of large intramural myomas: preliminary results. Hum Reprod. 1996;11:518–22.
7. Stovall DW. Clinical symptomatology of uterine leiomyomas. Clin Obstet Gynecol. 2001;44:364–71.

8. Coutinho EM, Maia HS. The contractile response of the human uterus, fallopian tubes and ovary to prostaglandins in vivo. Fertil Steril. 1971;22:539–43.

9. Deligdish L, Loewenthal M. Endometrial changes associated with myomata of the uterus. J Clin Pathol. 1970;23:676–9.

10. Farrer-Brown G, Beilby JO, Tarbit MH. Venous changes in the endometrium of myomatous uteri. Obstet Gynecol. 1971;38:743–6.

11. Ng EHY, Ho PC. Doppler ultrasound examination of uterine arteries on the day of oocyte retrieval in patients with uterine fibroids undergoing IVF. Hum Reprod. 2002;17:765–70.

12. Katz VL, Dotters DJ, Droegemueller W. Complications of uterine leiomyomas in pregnancy. Obstet Gynecol. 1989;73:593–6.

13. Eldar-Geva T, Meagher S, Healy DL, MacLachlan V, Breheny S, Wood C. Effects of intramural, subserosal and submucosal uterine fibroids on the outcome of assisted reproduction technology treatment. Fertil Steril. 1988;70:687–91.

14. Stovall DW, Parrish SB, Van Voorhis BJ, Hahn SJ, Sparks AE, Syrop CH. Uterine leiomyomas reduce the efficacy of assisted reproduction cycles: results of a matched follow-up study. Hum Reprod. 1998;13:192–7.

15. Hart R, Khalaf Y, Yeong CT, Seed P, Taylor A, Braude P. A prospective controlled study of the effect of intramural uterine fibroids on the outcome of assisted conception. Hum Reprod. 2001;16(11):2411–7.

16. Oliveira FG, Abdelmassih VG, Diamond MP, Dozortsev D, Melo NR, Abdelmassih R. Impact of subserosal and intramural uterine fibroids that do not distort the endometrial cavity on the outcome of in vitro fertilization-intracytoplasmic sperm injection. Fertil Steril. 2004;81(3):582–7.

17. Jayakrishnan K, Menon V, Nambiar D. Submucous fibroids and infertility: effect of hysteroscopic myomectomy and factors influencing outcome. J Hum Reprod Sci. 2013;6(1):35.

18. Guo XC, Segars JH. The impact and management of fibroids for fertility. Obstet Gynecol Clin North Am. 2012;39(4):521–33.

19. Shavell VI, Thakur M, Sawant A, et al. Adverse obstetric outcomes associated with sonographically identified large uterine fibroids. Fertil Steril. 2012;97(1):107–10.

20. Bozzini N, Rodrigues CJ, Petti DA, Bevilacqua RG, Goncalves SP, Pinotti JA. Effects of treatment with gonadotropin releasing hormone agonist on the uterine leiomyomata structure. Acta Obstet Gynecol Scand. 2003;82(4):330–4.

21. Khan KN, Kitajima M, Hiraki K, et al. Changes in tissue inflammation, angiogenesis and apoptosis in endometriosis, adenomyosis and uterine myoma after GnRH agonist therapy. Hum Reprod. 2009;25(3):642–53.
22. Bizzarri N, Ghirardi V, Remorgida V, Venturini PL, Ferrero S. Three-month treatment with triptorelin, letrozole and ulipristal acetate before hysteroscopic resection of uterine myomas: prospective comparative pilot study. Eur J Obstet Gynecol Reprod Biol. 2015;192:22–6.

Chapter 19
Innumerable Fibroids

Kari Plewniak and Hye-Chun Hur

Clinical Case Presentation: Innumerable Fibroids

A 26-year-old gravida 0 female with discoid lupus presented to our minimally invasive gynecologic surgery (MIGS) clinic in consultation for increasing menorrhagia and dysmenorrhea. At initial presentation, she reported a lifelong history of regular but heavy menses with more recent patterns of increasing flow manifesting with cyclic menorrhagia without prolonged or intermenstrual bleeding. She also reported increasing dysmenorrhea that was no longer responsive to nonsteroidal anti-inflammatory medications. A thorough review of systems did not reveal further complaints. She was in a monogamous relationship with the same male partner for many years. Although she was not currently planning a pregnancy, she strongly desired future fertility.

K. Plewniak, MD • H.-C. Hur, MD, MPH (✉)
Division of Minimally Invasive Gynecology, Beth Israel Deaconess Medical Center, Harvard Medical School, Boston, MA, USA
e-mail: kmplewniak@gmail.com; hhur@bidmc.harvard.edu

N.S. Moawad (ed.), *Uterine Fibroids*,
https://doi.org/10.1007/978-3-319-58780-6_19,
© Springer International Publishing AG 2018

A thorough physical examination revealed no signs of anemia. A pelvic examination was unrevealing overall but was limited by her body habitus. Laboratory tests were drawn. A CBC revealed a hematocrit of 28.9% and a serum hCG was negative. A pelvic ultrasound showed a fibroid uterus measuring 8.1 cm × 4.7 cm × 5.4 cm. There were two FIGO type 1 submucosal fibroids; the anterior submucosal fibroid measured 2.4 cm × 2.1 cm × 1.5 cm and a fundal submucosal fibroid measured 1.4 cm × 1.2 cm × 1 cm. There was an additional left lateral intramural fibroid reported measuring 1.2 cm. The endometrial stripe measured 4 mm.

She was advised to undergo treatment given her symptomatic presentation with cyclic menorrhagia, significant anemia, and worsening dysmenorrhea. Iron supplementation was advised to ameliorate her anemia, but she was counseled regarding the need for fibroid treatment since the iron would not address the underlying cause of her anemia which was ostensibly, fibroid-related heavy bleeding. All medical and surgical treatments for fibroids and uterine bleeding were discussed along with the risks and benefits of each. In light of the patient's history of isolated discoid lupus, we also confirmed negative screening for antiphospholipid antibodies since these can be present in one-third of lupus patients and may increase one's risk of venous thromboembolism [1, 2].

After discussion of all treatment options, we advised a hysteroscopic myomectomy for resection of her two submucosal fibroids with expectant management of the smaller residual intramural fibroid in an effort to optimize both fibroid treatment and reproductive goals. This approach offers the possibility of improving fibroid-related symptoms (reduced uterine bleeding and dysmenorrhea) and decreasing fibroid burden while preserving fertility and optimizing future reproductive goals by normalizing the endometrial cavity.

After being thoroughly counseled at the initial MIGS consult visit, the patient declined any intervention and resumed care with her gynecologist. Over the course of 4 years, the patient's symptoms progressed with worsening symptomatic anemia and abnormal uterine bleeding. She had increasingly severe menorrhagia resulting in profound anemia, requiring in multiple hospitalizations at another institution. She received several blood transfusions as a consequence of her anemia. She underwent extensive evaluation for her bleeding and was started on oral medroxyprogesterone for medical treatment of her fibroids and uterine bleeding by her gynecologist. The patient then returned to our MIGS service to have her fibroid surgery.

Examination Findings

On initial presentation 4 years ago, the patient's examination was unremarkable. However, when the patient represented with worsening menorrhagia and symptomatic anemia, she had conjunctival pallor and the pelvic examination was notable for a 16 cm uterus with an irregular contour, suggestive of multiple fibroids. The uterus was mobile and nontender. There was a mass palpable in the left lateral lower uterine segment, possibly extending into the parametrium. There was no adnexal fullness or tenderness noted on examination. The remainder of her examination was unremarkable.

Diagnostic Workup

Laboratory

For all patients who report abnormal uterine bleeding we obtain a CBC. Additional tests are directed by the patient's history and medical profile. We obtain a pregnancy test for all reproductive-aged women and this was negative for our patient. Unless there are other indications, such as concurrent liver disease or a suspicious history or bleeding disorders, we do not obtain coagulation studies or testing for von Willebrand disease. All patients with life-threatening bleeding should get a type and screen with consideration of coagulopathy labs. During this patient's hospitalization at another institution, she had an extensive evaluation. There was no evidence of a coagulopathy and a CBC was only notable for anemia of 18%.

Imaging

For virtually all our patients, our primary mode of imaging is a pelvic ultrasound (PUS), specifically a transvaginal approach in conjunction with transabdominal. As a consultative practice receiving patients from numerous hospitals, we have found that the quality of the ultrasound can vary tremendously. It is our practice to routinely correlate imaging findings with pelvic examination. Many patients do not warrant additional imaging beyond a PUS. We may consider further imaging with a sonohysterogram or pelvic magnetic resonance imaging (MRI) for surgical planning on a case-by-case basis. A sonohysterogram is somewhat unique in its ability to define the potential cavitary involvement of uterine pathology. Many studies have shown superiority of a sonohysterogram or hysteroscopy over hysterosalpingograms for assessment of the endometrial cavity. In our practice, our preference is to perform an in-office hysteroscopy, rather than ordering a sonohysterogram, for a more direct endometrial assessment and surgical planning. However, if additional evaluation of the adnexae or myometrium is indicated, then a sonohysterogram may be superior to the office hysteroscopy. The plan should be tailored to the specific needs of each patient.

Pelvic MRI may offer additional information that can facilitate patient counseling and surgical planning preoperatively, especially if there is concern for adenomyosis, significant fibroid burden, or a challenging anatomical presentation. When there is particular concern for clinically significant fibroid bulk noted by limited uterine mobility and significant pelvic fullness on exam, or report of urinary dysfunction (e.g., urinary frequency or retention) by history, we order a renal ultrasound to assess for hydronephrosis or any other effects on the genitourinary system. The ease of access, convenience, cost, and technical skill of those performing and interpreting the results of these studies are all factors to consider when ordering imaging for fibroid evaluation.

In our practice, we typically start with a PUS and do not order additional imaging unless there is concern for concurrent adenomyosis or adenomyomas, a disproportionate fibroid growth rate concerning for malignancy, or examination findings concerning for challenging anatomical presentations such as large cervical fibroids. We find a thorough preoperative physical examination to be incredibly valuable. We couple the information gained from a pelvic examination with all available data to decide whether further imaging might be beneficial for surgical planning.

For this patient, all imaging including the pelvic ultrasound and MRI was obtained by the referring provider at an outside institution. The MRI reported a uterus measuring 10.9 cm × 10.8 cm × 9.9 cm with numerous fibroids but did specify the number of fibroids present. Four fibroids were described: a right bilobed fibroid measuring 5.8 cm × 5.3 cm × 4.5 cm, a left fundal fibroid measuring 5.3 cm × 4.8 cm × 4.2 cm, a left anterior fibroid measuring 2.2 cm × 2.9 cm × 2.9 cm, and a 1.8 cm largely intracavitary fibroid. A representative image from the PUS is shown in Fig. 19.1 below which illustrates a multifibroid uterus.

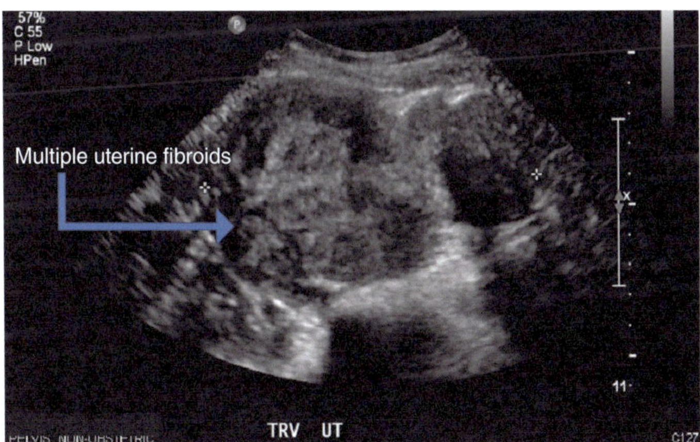

FIGURE 19.1 Pelvic ultrasound, transverse view of uterus with multiple fibroids

For the vast majority of our patients, due to their history of menorrhagia, we obtain sampling of the endometrium preoperatively to evaluate for endometrial hyperplasia or malignancy or infection as part of the abnormal uterine bleeding workup. An endometrial biopsy was obtained for this patient and it showed menstrual endometrium. While the endometrial biopsy has relatively good sensitivity to evaluate for endometrial cancer preoperatively, there are no preoperative tests to effectively assess for occult malignancy of fibroids [3, 4]. It is important to discuss the lack of preoperative fibroid cancer screening tests with patients who present with fibroids concerning for malignancy [5]. If the surgeon is planning to perform laparoscopic power morcellation then there must be careful patient selection and preoperative discussion of risks and benefits of this technique [6].

Treatment Options

Preoperative Counseling and Planning

At initial presentation 4 years prior, the patient was a candidate for several therapies including all medical treatment options as well as surgical treatments. A thorough discussion of all medical and surgical treatment options was done at that time. All medical options were reviewed including combined estrogen-progestin contraceptives (available by pill, patch, or vaginal ring), progestin-only hormonal therapies (available by pill, depot injection, intrauterine insert, or implant), as well as options like gonadotropin receptor hormone agonists. Additional medical treatments for fibroids include androgenic steroids such as danazol and gestrinone, and while they may have beneficial effects on fibroid symptoms, we do not typically prescribe these medications because of frequent side effects like weight gain, acne, hirsutism, and impact on mood. In addition, we reviewed surgical treatment options as well as procedural treatments such as uterine artery embolization. Given her nulliparity, young age, and desire for future fertility, the patient was not a candidate for hysterectomy or traditional uterine artery embolization. Based on PUS findings on initial consultation, we determined that the patient was a good candidate for hysteroscopic myomectomy. A laparoscopic myomectomy was less ideal given the location and small size of many of the fibroids, especially since deep fibroids with a submucosal presentation and small intramural fibroids are not always visible on laparoscopic survey. The patient declined treatment at that time and elected to maintain expectant management of her fibroids and bleeding. She was strongly advised to undergo hysteroscopic myomectomy before she conceived to normalize her uterine cavity and to minimize the risk of pregnancy complications such as pregnancy loss [7].

The patient subsequently represented to our minimally invasive gynecology clinic to discuss fibroid treatment options given the significantly increased fibroid burden, worsening symptoms, and severe blood loss anemia. She was strongly advised to undergo surgical intervention. In our experience, once patients have become transfusion dependent, the role for medical therapy alone is limited. Medical therapies, however, can be used for interim treatment of bleeding as a bridge to surgery. In this case, the patient was started on progestin therapy by her gynecologist with oral medroxyprogesterone 10 mg daily. We increased the dosing to 10 mg twice a day to further stabilize the endometrium and inhibit bleeding. Oral progestin was administered in conjunction with iron infusions to address her severe iron-deficiency and blood-loss anemia. With a combination of blood transfusions, iron infusions, and oral medroxyprogesterone, her hematocrit was increased from 18 to 32.9%. Other preoperative methods to inhibit uterine bleeding and allow for improvement in blood count include GnRH agonists; however, for myomectomy patients we do not advise this treatment since it may compromise the pseudo-capsule dissection planes for the fertility-sparing myomectomy surgery. Autologous blood transfusions are another option, but we do not use it widely in our practice. Our preference is to optimize preoperative hematocrit with IV iron infusions if appropriate, decrease preoperative blood loss, and minimize intraoperative blood loss.

For patients desiring future fertility, we do not typically advise uterine artery embolizations (UAE) for fibroid treatment given the theoretical risk to future pregnancy and placental complications. There have been small case series of pregnancies following UAE; however, the numbers are small, and the embolization material is not uniform across studies and therefore may not be completely generalizable. A case-control study examining UAE for fibroid treatment by Dobrokhotova et al. does not show an increase in adverse outcomes after UAE. Although it is one of the larger studies, it only includes 59 pregnancies after UAE [8]. There are several additional reports of successful pregnancies after UAE treatment for postpartum hemorrhage, but whether this data can be extrapolated to fibroid patients who undergo UAE is yet to be determined [9]. In addition, some data suggest that UAE may cause temporary ovarian failure [10, 11]. Most patients, however, eventually recover normal ovarian function [12, 13]. In our practice, we offer UAEs to patients with symptomatic fibroids who have completed childbearing. We do not typically recommend UAEs to reproductive-aged women who have not completed their family planning. Instead, we prioritize alternative treatments to UAE in order to maintain the uterine blood supply. This recommendation may change as we are able to follow more pregnancies after UAE [14]. Similarly we do not recommend the various other methods of minimally invasive ablation techniques including radiofrequency myolysis or magnetic resonance-guided focused ultrasound for women seeking future fertility as the data to support its safe use in this population is lacking.

We occasionally utilize a preoperative UAE for patients undergoing myomectomy with extreme fibroid presentations or significant fibroid burden, which may place the patient at high risk for an unplanned hysterectomy. Significant fibroid burden may reflect numerous, sizeable, or anatomically challenging fibroids such as large cervical fibroids compressing the

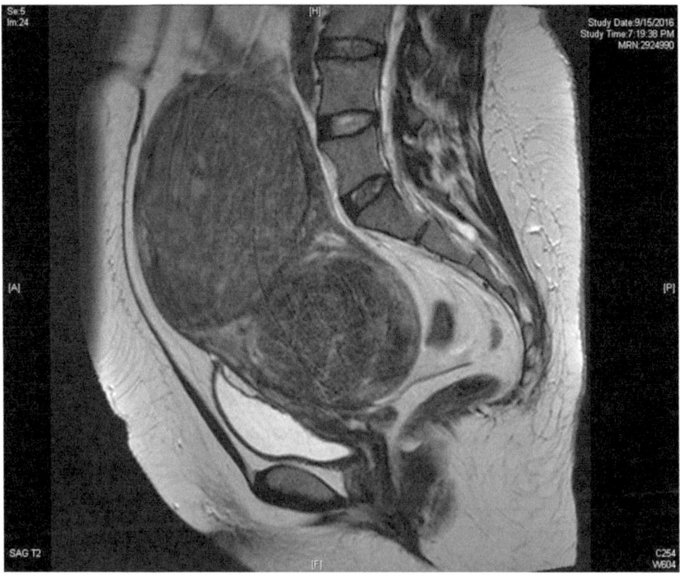

FIGURE 19.2 Enlarged uterus with significant fibroid burden that may benefit from preoperative UAE

bladder. See Fig. 19.2 above. Although these cases may be better served with hysterectomy, this may not be an option for nulliparous patients trying to reproduce. In these extreme cases, we coordinate with the interventional radiology service to utilize temporary occluding agents, typically gel foam at our institution, for reversibility of the embolization effect. For this very select patient population we coordinate to have the gel foam UAE performed on the day prior to the myomectomy. Again this is for individuals where every heroic effort is made to accomplish a fertility-sparing surgery while avoiding excessive blood loss and unplanned hysterectomy [15].

If a patient with innumerable fibroids does not have plans for future childbearing and opts to have fibroid surgery, then we would strongly recommend hysterectomy, especially if one has become dependent on transfusions of blood products. For patients who select uterine-sparing fibroid surgery, we counsel them about the risk of future fibroid growth after myomectomy with recurrent symptoms and need for further intervention that can be greater than 20% at 5 years and 30% at 7 years [16, 17]. We also discuss the mode of incision, which is best determined by the location and number of fibroids present. Patients with submucosal fibroids are best served with a hysteroscopic approach, which is what we offered this patient on initial presentation. However, when the patient represented with an increased fibroid burden manifesting with innumerable fibroids riddled throughout the uterus, a hysteroscopic approach was no longer appropriate.

Patients with fibroids in multiple different locations requesting fertility-sparing myomectomy require careful surgical planning to balance both fibroid treatment and reproductive goals. Some patients may benefit from a hybrid approach where a hysteroscopic myomectomy is performed to resect the submucosal fibroids and a concomitant laparoscopic or abdominal myomectomy is done to remove the intramural and/or subserosal fibroids. This may offer optimal preservation of the myometrium and endometrial cavity in select patients. Alternatively, a partial myomectomy may be appropriate for those prioritizing fertility while addressing fibroid-related symptoms: either with a hysteroscopic myomectomy for removal of only submucosal fibroids to normalize the endometrial cavity and avoid a myometrial incision altogether or with a partial laparoscopic myomectomy for removal of only the largest fibroids to avoid numerous myometrial incisions and minimize adhesion risks. Both these options leave residual smaller intramural/subserosal fibroids behind, posing the potential for increased risk of needing additional fibroid treatment at a future date. Partial myomectomies, or procedures with planned residual disease, may be better suited for women planning to conceive in the near future, but may be less ideal for those planning to have multiple children over the span of many years. If patients desire future fertility, but do not have an immediate timeline, the risk of leaving residual pathology and developing symptoms in the interim before conception may not be insignificant. Because our patient had many deeply intramural fibroids and several large submucosal fibroids, and was not planning immediate conception we advised an abdominal myomectomy for complete removal of all fibroids present.

Patients like this require careful preoperative evaluation and planning and the importance of thorough counseling cannot be overemphasized. At times this requires the preoperative discussion regarding possible purposeful retention of pathology because of the presenting fibroid anatomy. If, for example, there is an intimate relationship between a fibroid and the blood supply to the uterus or ovaries, the risk of unplanned hysterectomy or oophorectomy increases with removal of such fibroids. This is illustrated well in Fig. 19.3, which shows a fibroid that intimately involves the utero-ovarian ligament. Resection of this fibroid would risk the cornua, ostia, and some of the vascular supply to the ipsilateral ovary. This risk must be understood by the patient, and the provider must understand the patient's preference for either total removal of all possible pathology or minimizing the risks to future fertility. We did remove the utero-ovarian ligament fibroid for this patient while conserving her adnexae and utero-ovarian ligament blood supply.

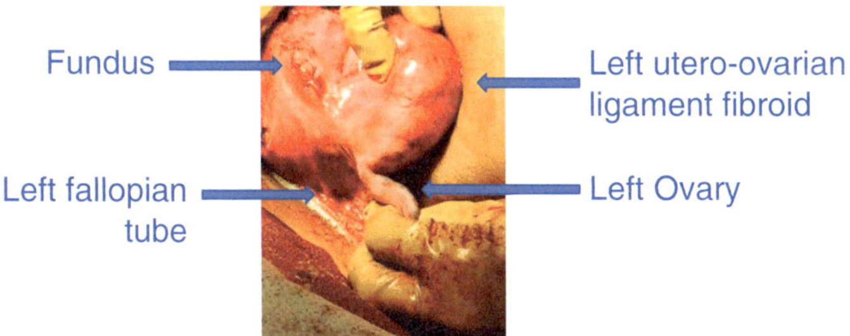

FIGURE 19.3 Anatomically challenging fibroid presentation, left utero-ovarian ligament fibroid

Operative Management

Myomectomies can be technically challenging due to the anatomical location, number, size, and vascularity of the fibroid. Good surgical technique and an intimate knowledge of pelvic anatomy and fibroid anatomy are essential to minimize blood loss and optimize outcomes during fibroid surgery. Differentiating between a leiomyoma, an adenomyoma, and adenomyosis is critical since the surgical approach for adenomyomas and adenomyosis is vastly different from a traditional leiomyoma that has a pseudo-capsule plane. Although we do not routinely order preoperative MRIs, an MRI may offer a higher sensitivity for detecting adenomyosis and adenomyomas which may offer the patient more detailed preoperative counseling, which can facilitate with preoperative counseling and help set appropriate postoperative expectations. Concurrent adenomyosis or adenomyoma can be difficult to differentiate intraoperatively from degenerating fibroids and all of these abnormalities can pose technical difficulties. Anatomical planes can be difficult to identify among degenerated fibroids or may not exist among adenomyomas or uteri with adenomyosis, thereby increasing the chance of greater blood loss, incomplete treatment, ongoing symptoms, and unintentional removal of excess myometrium.

For this patient, we achieved abdominal entry via a small low transverse abdominal incision that was "cut to size" based on our bimanual examination and pelvic ultrasound findings that assessed for uterine mobility and largest fibroid size. The abdominal incision was approximately 8 cm in width, just large enough to fit one hand through the abdominal incision. The abdominal-pelvic cavity was first palpated to verify that there were no surrounding uterine or adnexal adhesions, and then the uterus was delivered one fibroid at a time, rather than as a whole, to optimize removal of large masses through the smallest possible incision. Diluted vasopressin was injected at the myomectomy site and a perforating towel clamp was used to grasp the fibroid where the myometrial incision would be made. We were able to deliver the uterus through this small incision by using perforating towel clamps for traction on the uterus while applying countertraction on the abdominal wall to squeeze the uterus out thorough an incision smaller than the smallest dimension of the uterus.

Prior to making the myometrial incision and enucleating the fibroid, we typically inject a dilute solution of vasopressin into the pseudo-capsule plane to assist with hemostasis. We always withdraw the syringe prior to injection to avoid an intravascular injection and communicate with the anesthesiology team when injecting vasopressin, as intravascular injection can manifest clinically as profound bradycardia and/or cardiovascular compromise. Vasopressin is a synthetic form of antidiuretic hormone, and, when used locally, produces temporary and somewhat local vasoconstriction. There is no high-quality evidence to support the use of uterotonics such as misoprostol or oxytocin, and we do not routinely use it in our practice [18, 19].

In addition to the vasopressin, a uterine vessel tourniquet was placed using a 0.25 Penrose drain, effectively decreasing uterine perfusion and total EBL (Fig. 19.4). Although no blinded studies exist to support the practice of a uterine tourniquet, multiple studies have shown good effect. In our experience clinically, the tourniquet is quite valuable and we use the tourniquet technique routinely. We start by incising an avascular peritoneal window in the lower broad ligament bilaterally, threading and wrapping the Penrose drain around the uterine vessels, and then tying the drain anteriorly at a level above the bladder but below the fibroids, i.e., at the "neck of the uterine head" (see Fig. 19.4). The tourniquet is removed as soon as possible to avoid prolonged devascularization of the uterus.

There are some cases in which the anatomic distribution of disease precludes the proper placement of a tourniquet. Usually these patients can be found preoperatively by a careful physical examination. We find that the most difficult cases are with bulky lower uterine segment disease or large distorting cervical fibroids. In these cases we carefully consider the use of a gel foam UAE preoperatively. Again there is limited data, but at least in the case of peripartum hemorrhage there seems to be reasonable data supporting the safety of gel foam in regard to subsequent pregnancy. There

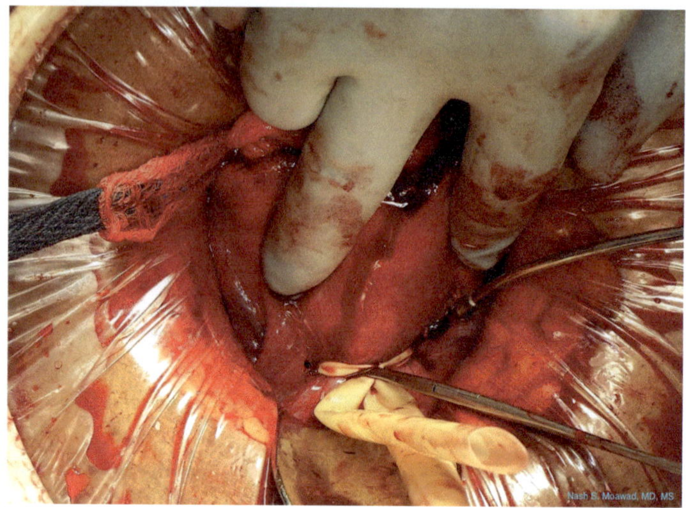

Figure 19.4 Uterine vessel tourniquet

are several case reports of pregnancies after embolization but due to the paucity of data we still do not routinely recommend embolization in a patient planning or considering future fertility [20, 21].

When making the myometrial incision, we make every effort to identify the correct pseudo-capsule plane and to minimize overdissection of the myometrium to avoid excessive tissue necrosis. Performing a dissection within the pseudo-capsule layer requires a careful understanding of fibroid anatomy. The pseudo-capsule is called such because it is easy to misinterpret this layer as the fibroid capsule when in reality it is part of the normal myometrium that should not be removed.

When enucleating the fibroid, we perform an "in-plane" dissection within the pseudo-capsule layer that has a significant clinical impact—to help minimize blood loss and maximize preservation of residual myometrium. This is shown in Fig. 19.5, showing that the pseudo-capsule should be carefully dissected away from the fibroid and left in situ. Dissecting within the pseudo-capsule plane also minimizes the risk of entering the endometrial cavity even among fibroids abutting or indenting into the endometrial cavity. We find anecdotally that this reduces the risk of iatrogenic intrauterine adhesions (Asherman's syndrome) or iatrogenic adenomyosis related to the myomectomy. Reducing the risk of myometrial hematomas, preserving myometrium, minimizing tissue necrosis to optimize healing, and minimizing entry into the endometrial cavity to reduce the risk of intrauterine adhesions are factors that are especially important among women undergoing fertility-sparing fibroid surgery with long-term reproductive goals in mind.

For this patient in particular, given her young age and nulliparity, and given the unclear interval to planned pregnancy, our goal was to remove as much pathology as possible in the hope of minimizing the risk of needing a second fibroid surgery during the next 5 years while she might achieve a pregnancy. Figure 19.6 illustrates the size and number of fibroids removed in this case. We find that with increasing interval to

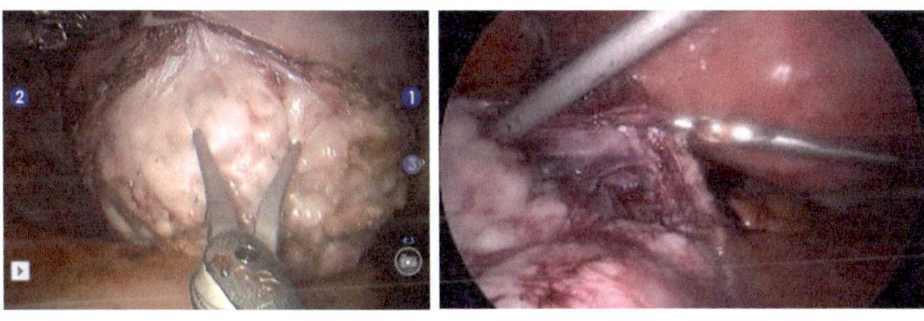

FIGURE 19.5 Example of fibroid pseudo-capsule anatomy

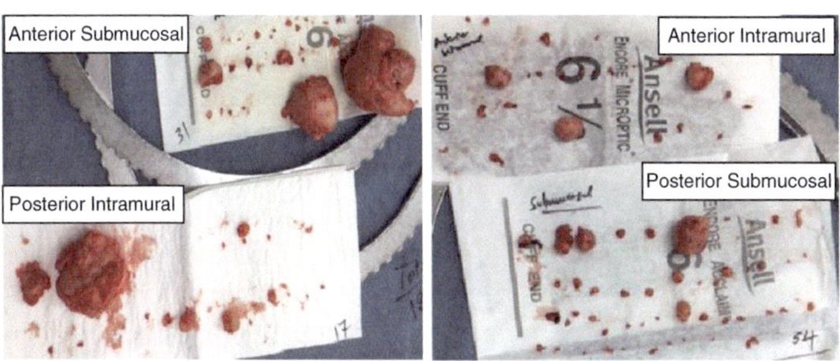

FIGURE 19.6 Abdominal myomectomy specimen, with significant submucosal and intramural fibroid components

pregnancy, there is an increased chance of recurrent pathology. This is likely analogous to the increase in reoperation rates with time, as between 20 and 30% of patients choosing myomectomy will have another procedure by 5 years [13, 16].

For patients like ours, if the endometrial cavity is entered, we recommend a careful multilayer closure of the endometrium and myometrium to minimize the risk of iatrogenic adenomyosis and to ensure tissue integrity, hemostasis, and strength of the myometrial closure. The myomectomy closure should be carefully inspected once the uterine vessel tourniquet has been removed and the uterus has been delivered back into the pelvis so the areas of dissection can be carefully inspected off-tension to ensure hemostasis.

Postoperative Management

All patients should be monitored closely after surgery to ensure that there are no surgery-related complications. Patients who undergo a multiple myomectomy procedure with significant fibroid burden are at greater risk for transfusions, uterine hematomas, delayed bleeding, infection, postoperative adhesions, bowel obstruction, etc. We advise all providers to maintain a high level of awareness for these potential risks among patients who undergo myomectomy for removal of numerous and sizeable fibroids.

Like our patient, those who present with extensive submucosal fibroids where a significant proportion of the surface endometrium is affected requiring submucosal myomectomy, we advise insertion of a device in the uterus to minimize the risk of intrauterine adhesions. An IUD, Foley catheter, Malecot catheter, or alternative intrauterine devices available on the market can be inserted intraoperatively. The advantage of the IUD over the intrauterine Foley is that the IUD can provide interim contraception while offering endometrial protection by separating the anterior endometrium from the posterior endometrium in the hopes of minimizing intrauterine adhesions during the myomectomy healing period. There is again a paucity of high-quality data comparing these methods in this patient population [22–25].

We advise patients to wait a minimum of 3–6 months (our preference is 6 months) before conceiving to allow uterine healing. For patients whose surgeries required numerous, sizeable, and/or deep incisions into the myometrium for fibroid removal, we advise cesarean delivery to minimize future risk of uterine rupture or myomectomy scar dehiscence [26, 27].

For patients with extensive submucosal fibroids involving a significant portion of the endometrial cavity, a postoperative sonohysterogram may be indicated to assess for intrauterine adhesions (Asherman's syndrome). If either cornua/ostia is affected by the intrauterine adhesions, this may result in proximal tubal occlusion. In addition, patients who undergo removal of intramural or subserosal fibroids in close proximity to the fallopian tubes may be at risk for compromised proximal tubal patency. For patients who undergo myomectomy and develop adhesions, they may also be at risk for distal tubal occlusion. If there is any concern for a patient's tubal status after myomectomy, a hysterosalpingogram should be considered. We do not routinely obtain sonohysterograms or hysterosalpingograms for myomectomy patients at baseline. For select patients who would benefit from further assessment of the endometrial cavity or fallopian tubes after fibroid removal, testing should be done before the patient tries to conceive. Given the extent of submucosal fibroid removal in our patient, we obtained a postoperative hysterosalpingogram to assess for possible intrauterine adhesions. The hysterosalpingogram showed a normal-appearing uterine cavity without intrauterine adhesions, a patent left fallopian tube, but no fill of the right fallopian tube due to either spasm or proximal occlusion; see Fig. 19.7. At the time of the writing of this chapter, the patient had yet to attempt conception, which may be the most important follow-up test.

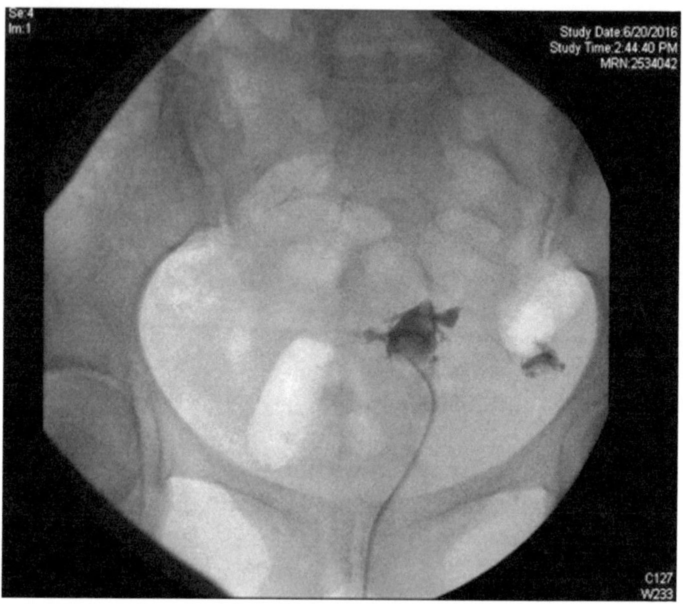

FIGURE 19.7 Hysterosalpingogram postmyomectomy

Conclusion

There is a wide range of treatment options for patients with fibroids. For symptomatic patients who want to maintain their reproductive options, myomectomy is the surgery of choice. The surgical plan for reproductive women with fibroids should be tailored to each individual patient—factoring in the patient's age, family planning goals, reproductive timeline, fibroid presentation, and symptoms. This requires careful planning and discussion with the patient as detailed in this chapter.

References

1. Ruffatti A, Veller-Fornasa C, Patrassi GM, Sartori E, Tonello M, Tonetto S, et al. Anticardiolipin antibodies and antiphospholipid syndrome in chronic discoid lupus erythematosus. Clin Rheumatol. 1995;14(4):402–4.

2. Kind P, Schuppe HC, Jung KP, Degitz K, Lakomek HJ, Goerz G. Cutaneous lupus erythematosus and cardiolipin antibodies. Incidence and clinical significance. Hautarzt. 1992;43(3):126–9.

3. Kanis MJ, Rahaman J, Moshier EL, Zakashansky K, Chuang L, Kolev V. Detection and correlation of pre-operative, frozen section, and final pathology in high-risk endometrial cancer. Eur J Gynaecol Oncol. 2016;37(3):338–41. PubMed

4. Fakhar S, Saeed G, Khan AH, Alam AY. Validity of pipelle endometrial sampling in patients with abnormal uterine bleeding. Ann Saudi Med. 2008;28(3):188–91. PubMed

5. Hinchcliff EM, Esselen KM, Watkins JC, Oduyebo T, Rauh-Hain JA, Del Carmen MG, et al. The role of endometrial biopsy in the preoperative detection of uterine leiomyosarcoma. J Minim Invasive Gynecol.2016;23(4):567–72.doi:10.1016/j.jmig.2016.01.022.

6. Harris JA, Swenson CW, Uppal S, Kamdar N, Mahnert N, As-Sanie S, Morgan DM. Practice patterns and postoperative complications before and after US Food and Drug Administration safety communication on power morcellation. Am J Obstet Gynecol. 2016;214(1):98.e1–98.e13.

7. Pritts E, Parker W, Olive D. Fibroids and infertility: an updated systematic review of the evidence. Fertil Steril. 2009;91(4):1215–2.

8. Dobrokhotova J, Grishin I, Ibragimova D, Knysheva I, Ilchenko V. Uterine artery embolization and pregnancy: actual and controversial issues of gestation terms and delivery. Int J Biomed. 2016;6(1):33–7.

9. Eriksson LG, Mulic-Lutvica A, Jangland L, Nyman R. Massive postpartum hemorrhage treated with transcatheter arterial embolization: technical aspects and long-term effects on fertility and menstrual cycle. Acta Radiol. 2007;48(6):635–42.

10. Sentilhes L, Gromez A, Clavier E, Resch B, Verspyck E, Marpeau L. Fertility and pregnancy following pelvic arterial embolisation for postpartum haemorrhage. BJOG. 2010;117(1):84–93. doi:10.1111/j.1471-0528.2009.02381.x.

11. Salomon LJ, deTayrac R, Castaigne-Meary V, Audibert F, Musset D, Ciorascu R, Frydman R, Fernandez H. Fertility and pregnancy outcome following pelvic arterial embolization for severe post-partum haemorrhage. A cohort study. Hum Reprod. 2003;18(4):849–52.

12. Soyer P, Dohan A, Dautry R, Gueurrache Y, Ricbourg A, Gayat E, et al. Transcatheter arterial embolization for post partum hemorrhage: indications, techniques, results, and complications. Cardiovasc Intervent Radiol. 2015;38:1068–81.

13. Deux JF, Bazot M, Le Blanche AF, Tassart M, Khalil A, Berkane N, Uzan S, Boudghène F. Is selective embolization of uterine

arteries a safe alternative to hysterectomy in patients with post-partum hemorrhage? AJR Am J Roentgenol. 2001;177(1):145–9.

14. Spies JB. Current role of uterine artery embolization in the manadgement of uterine fibroids. Clin Obstet Gynecol. 2016;59(1):93–102.

15. Goldman K, Hirshfeld-Cytron J, Pavone M, Thomas A, Vogelzang R, Milad M. Uterine artery embolization immediately preceding laparoscopic myomectomy. Int J Gynaecol Obstet. 2012;116(2):105–8.

16. Reed SD, Newton KM, Thompson LB, Mccrummen BA, Warolin AK. The incidence of repeat uterine surgery following myomectomy. J Womens Health (Larchmt). 2006;15(9):1046–52.

17. Sharp HT. Assessment of new technology in the treatment of idiopathic menorrhagia and uterine leiomyomata Obstet Gynecol 2006108(4):990-1003.

18. Kongnyuy EJ, Wiysonge CS. Interventions to reduce haemorrhage during myomectomy for fibroids. Cochrane Database Syst Rev. 2011;11:CD005355.

19. Kongnyuy EJ, van den Broek N, Wiysonge CS. A systematic review of randomized controlled trials to reduce hemorrhage duringmyomectomy for uterine fibroids. Int J Gynaecol Obstet. 2008;100(1):4–9.

20. Lee HY, Shin JH, Kim J, Yoon H-K, Ko G-Y, Won H-S, et al. Primary postpartum hemorrhage: outcome of pelvic arterial embolization in 251 patients at a single institution. Vasc Interv Radiol. 2012;264(3):903–9.

21. Chauleur C, Fagnet C, Levy R, Larchez C, Seffert P. Serious primary post-partum hemorrhage, arterial embolization and future fertility: a retrospective study of 46 cases. Hum Reprod. 2008;23(7):1553–9.

22. Papoutsis D, Georgantzis D, Daccò MD, Halmos G, Moustafa M, Mesquita Pinto AR, Magos A. A rare case of Asherman's syndrome after open myomectomy: sonographic investigations and possible underlying mechanisms. Gynecol Obstet Invest. 2014;77(3):194–200.

23. AAGL Advancing Minimally Invasive Gynecology Worldwide. AAGL practice report: practice guidelines for management of intrauterine synechiae. J Minim Invasive Gynecol. 2010;17(1):1–7.

24. Gambadauro P, Gudmundsson J, Torrejón R. Intrauterine adhesions following conservative treatment of uterine fibroids. Obstet Gynecol Int. 2012;2012:853269.

25. Asgari Z, Hafizi L, Hosseini R, Javaheri A, Rastad H. Intrauterine synechiae after myomectomy; laparotomy versus laparoscopy: non-randomized interventional trial. Iran J Reprod Med. 2015;13(3):161–8.
26. Gambacorti-Passerini Z, Gimovsky AC, Locatelli A, Berghella V. Trial of labor after myomectomy and uterine rupture: a systematic review. Acta Obstet Gynecol Scand. 2016;95(7):724–34. doi:10.1111/aogs.12920.
27. Koo YJ, Lee JK, Lee YK, Kwak DW, Lee IH, Lim KT, Lee KH, Kim TJ. Pregnancy outcomes and risk factors for uterine rupture after laparoscopic myomectomy: a single-center experience and literature review. J Minim Invasive Gynecol. 2015;22(6):1022–8. doi:10.1016/j.jmig.2015.05.016.

Erratum to: The Prolapsed Myoma

Richard Guido, Mallory Stuparich, and Nash S. Moawad

Erratum to:

Chapter 9 in: Nash S. Moawad (ed.), Uterine Fibroids: A Clinical Casebook, DOI 10.1007/978-3-319-58780-6_9

The original version of Chapter 9 was inadvertently published with two author names "Richard Guido and Nash S. Moawad" instead of three "Richard Guido, Mallory Stuparich, and Nash S. Moawad". The chapter has been updated.

The updated online version of this chapter can be found at
10.1007/978-3-319-58780-6_9

R. Guido, MD, CIP (✉) • M. Stuparich, MD
Department of Obstetrics, Gynecology and Reproductive Sciences,
University of Pittsburgh, Magee-Womens Hospital of the UPMC
Health System, 300 Halket St, Pittsburgh, PA 15213, USA
e-mail: rguido@mail.magee.edu

N.S. Moawad, MD, MS, FACOG
Minimally Invasive Gynecologic Surgery, Department of Obstetrics
and Gynecology, University of Florida College of Medicine,
Gainesville, FL, USA
e-mail: nmoawad@ufl.edu

N.S. Moawad (ed.), *Uterine Fibroids*,
https://doi.org/10.1007/978-3-319-58780-6_20,
© Springer International Publishing AG 2018

Index

N.S. Moawad (ed.), *Uterine Fibroids*,
https://doi.org/10.1007/978-3-319-58780-6
© Springer International Publishing AG 2018